EUROPEAN ARTS THERAPY

GROUNDING THE VISION
to advance theory and practice

Other ECArTE publications:

Line Kossolapow; Sarah Scoble; Diane Waller (eds.)
Arts – Therapies – Communication, Volume I
On the Way to a Communicative European Arts Therapy
Published by LIT Verlag Munster – Berlin – Hamburg – London – Wien
ISBN 3-8258-5728-X

Line Kossolapow; Sarah Scoble; Diane Waller (eds.)
Arts – Therapies – Communication, Volume II
On the Way to a Regional European Arts Therapy
Published by LIT Verlag Munster – Berlin – Hamburg – London – Wien
ISBN 3-8258-5729-8

Line Kossolapow; Sarah Scoble (eds.)
Arts Therapy: Recognized Discipline or Soul-Graffiti?
Approaches, Applications, Evaluations
Abstract Book of the 7th European Arts Therapies Conference
Published by LIT Verlag Munster – Berlin – Hamburg – London – Wien
ISBN 3-8258-7182-7

Line Kossolapow; Sarah Scoble; Diane Waller (eds.)
Arts – Therapies – Communication, Volume III
European Arts Therapy – Different Approaches to a Unique Discipline.
Opening Regional Portals
Published by LIT Verlag Munster – Berlin – Hamburg – London – Wien
ISBN 3-8258-8935-1

EUROPEAN ARTS THERAPY

GROUNDING THE VISION
to advance theory and practice

Edited by Sarah Scoble
Preface by Christine Lapoujade

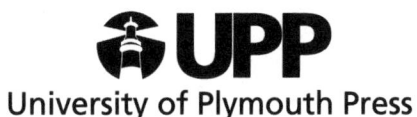

University of Plymouth Press

Paperback edition first published in the UK in 2006
by University of Plymouth Press,
Scott Building, Drake Circus, Plymouth,
Devon, PL4 8AA, United Kingdom

Copyright © 2006,
ECArTE (European Consortium for Arts Therapies Education)

A catalogue record of this book is available from the British Library

ISBN 10: 1-84102-164-4
ISBN 13: 987-1-841021-64-5

Library of Congress Cataloging in Publication

European Arts Therapy – Grounding the Vision to advance theory and practice
Edited by Sarah Scoble
Preface by Christine Lapoujade

All rights reserved. No part of this publication may be reproduced,
stored in a retrieval system or transmitted in any form or by any means
electronic, mechanical, photocopying, recording, or otherwise,
without written permission.

Printed by Short Run Press Limited, Exeter, UK
www.shortrunpress.co.uk

CONTENTS

Acknowledgements	ix
European Consortium for Arts Therapies Education (ECArTE)	xi
Foreword: The Eighth European Arts Therapies Conference	xiii
Preface, *Christine Lapoujade*	xvii

I. Grounding our vision

The Greek Tragedy as a Model for the Arts Therapies *Jan Van Camp*	2
Between the Arts Therapies: How different is different? How similar is similar? *Phil Jones*	13

II. Concepts and debates

On the Flow of Inner Images and the Borders of Consciousness . . . *Ralf Bolle*	28
Lead Pipe in the Library: art, creativity and consciousness – so what? *Michael Barham*	42
Breaking New Ground – expanding our vision *Pauline Mottram*	54
Art as the Centre of Art Therapies Education *Peter Sinapius*	64
On the Symptomatology of the Image *Peter Rech*	69

III. Practitioner research and assessment of practice

Introducing a New Method of Arts-based Therapeutic Research: narrative phenomenological analysis *Martin Cope*	78
Aristotle's Poetics in Dramatherapy Assessment and Evaluation *Lambros Yotis*	91

Dance Movement Therapy for Depressed Teenage Girls 103
 Erna Grönlund, Barbro Renck and Nita Gyllander Vabö

Grounded Vision: a matter of 'making explicit', or how to bridge the gap 110
between practice and theory
 Mathilde Tubben

Research in Analytic Group Music Therapy: analysis of a workshop in 120
Argentina. The foreign leader and the question of tuning the emotional
instrument in the group
 Edith Lecourt and Violeta Hemsy de Gainza

Passages to Transformation: play therapy with a young girl who avoided 131
body contact
 Vicky Zerva-Spanou

In Search of an Identity: individual dramatherapy with a client suffering 140
from panic attacks
 Katerina Couroucli-Robertson

The Drama of Addiction and Recovery : applying the ritual model of 149
dramatherapy in qualitative research with members of narcotics
anonymous
 Lia Zografou

IV. Essays in theory and practice

Does Engaging with their Own Artwork Protect Art Therapists, 162
Working with Childhood Sexual Abuse from Vicarious Traumatisation?
 Pauline McGee

Art in Times of War and Political Conflicts 172
 Simone Alter-Muri

Art as a Vehicle: performing arts and arts therapies between ritual and 179
aesthetics
 Aleksandra Schuller

Embodiment and Creative Arts Therapy: from phenomenology to cognitive 186
science
 Sabine Koch

V. Developments in training and education

Listening to the Music of the Words and the Words behind the Music: 196
reflections on the selection and assessment procedure for students
applying to a music therapy training programme
Alison Levinge

Permission to be Seen: art therapy in Finnish education settings 202
Päivi-Maria Hautala

A Study into the Individual's and the Director's Experience of Training 208
and Presenting Forum Theatre
Mezzi Franklin

The Fascinating Dialogue between Photography and Therapy: 219
The Phototherapy Institute in Jerusalem
Brigitte Anor

The Contributors 223
Author Index 228

ACKNOWLEDGEMENTS

First, I should like to thank Christine Lapoujade, from the University of Rene Descartes, Paris, for writing the Preface for this publication and for her valuable and enthusiastic support throughout the editing process.

I should like to extend my thanks to Dorothy and Gordon Langley for their diligence as members of the scientific selection committee and for their willing support, focused expertise and camaraderie throughout the process of shaping this publication. Gordon has offered me much advice and has been tireless in contributing to the task of proof-reading.

My personal thanks also to Dianne Gammage for gladly assisting in editing one of the papers, and for the support of colleagues on the Executive Board of ECArTE: Christine Lapoujade, Egbert Hulshof, Albrecht Lampe and Jan-Berend van der Wijk.

I gratefully acknowledge the extensive work of two members of the Local Conference Organising Committee, 2005 – Professor Anastasia-Valentine Rigas (Chair) in Rethymno, Crete, and Katerina Robertson, in Athens – without whom the 8th European Arts Therapies Conference could not have taken place in Greece and, in turn, this publication could not have been realised.

As Editor, I am grateful to all those who have contributed interesting papers to this international publication and for your patience as we worked conscientiously through the editing process.

Sarah Scoble

Publication Selection Committee:

Dorothy Langley
Gordon Langley
Christine Lapoujade
Sarah Scoble

This publication comprises selected papers from: Argentina, Belgium, Finland, France, Germany, Greece, Holland, Jerusalem, Slovenia, Sweden, UK, USA.

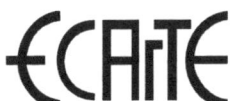

EUROPEAN CONSORTIUM FOR ARTS THERAPIES EDUCATION
14th-17th September 2005

The European Consortium for Arts Therapies Education is a non-profit making organisation. It is a consortium of universities, which was founded in 1991. Its primary purpose is to represent and encourage the development of the arts therapies at a European level, in particular courses offering nationally validated and professionally recognised education for arts therapists. (The arts therapies include art therapy, dance-movement therapy, drama therapy and music therapy). The Consortium currently comprises 32 member institutions from 14 European countries.

The Consortium's work includes:
- creating stronger European links in the arts therapies through the international exchange of staff and students
- promoting research into methods of arts therapies practice within Europe
- developing opportunities for international study in arts therapies education programmes
- promoting recognition of qualifications in the arts therapies at a European level;
- supporting the development of appropriate, academically recognised, nationally validated University courses for the arts therapies.
- offering opportunities for professional communication at its international conferences.

Honorary President
Prof. Dr. Line Kossolapow, University of Münster, Germany

ECArTE Executive Board

Chair: Christine Lapoujade, Université René Descartes, Paris, France

Vice Chair: Sarah Scoble, University of Plymouth, United Kingdom

Co-ordinator: Albrecht Lampe, University of Applied Sciences, Ottesberg, Germany

Treasurer: Egbert Hulshof, HAN University, Nijmegen, The Netherlands

Current Member Institutions of ECArTE

Belgium: Hogeschool voor Wetenschap en Kunst, (Lemmensinstituut), Leuven

Croatia: Sveuciliste U Zagrebu

Finland: Pohjois-Karjalan Ammattikorkeakoulu, Outokumpu
Satakunnan Ammattikorkeakoulu, Kankaanpää

Estonia: Tallinn University

France: Université René Descartes, Paris
Université de Nantes

Germany: Westfälische Wilhelms-Universität, Münster
Fachhochschule für Kunsttherapie, Nürtingen
Universität zu Köln
Fachhochschule für Kunsttherapie, Kunstpädagogik und Freie Kunst, Ottersberg

Ireland: Crawford College of Art and Design, Cork

The Netherlands: HAN University, Nijmegen
CHN University, Leeuwarden
Zuyd University, Sittard
University of Utrecht, Amersfoort
Codarts, Hogeschool voor de Kuusteu, Rotterdam

Poland: Uniwersytet Wroclawski

Russia: St Petersburg Academy for Postgraduate Pedagogocal Training

Slovenia: Univerza v Ljubljani, Ljubljana

Spain: Universidad Complutense de Madrid
Universitat de Barcelona
Universitat de Ramon Lull, Barcelona

Sweden: Universitet Umea
Universiy College of Dance, Stockholm

United Kingdom: University of Hertfordshire
University of Derby
The Central School of Speech and Drama, London
University of Plymouth
Goldsmiths' College University of London
Roehampton University
Queen Margaret College, University of Edinburgh

FOREWORD
The Eighth European Arts Therapies Conference

This volume contains selected papers presented at ECArTE's Eighth European Arts Therapies Conference. The conference took place from 14th to 17th September 2005 and was hosted by the University of Crete, Rethymno, Greece. Delegates attended from thirty countries from across the world.

CONFERENCE DIRECTORS:
Christine Lapoujade,	Université René Descartes, Paris, France
Sarah Scoble,	University of Plymouth, UK
Jan-Berend van der Wijk	University of Professional Education of CHN, Leeuwarden, The Netherlands

LOCAL CONFERENCE ORGANISING COMMITTEE:

In Rethymno, Crete:
Ass. Prof. Anastasia-Valentine Rigas (Chair)
Prof. Joannis Nestoros
Prof. George Galamis
Irene Katsogianni
Elina Brouhatska
Tassos Charalambakis

In Athens:
Katerina Robertson
Vicky Zerva

REGIONAL REPRESENTATIVES:
Austria
Ernst J. Wittkowski

Belgium
Jan van Camp

Croatia
Miroslav Prastacic

Denmark
Vibeke Skov

England and Ireland
Richard Hougham

Estonia
Alice Pehk

Finland
Päivi-Maria Hautala

France
Anne-Marie Dubois

Germany
Peter Rech

Greece
Katerina Robertson

Hungary
Ladislaus Vértes

Iceland
Anna Rögnvaldsdóttir

Italy
Mimma Della Cagnoletta

Lithuania
Danguole

Luxembourg
Marie-Claude Schmit

Netherlands
Egbert Hulshof

Norway
Astri Aakrann-Ziesler

Poland
Wita Szulc, e-mail: wszulc@amu.edu.pl

Portugal
Isabel Figueira

Russia
Alexander Kopytin

Slovenia
Breda Kroflic

Spain
Marian Lopez Fernandez

Sweden
Birgitta Englund

Switzerland
Fausto Sergej Sommer

Turkey
Melike Güney

GLOBAL PARTNERS:
Australia
John Henzell

Brazil
Cristina Dias Allessandrini

Canada
Suzanne Lister
Israel
Avi Goren-Bar
Japan
Tamae Okada
USA
Christine Kerr

PREFACE
by Christine Lapoujade

One of the particularities of modern art consists of bringing together different artistic disciplines. As in ancient Greek theatre, music is again finding its place among the actors on the stage, paintings at exhibitions are being commented on by live dancing figures, video artists are projecting their images on the backstage of operas and so on.
ECArTE considers the bringing together of all these artists in the context of a therapeutic concern as one of its particular and exceptional tasks. In so doing, it is indicating that the arts have their rightful place in those places where people take care of others. Creating fiction (*poièsis*) is always considered as the core activity of humans as symbolising beings.
During ECArTE's 8th 'Arts Therapies Conference' at the Rethymnon, University in Crete, entitled "Grounding the Vision – to advance Theory and Practice", this age-old symbolising task of the arts is confronted – or "grounded" – with the demands of contemporary "evidence-based" therapeutic activity. You can find in this publication the results of this confrontation.

In the first chapter (**Grounding our vision**), the basic issues of art-therapies are marked off. Jan Van Camp evokes the 'uncanny' experience of Freud when for the first time in his life he set foot on the consecrated ground of the Acropolis. He feels as if he meets something that suddenly withdraws from the 'representation' he had of the monuments before and touches a 'presence' that hardly can be captured in words or images. The analysis of this 'derealising' event leads to the idea that the art-therapies are engaged in a specific area which is between 'presence' and 'representation' or, in the terms of Nietzsche, between the Dionysian and the Apollonian, an area which is explored in an inimitable way by the tragic experience of Greek theatre. Can we posit that the proper task of the art-therapies, although always embedded in a process of shaping (*Gestaltung*), lays in giving room to this unsayable and unimaginable 'presence'?
In spite of the fact that we speak about multiple art-therapies, every single artistic therapy has its own way of *Gestaltung*. Phil Jones, in providing an overview on the different disciplines of arts therapy and their current practice and thinking, stresses the differences and similarities between these disciplines and suggests that each can benefit from the other and that it would be possible to develop a sort of interdisciplinary "Ecartovision" on the art-therapies. His proposal is not an "integrationist" vision but a way through which light could be cast into each individual discipline and making clearer the respective places of the art therapists. Providing the concepts of "foreground" and "background" to create a dialogue which engages difference and similarity, he attempts to facilitate the understanding of the artistic form and process in the way they could affect the relationship between client and therapist. To conclude, he invites the art therapists to think about a model for core processes across the arts-therapies.

In the second chapter (**Concepts and debates**), different authors do honour to the title of the conference by trying to reconcile philosophical ideas about symbolising and fictionalising processes in the human psyche with modern neurological findings, giving them a so called 'scientific grounding'. Ralf Bolle confronts the Jungian approach of "Inner Images" as the expression of archetypal experiences with modern brain research, which proves the importance of such images for psychic development. Michael Barham calls upon the hypothesis of Noam Chomsky, which assumes that the human brain is well equipped with the neurological structures to generate symbolic and fictional systems, which corresponds, so asserts the author, with our social narratives. Pauline Mottram is concerned about the danger that a quite dominant psychoanalytic theory could obscure the tacit knowledge that works in the practice of art therapy. Art therapists have to elaborate concepts which emerge more directly from their practice, such as for example the notion of "dialogical self", which helps immensely to describe accurately that which happens during an art therapeutic session. This movement of 'going back to the art itself' is also perceptible in the following articles. Peter Sinapius stresses for example that artistic training has to be central in the education of art therapists and Peter Rech cautions us about adopting a predominantly 'psychologising' attitude towards pictures. Images are as ambiguous as symptoms, they may reveal and hide at the same time and so mislead the art therapist.

The presenters in the third chapter (**Practitioner research and assessment of practice**), by putting the nature of their works in the context of a theoretical framework, enlighten and facilitate the understanding of what is going on in the session and make it possible to develop the methodologies of assessment to evaluate those practices. The efficacy of the clinical work in art-therapies has been explored at different levels. Three of the authors stress that it is important to take as one's starting point methods derived from therapeutic practice, rather than trying to improve the traditional methodology used in therapeutic research. The aim of Martin Cope's research is to set the foundation for a new "Narrative Analysis" approach in dramatherapy research and, in so doing, to bridge the gap between the therapist's interpretation of a process and the client's experience of dramatherapy. Lambros Yotis uses Aristotle's Poetics in a therapeutic context, not only to create an evaluation system for drama therapy, but also to build up structure and meaning in the chaotic experience of his psychotic patients. Erna Grönlund, Barbro Renck and Nita Gyllander Vabö present the findings of an assessment of the effects and value of dance therapy with young depressed girls. As for Mathilde Tubben, she proves that even "The building of a hut" can be applied as an instrument to measure the ego strength of children.
The second part of this chapter presents two experiences of group-sessions. In the first, Edith Lecourt and Violeta Hensy de Gainza analyse the role of language and cultural differences through the use of sonorous communication in groups when the therapist does not share the culture of her client. In the second one, Lia Zografou presents the findings of a method based on a ritual model of dramatherapy in a group with addictive problems. Katarina Couroucli-Robertson

presents a case of an individual drama therapy with a client suffering from panic attacks and Vicky Zerva-Spanou describes the process of a play therapy, showing how the development of artistic abilities in a sexually abused young girl can give access to unsayable traumatic experiences and contributes to the reconstruction of the body-image.

The fourth chapter (**Essays in theory and practice**) enlarges the debate. The two first articles deal with the pre-eminently art-therapeutic theme of trauma. When the therapist him/herself becomes traumatised by the penetrating images produced by the client, it can have onerous consequences on the client as well as on the therapist. For Pauline McGee, coping with this "vicarious traumatisation" is the real sense of 'grounding' our vision. She suggests preventive strategies, which would enable the art therapists to have an ethical and balanced engagement in their work. Simone Alter-Müri presents one of the possible means to support such preventive activities: namely, the study of pictures and music created in response to crisis and war. This implies that art protects us against art. A well-shaped artistic form protects us against the cruelty of its traumatic kernel. The "théatre de la cruauté" of Antonin Artaud and Jerzy Grotowski's "Art as presentation" touch, in the sharpest of ways, this ambiguous status of art, as stated in the article by Aleksandra Schuller. Her article explores the enduring importance of ritual in western theatre, culture and arts therapy. Sabine Koch draws together art and science and discusses new interdisciplinary perspectives on embodiment in arts therapy.

The last chapter (**Developments in training and education**), brings up different views on the selection and education of arts-therapy students. During the selection procedure a balance has to be kept in mind between artistic and therapeutic talent. Alison Levinge describes the admission procedure in her music therapy department and draws attention to the importance of 'listening' to the candidate's words and music and to the relevance of the order in which each part of the process is carried out (first music, then words). In the context of dramatherapy, a study by Mezzi Franklin, demonstrates that it is important for a director to understand adult learning and group dynamics and not to underestimate the powerful impact of improvisation. That art therapists too have to improvise, is something Päivi-Maria Hautala figures out in her study regarding the integration of art therapy in the Finnish schooling system. The art therapists in question show their talents for improvisation more on the level of their capacity to assume a pedagogical discourse in their therapy. Finally, Brigittte Anor from Israel breaches the traditional Jewish prohibition on images by founding and leading a Masters course in Photo Therapy.

The different articles show the progress of the profession through various disciplines and in very diverse settings. Twelve countries brought contributions, which reflect the already established research issues as well as showcasing the new ones. Undoubtedly, this manifestation bears a tribute to ECArTE's promotion of dialogue and learning from each other. Only through cooperation at the level of research, can we give our therapies a strong foundation in the world of healthcare and psychotherapy. The different papers of this scholarly publication point to the growing level of theoretical grounding and research programmes in the arts therapies. They demonstrate that, in the face of suffering, the arts is our strongest ally.

1st December, 2006

I
GROUNDING OUR VISION

JAN VAN CAMP

THE GREEK TRAGEDY AS A MODEL FOR THE ARTS THERAPIES

It is a particular experience to be confronted *in reality* with something that we knew until then only by means of a *representation*. When suddenly we can see, feel and touch that with which we were familiar for a long time in an imaginary way, an experience of shudder and *Unheimlichkeit* (uncanny) emerges.

Such a shivering experience came over Freud (1926: 553), when at the age of forty-eight he visited Greece for the first time. He initially planned to set out for the island of Corfu together with his brother Alexander, but when in Trieste, preparing for the crossing, they were advised against it by a friend, telling them Corfu would be too hot. He suggested instead going to Athens. But Freud and his brother objected and thought it would present too many insurmountable obstacles to change their travel plans. Freud wrote that, the day before they had to make a decision, spirits were low. Remarkably enough, they almost automatically and without breathing a word about it, went to the ticket-service for a boat destined for Athens.

When in Athens, they obviously visit the Acropolis and it is there that Freud has a remarkable thought – or a flash as he calls it: "So", he observed, "all this really exists like we learned at school!?", and at the same time he had the feeling that what he saw there was not real, not true. This expression of disbelief continues to intrigue Freud, so much in fact that even thirty-two years later he writes a text about it on behalf of a commemorative book for his friend Romain Roland. He is fascinated by the fact that such a pleasant experience of finally seeing with his own eyes what had fed his imagination and desire since secondary school, gave rise to this experience of disbelief and denial of the reality of what he beholds. He says it is a case of 'too good to be true', which can overtake people when they, bothered by feelings of guilt and inferiority, cannot grant themselves any happiness and deny the reality of the happiness that falls to their lot.

But, even more decisive for the feeling of *derealisation* (*Entfremdung*) is the fact that it is unconsciously connected to a prohibition, namely the prohibition to surpass his father and to behold something that his father was not granted to behold, because of lack of money or classical education.[1] So it's about an oedipal conflict.

This is how the unconscious works: you don't have to want to go to Athens, but to

---

[1] We don't take up here the idea that Freud's derealisation can also be considered as the expression of a reactivation of an old conflict between Freud, who as a scholar admired largely the bourgeois culture of Vienna and was strongly fascinated by classical civilisation, and Freud, as the grandson of "Rabi Schlomo", an eminent representative of the traditional Jewish culture for whom Athens and its monuments didn't have any value. This approach emphasizes the 'splitting of the ego' as a result of the existence of two contradictory attitudes to reality, those of acceptance and disavowal (see Rey-Flaud, H., 2006 :113-119).

Corfu, to be able to end up in Athens, and then, once you have arrived at the Acropolis, say that what you see there is 'not true', 'not real'. Freud interprets his unconscious avoidance of mounting the Acropolis as an attempt to prevent competing with his father, to prevent exceeding him intellectually and geographically, or in oedipal terms: he did not want to eliminate him as an obstacle to reach the most desirable object, the mother.

Freud's every act before he at last ends up at the Acropolis – to choose Corfu as his destination, his bad mood concerning the possible cancellation of the destination, the unthinking purchase of steamboat tickets that would bring him to Athens – are 'deeds' which in a certain sense let the original Oedipal constellation, with defence and all, happen again.

From mirror to double, from representation to image

One could compare Freud's experience of estrangement to the alienation that occurs when the image in a mirror ('reflection') changes into the image of a 'double', which is, for example, the case in the famous painting by René Magritte 'La reproduction interdite'(1937, Boymans-Van Beuningen, Rotterdam). Instead of the familiar reversal by which left becomes right and right left, a double appears, along with the uncanny sensation of disbelief, the *unheimliche* sensation of disbelief.

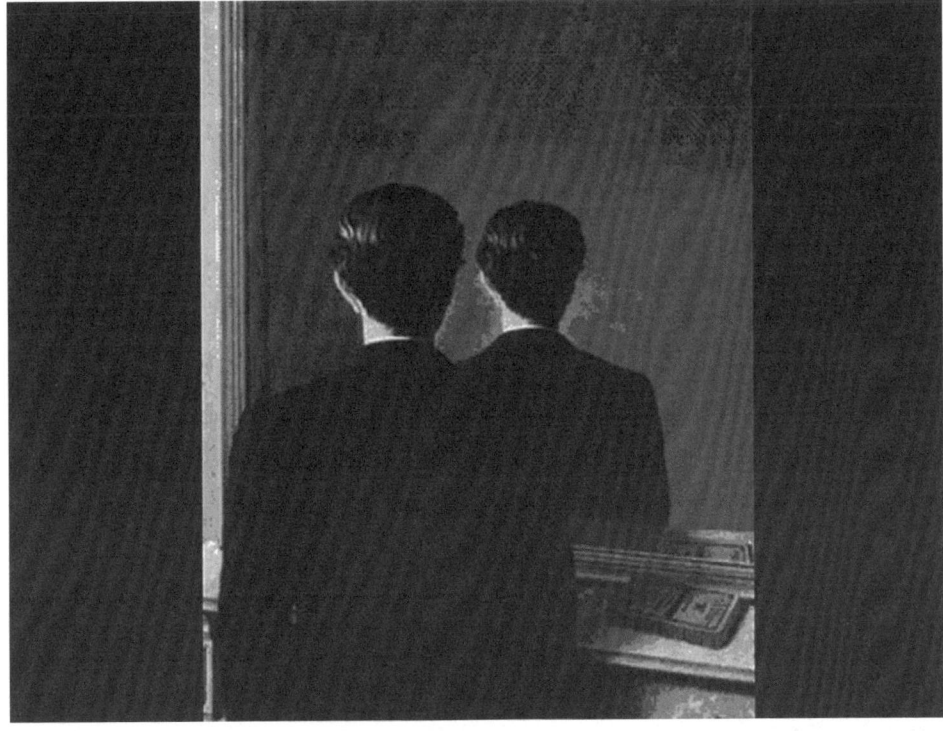

René Magritte, (1937), *La reproduction interdite (portrait d'Edward James)*, Rotterdam, Museum Boymans-Van Beuningen.

In his famous text 'Das Unheimliche' (Freud, 1919: 227) Freud describes a similar experience which he had in the sleeping compartment of a train when he saw the shape of a man who suddenly entered his compartment. Immediately after, he realised in amazement that what he saw was his own image, reflected in the mirror of a cupboard which had fallen open. The strange thing, Freud says, is in fact always the familiar, but a familiarity of which we'd rather know nothing about and which we cover with representations that keep the abject at a distance.
In that sense it is interesting, following P. Fédida (2001) and G. Didi-Huberman (2004), to make a clear distinction between an *image* and a *representation*. An image is a figure that is hardly figured, a form which is gradually shaping into a form, an inconceivable sensation which is quickly sketched and which, when at the point of observation, is already gone.
Although images may possess a substance and therefore are material or organic, the element they are made of is rather air or breath. It is the same breath of which Paul Celan (2003) speaks (*Atemwende*) when he wants to describe the movements and caesura in his poetic texts, texts that indeed form figures, but which hardly refer to some imaginable or represantable reality outside the text. Images emerge from a memory (*Gedächtnis, mémoire*) that can't be remembered (*Erinnerung, souvenir*) because it is not composed of representations that can be recollected. Although the traumatic experiences of the concentration camp of Paul Celan are registered in an unconscious memory, they cannot be called up as recollection, as representation, since the most proper aspect of a traumatic experience lies in the fact that it is situated outside any world of representation. Even though images may be extremely sketchy and unstable and may not do more than occasionally blow along so that sometimes we can catch a glimpse of them, they probably do form the core of what we are and they can be seen as a necessary condition for every one of us to be able to live. Lacan (2005) would say that they form our *sinthome*, sinthome written in this old-French manner to distinguish it from the neurotic *symptom*. The neurotic symptoms built themselves around the *sinthome* like a fence ('enclosure') and the purpose of the treatment is to realize a gradual removal of that fence whereby the *sinthome* stands free again. What stands free, however, possesses no single representation, evades every meaning and can as such no longer be interpreted.
Could it be that art therapists are mainly occupied with this matter, with this 'core of enjoyment' which surfaces behind the symptoms, the world of unrepresentable images which deal with the fundamental way in which we stand in the world?

Returning to Freud who is still amazed when he is standing at the Acropolis, we could now say that something like this must have happened to him, namely that the covert 'representation' of the Acropolis had been replaced by an 'image' of the Acropolis. As if everything he had witnessed before was spectacle (*opsis*), simulacrum, appearance, comforting representation which kept the thing itself at a certain distance, as if it were reflected in a mirror.

Medusa and anxiety
The mirror-theme and its necessity are represented in mythology by the monstrous face of Medusa and the measures that had to be taken to protect

oneself against her petrifying gaze. Medusa, with her large round head covered with snake hair, dilated eyes and an open mouth with her tongue out, transforms every living creature that crosses her sight into solidified rock. The sounds she makes are guttural and sharp, as an animal-like scream mixed with gnashing of teeth. She is the outstanding example of the inconceivable, since everyone who tries to form an image of her by looking at her and hearing her hideous sounds, is already dead. The Medusa can only be conquered with a mirror and a musical instrument, the *aulos*. By means of a glittering, reflecting shield that he got from Athena and in which Medusa's sight is refracted, Perseus succeeds in looking at her through the representation in the mirror and killing her. Athena herself knows how to construe a wind instrument, the aulos, out of the unbearable sounds the monster utters the moment it is being decapitated. The aulos in an instrument that is not known for its harmonic qualities, but for its power to integrate dissonant sounds into a musical form.

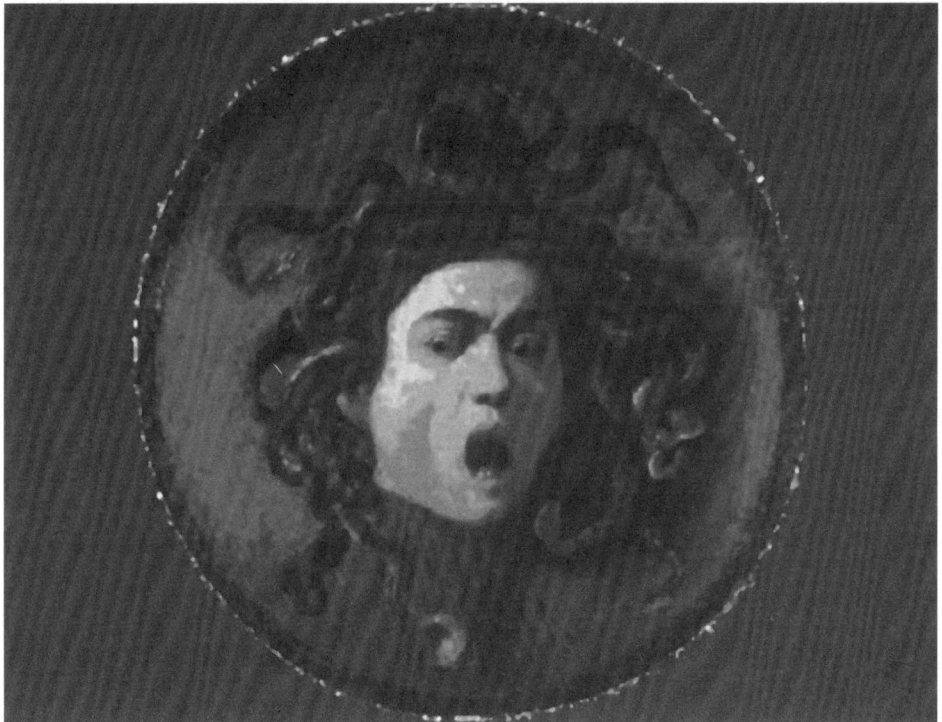

Caravaggio (1573–1610), *Medusa*, Florence, The Uffizi Gallery.

Consequently, we can say that the Acropolis was only the *signifier* for Freud, connected with all sorts of specular representations, photographic images of the Parthenon, the Propylaea, the Nike-temple and the Erechteion. But the Thing itself appears as nothing in the representation, like the *real* which languishes under the signifier. Suddenly, standing there in front of these temples, he is confronted with the idea that these representations are no fiction, that he sees them here and now and that he can touch them in their original substantiality, as a genuine presence, as if they were not representations (*mimesis*) of something else that is inconceivable. As if there would be a reality outside of the representation, a reality that can present itself as such, a full, complete, virginal, unaffected and inviolable presence. It is probably only anxiety which can originate such thought. Is it the human anxiety which haunts the whole of Western thinking when the idea is put forward of a reality without theatre, a real without representation? That there would be a place where we could be our complete self, not alienated and not dissociated, perfect innocent subjects, without tragic fault and without prohibition, freed from war and rivalry and free from any institution. And that we could say that art has the capacity of representing the real, that it could make something take place in an original manner, outside of any representing arrangement. Does for example not Sophocles show us such an innocent subject in the shape of Antigone? Can theatre show us the inconceivable, can it show us for example the most inconceivable thing of all, namely death? Does the inconceivable take place there, upon the scene and is that scene necessary as to we can observe it with fear (φοβος) and compassion (ελειος)? Does the scene give us access to the inconceivability of death, of incest, of maternal sexuality, of trauma, or does it make us immune to these things, does it hypnotise us and does it stupefy us with its shining representations?

Back to the Acropolis. Freud is shuddering when setting foot on the Parthenon. This is not real, he thinks, this can not be true. In fact, he is right, because the Parthenon is in a certain sense only a representation of the earlier temple, the sixth century Hekatompedon, which by order of Xerxes was destroyed by the Persians and which for its part is a representation of the earlier temples that had been built for the goddess Athena. These temples which were built and destroyed are representations of the way the architects represented them in their imagination and drew them in their plans. These representations and drawings are undoubtedly inspired by models of places of sacrifice, which, since time out of mind, were established.

The most interesting, however, is the explanation Freud gives for his destabilizing experience at the Acropolis. He says that his sight was crossed by a forbidden pleasure causing him to see no more, that is, that he designates what he sees as 'untrue', 'unreal'. His look is haunted by an immemorial pleasure that causes the spectacle on the Athens hilltop to withdraw itself from his sight. This phantom disrupts his observation so much that he cannot appropriate the sight of the temples. It is a look that not only determines his way of watching, but is just as much hidden inside the field of the visible and it renders unreal the scene on the top of the hill. Freud is, unconsciously and opposed to everything, driven into seeing the Acropolis, as if in the observation of the temple complex something were hidden, something he can't figure out at first glance. The temples are a kind of screen in which something of a reflected object is hidden, an object that Lacan (2004) calls an object which causes Freud's desire. Freud says that the fascination for the Acropolis protects himself against an incestuous desire. The fact that the shining beauty of Greek architecture is a good protection is proof of the fact that it took Freud thirty-two years to be on the trail of the actual cause for his fascination and for his 'memory defect' which was connected with it. For this classical, Apollonian architecture did not prove to give so much protection that it could have prevented Freud's depersonalizing and derealizing experience. The brilliance of beauty blinds the spectator, but at the same time illuminates and transfigures the object. The fact that the clear, tight and harmonic forms of Greek architecture could still not prevent the outbreak of anxiety Freud suffered from, explains undoubtedly why he has always had an aversion to the more baroque, vague and endless forms which appear in theatre, dance and music.

Time and representation
It is a traditional idea to situate theatre, dance and music as arts of *time* as opposed to the arts of *representation*, represented by the art of painting, sculpture, architecture and literature. Arts of time do not immediately appeal to representation, but to an *event* which takes place in time. Like in ritual and music, dance also is carried by a specific succession of events which cannot be reduced to an idea or a representation. The essence of what's happening lies not in the representation, but in the occurrence itself. That which takes place is not the accidental more or less successful incarnation of something that had already received a more intelligible form, but it is the unique matter itself which merely by taking place is at the basis of some form. To give a simple example: the funeral ritual is not the accidental expression of respect for the dead which precedes the ritual. This and all other possible representations (like, for example, the belief in immortality) arise rather from the *as such* meaningless act of the ritual which came first.
'Im Anfang war der Tat', Freud (1912-13) says. We cannot replace the acting of Sophocles' Antigone by some summarizing interpretation, how ever interesting that may prove to be. Antigone has to be played over and over again because the essence of Antigone lies in the terrifying intensity of the play itself. Every interpretation or representation destroys to a certain extent the event (the ritual), not only because every interpretation fails to capture the whole richness of the event, but especially because an interpretation succeeds only when it is impregnated by the effectful resonance of the event itself.
Consequently, the so called arts of time are characterized by the fact that they have to take place time and time again, that they have to occur and cannot be represented in any other way than through this original coming about itself. But is this coming about not also a representation of something which has occurred earlier? Every theatrical and musical performance, are they not the somewhat varied repeats of an earlier play or performance?

To explore the strained relationship between time and representation, Didier-Weill (1995, 1998) introduces a series of oppositions which can be found in philosophy, history of art and mythology. He speaks of a structural tension between a philosophy of *becoming* (Heraclites) and a philosophy of *being* (Parmenides), between baroque and classicism and between the mythological figures Dionysus and Apollo (Nietzsche). Heraclites looked at the world from the flowing of becoming, as a continuing movement of succeeding and not recoverable events (Παντα ρει κ'ουδευ μενει, and: we step not twice in the same river), whereas Parmenides created with his philosophy the foundation of Western philosophical thinking which since Plato orientates itself for the most part on stability and the unchanging nature of ideas. That is why Nietzsche (1881) speaks about music as 'the night of philosophy'.

Baroque, not only as an historical situated period of style, but as a structural position in art in general, emphasizes continuity, movement and evanescence. Classicism, by contrast, is the art of the plain, visible, clear-cut form. It is born in Greece with the vertical lines of the Doric pillars and the discovery of the perfect contours which distinguish sculpture. Baroque art is fascinating, ravishing and passionate, because it resists the straightforward limits of classicism and wipes them away with a brilliant light which originates more from the colour than from the form.

Didier-Weill (2002) thinks baroque can be seen as the reflection in art of the constant insistence of drive, which it tries to incarnate into form. Eugenio d'Ors (2000) says baroque is essentially musical. As in music, he places movement in the forefront, a movement which suddenly arises and of which one can only be receptive to, when surrendering to it. The enjoyment that is experienced by losing oneself in such unlimited movement is, in Lacanian psychoanalysis, indicated with the term 'jouissance'. It is an enjoyment beyond pleasure, an ambiguous enjoyment which can not be described in terms of emotion or feeling, precisely because it withdraws itself from the world of representation, and which lies closer to the pure body-like attitudes, movements and sensations which in music were formerly called *affects*.

The subject which relates itself to the real, in this baroque way, has the tendency to merge into the object, to lose its own contours and to give up its position of desiring subject. There is only one possible way to ascertain that such abandonment of the subject position is threatening, which is the appearance of the affect of anxiety or the experience of *Unheimlichkeit*. The anxious affect of unreality that Freud experiences on the Athens Acropolis, signals that the object which is at the basis of its looking forward to this meeting, is starting to shine through too much, and becomes all too present in the sight of these antique temples.

That what normally should stay concealed behind the blinding beauty of the aesthetic form and which rouses fascination for it, will then so prominently stand out that looking becomes unbearable and that one has to avert his eyes to become oneself again. Anxiety, as Lacan (2004) puts it, does not appear when the child loses or threatens to lose his mother, but on the contrary when she comes too close and is no longer the lost object which carries his desire. Art, especially when it strikes us, always evokes this strange bond between desire and *Unheimlichkeit*. Since Kant, this specific aesthetic experience has been called 'the sublime'. In the Lacanian terminology the object, the lost object, is said to be elevated into the dignity of the Thing. Only that way a work of art can acquire an irreplaceable significance, overwhelm us with its timeless presence, and withdraw itself from its status as cultural product (Lyotard, 1988). At the same time this sublime aspect of art warns us, art therapists, of the fact that dealing with aesthetic objects is a delicate, sometimes dangerous and frightening venture. Every art therapist, and surely those who work with neurotic and borderline patients, knows the phenomenon whereby their patients at first instance draw back when they are asked to surrender to musical improvisation or freely to express themselves in art therapy. It takes a whole lot of preparation gradually to appropriate musical or plastic forms which allow patients get into a sound or a colour safely, to let them be affected by something of which the destination or result is uncertain.

The sirens and the *apotropaion*
Greek mythology offers us brilliant stories about how the human being must resist the devastating power of that which fascinates us in beauty and where, at the same time, beauty protects us. Odysseus has to tie himself to the mast of the ship and his crew have to cover their ears so as not to get carried away by the sublime singing of the sirens. To surrender to it would mean their death, the loss of themselves. In the story about the return of the Argonauts, it is Orpheus, singing and being accompanied by a lyre, who must offer resistance to the call of the sirens. Orpheus proceeds to neutralize the deadly singing with his music. What is this Orphic addition, this Orphic *farmakon*, this *apotropaion* which protects people against the irresistible terror that is the singing of the sirens? How does music protect us against music?

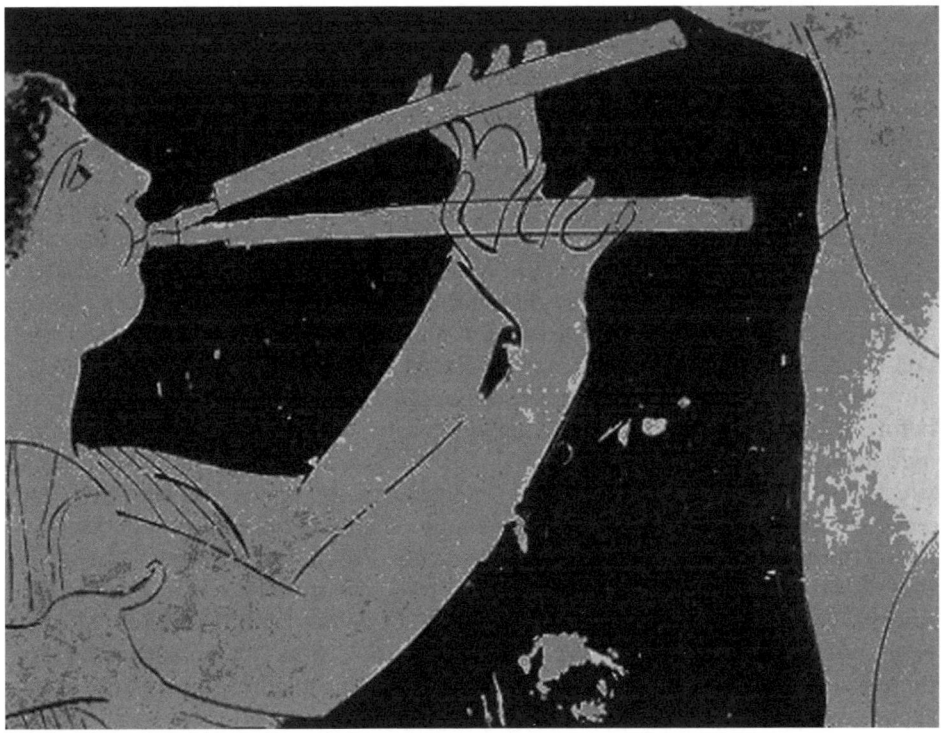

Aulos, Ancient Greek pottery, 5th cent. B.C., British Museum.

The moment when the ship's company is at the verge of surrendering to the call, of letting in the *jouissance* and losing themselves, Orpheus offers us a possibility to create a certain *distance* regarding the domain of the 'thing'. The Orphic musical form offers a sort of representation, a figure which transforms the timeless sacral singing of the sirens to a representation in which the human being recognizes itself in his temporary, mortal condition. A form with a beginning and an ending, in which every part arranges itself in a symbolic way into a whole in which nothing lasts forever, but everything is no more than a nostalgic repeat of what has been. That is probably the core of what the Greek call the 'tragic': that we are condemned to representation, that we are irrevocably captured within a mimetic structure and that there is nothing, neither belief, nor philosophical thinking that can set us free from this. As speaking and desiring creatures we are subjected to the Delphic γνωτι σεαυτον᷅ (know yourself), namely the awareness that from the moment we start to speak and desire, we are subjected to time and representation and that we have to accept our mortality.

Greek tragedy

But the Greek tragedy is of course much more than an urge to accept our mortality with a certain resignation. When Antigone enters the scene with a lot of daring and declares: 'I am already dead', she shows as a living dead that the essence of her desire does not consist of a passive acceptance of the *gnôti seauton*, of her mortality, but also precisely in the resistance against it, in being attracted by a point which withdraws itself from representation. That the human desire is characterized by a tragic understanding means that it is captured in an insolvable opposition and strained relation between Thing and representation, between the sacral and the human, between the continuous time and the historical time. The Orphic music may indeed be a *lamento*, an elegy on the inevitability of loss, but it draws its strength from its shaking and pulsating snatching away from the deadly atmosphere of the inaudible singing of the sirens, from a rhythmic unfolding of reflections, echoes which create an in-between space, a distance, a reprise. It is thanks to the power of the sirens that the Orphic elegy obtains a glorious beauty, a beauty which explodes because in that outburst there still appears to be a glimpse of what it was before it erupted, when it was still concealed in an unsuspecting, unlocatable silence. By the grace of the Muses it unexpectedly breaks out, and in the gifted moment of the outbreak itself, originates an assumption of what it was before it broke out, when it was that mythical inaudible 'nothing', that *musica mundana* that lies now at the basis of the twisted and pulsating movements in which the sounds start to recognize themselves, in which for the first time something audible emerges and in the shape of that audible music something of a non recollectable origin seems to resonate. From the singing of the sirens that cannot be heard, nor staged, we can only see the *effect* in the irresistible fascination, the threatening acknowledgement of defeat from the sailors. Music is never fascinating because it is the imitation of a fine form, but because in its form there is a memory resonating of her formless, chaotic, inaudible and deadly origin: silence. Only the ear that is recast by the desire is able to hear this silence and the 'grace' it grants to the music.

This strained relationship between Thing and representation, or, in analytical terms, the issue of desire is, in the context of the tragedy, translated by Nietzsche (1872) as the opposition between Dionysus and Apollo. Nietzsche's originality lies in his intuition that the transition of the invisible or inaudible essence of the real (the Thing) to the visible and audible incarnation in the form, or in the *appearance* (emerging) as such, takes place through music, personified by the god Dionysus. Dionysus is known to be the god of immoderateness and fuddle,of that which we call *enthusiasm*, that is, the singing and dancing ecstasy and so being absorbed in the god himself (ενθεος). It is said that his followers, the Menades or Bacchantes, in real life good housewives, daughters or wives, would tear themselves away from their social identity and transform into delirious dancers who surrendered themselves to singing Dithyrambs, the hymns to Dionysus. The godhead thus takes possession of the women in town, for he calls on that part in them – analytically speaking their 'real' part – that is not supported by a written law and is irresistibly recognized by music. This assembly of Menades, the thiasos of Dionysus, would become the predecessor of the choir in the tragedy. But this group only exists as a choir in as far as one member withdrew himself to perform as a speaking actor. From that moment on one can speak of the basic structure of theatre, in which choir and actor are separated from each other by the tragic scene and in which a transformation has taken place from a collective celebrated ritual between the initiates to a spectacle with spectators who observe the whole event from a distance. The actor, who initially figures as choirmaster, who improvises a set of stanza's (couplets) to which the choir responds, will gradually base himself on texts that are written by others. He's but an actor in the full meaning of the word, that is, a player instead of a narrator, as soon as he is individualized by wearing a mask and other actors are brought onto the scene with whom he goes into dialogue. That is how play and illusion are born.

The speaking and playing actor makes a decisive move from Dionysus to Apollo, from the god of the immoderateness of the real to the god of measure and language and it is essential for the actor's play that, in his speaking and in his presence, the enthusiasm of the Menades is not forgotten. The chant of the choir of the Menades, although inaudible by the actor's speech, is still resonating in the graciousness and presence of his play. As Nietzsche (1872) notes, in classical tragedy, a unique reconciliation originates between Dionysus and Apollo, between a chthonic musicality and the Olympic 'logos'. By the tragic actor, word and music are brought into continuity with each other, his speech remains inhabited by the music from his archaic, sacral origin. The tragic guilt of the actor is therefore not as much the result of a delinquent act or a misjudging, but is due to the fact that it is contesting the written laws of the city, because of its recognition of another power – a power which can not be assumed by the symbolic law.

This other power is invoked by Oedipus and Antigone when, at the end of the play, they don't have anything left to say, because everything that had to be said has already been said. When they have lost everything and no hope is left, when there's nobody who understands their words, they don't fall into a melancholic abandonment, but direct themselves to *another* (Alter), which is receptive for a significance which cannot be put into words and can only be transferred by music. They sing, supported by the aulos, a recitative on the vowels 'o', 'a'.

Bibliography

Celan, P. (1967). *Atemwende*, Frankfurt am Main: Suhrkamp Verlag.
Didier-Weill, A. (1995). *Les trois temps de la loi*, Paris : Seuil.
Didier-Weill, A. (1998). *Invocations. Dionysos, Moïse, Saint Paul et Freud*, Paris: Calman-Lévy.
Didier-Weill, A. (2002). *L'amour fou*, in : Balestriere, L. (e.a.), *Parler d'amour*, Bruxelles: La Lettre volée.
Didi-Huberman, G. (2004). *Geste d'air et de pierre. Corps, parole, souffle, image*, Paris: Minuit (Collection « Paradoxe »).
Fédida, P. (2001). *Les bienfaits de la dépression. Eloge de la psychothérapie*, Paris : Ed.Odile Jacob.
Freud, S. (1912-13). *Totem und Tabu*, in: Gesammelte Werke, Bd.9, , Frankfurt am Main: Fisher Verlag, 1960.
Freud, S., (1919). *Das Unheimliche*, in: Gesammelte Werke, Bd.12, p.227, Frankfurt am Main: Fisher Verlag, 1960.
Freud, S. (1926). *An Romain Rolland*, in: Gesammelte Werke, Bd.14, p.553, Fisher Verlag, Frankfurt am Main, 1960.
Lacan, J. (2004). *Le Séminaire*, Livre X, *L'angoisse*, Paris: Seuil.
Lacan, J. (2005). *Le Séminaire*, Livre XXIII, *Le sinthome*, Paris: Seuil.
Lyotard, J.-F. (1988). *L'inhumain. Causeries sur le temps*, Paris: Galilée.
Nietzsche, F. (1872). *Die Geburt der Tragödie aus dem Geiste der Musik*, in: Sämtliche Werke. Kritische Studienausgabe in 15 Bänden. Eds. Giorgio Colli und Mazzino Montinari, München, Berlin, New York: (DTV und Walter de Gruyter), 1980.
Nietzsche, F. (1881). *Morgenröte*, in: Sämtliche Werke. Kritische Studienausgabe in 15 Bänden. Eds. Giorgio Colli und Mazzino Montinari, München, Berlin, New York (DTV und Walter de Gruyter), 1980.
Ors, E. d', (2000). *Le Baroque*, Paris: Gallimard.
Rey-Flaud, H. (2006). « *Et Moïse crea les Juifs..* ». *Le Testament de Freud*, Paris: Aubier.
Van Camp, J. (2000). *Musik, Wiederholung und Affekt*, in: *Musiktherapeutische Umschau*, Band 21.

Picture references

René Magritte, (1937), *La reproduction interdite (portrait d'Edward James)*, Rotterdam, Museum Boymans-Van Beuningen.
Caravaggio (1573–1610), *Medusa*, Florence, The Uffizi Gallery.
Aulos, Ancient Greek pottery, 5th cent. B.C., British Museum.

PHIL JONES

BETWEEN THE ARTS THERAPIES: HOW DIFFERENT IS DIFFERENT? HOW SIMILAR IS SIMILAR?

Key Note ECArTE Conference 2005
Dedicated to the memory of Neil Walters

Introduction
Do the different art forms in the arts therapies make any difference to the client within these processes? Does research indicate different findings in terms of the aims, forms and efficacy within the separate art forms?
In my experience of working with students and trained arts therapists within the different disciplines over the past 20 years, there are three responses arts therapists often make in relation to participating in each others' arts in workshops. One is suspicion, that the other art forms are anxiety provoking, that it's 'not their language': they feel de-skilled and unable to express themselves as they would do in their 'own' art form and they are reluctant to engage. The second is that in response to potential difference they say 'but we do that too' or 'that's no different from when we...': which is often a quick hand to politely nod and note a family resemblance whilst, like many extended family interactions, really being a brief duty acknowledgement and visit before getting safely away home again. The third, and the one of which this presentation based on my new book 'The Arts Therapies' (Routledge 2005) is a part, is interest in the others' forms and practices, as a way forward for mutual discovery about the arts and change in therapy.
In the way they have evolved to date, the individual arts therapies have both things in common, and elements of difference. This keynote presentation looks at the way in which some aspects of the arts forms emphasise, or foreground, some processes, experiences and kinds of language over others in the client's participation. It will examine issues in training and writing within the arts therapies, and will review research approaches and developments in methodology across and between the disciplines.
It will offer a critical review of the different responses within the arts therapies to interdisciplinarity. Areas include: the way the arts therapies connect to the general provision of services for clients; how arts therapists communicate and work within multidisciplinary teams; and the understanding of client change in relation to existing systems and procedures. A part of this process can be seen in terms of the different worlds that the arts therapist connects with. These are both where the potential of the arts therapies lies, in bringing connection between art making and healing contexts, but also where tensions can exist. Peters, in writing about sharing responsibility for patient care, has pointed to the potential for tension between different professions in areas such as referral, treatment plans and collaboration

regarding 'discourse about health...(and) different languages in health care' (Peters, 1994 : 189). Reason echoes this,

> 'Clinicians from different disciplines clash because while they may agree about what the patient needs, they interpret those needs through different frameworks [with]...different assumptions about what an intervention may do...'(Reason, 1991 : 144).

The presentation will draw upon material from 'The Arts Therapies' (Jones 2005) which involves analysing working practices, case studies, the discussion of theory and practice and, crucially, the understanding of different clinical models and languages to offer a way of examining difference and similarity in the arts therapies.

The extent of interdisciplinity: Ecartovision

Some people will, of course, deny that there's any issue or problem here. They'll say – 'but I speak with my colleagues' or 'but there's book on...' or 'when I was training we did some role play'. But I suggest you have a look at any book in your own discipline, or examine any issue of your professional journal, or, indeed, any article in 'The Arts In Psychotherapy' to see what the proportion of references are to writing or research outside of the specific arts therapy discipline. As this is a European Conference and as a theme is collaboration, I've drawn on a great tradition of international collaboration. I've created this game for us, based on the Eurovision Song Contest. It's called *Ecartovision*.

Ecartovision: how to play

Imagine if we took any edition of an arts therapy journal, from music therapy or dramatherapy say, and just as countries vote for each other's songs, we took a reference to another discipline as being a vote....what do you think we would get? That's the basis of *Ecartovision*.

So, as an example I'm going to take the most recent edition of the art therapy journal *Inscape*. For every reference to a discipline we award a point. There are 85 references in all, so there are 85 votes. So how many out of 85 possible votes do art therapy authors give to music therapy, how many to dramatherapy, how many to dance movement therapy and how many to art therapy and non arts therapy disciplines such as psychotherapy?

Well, you have to guess – there's a lot of money spent on betting for the Eurovision contest. Let's see how well you do here anticipating the votes of Inscape's Art Therapy Profession Jury in *Ecartovision*. I'd like you to decide for yourself how the 85 references or 'votes' are divided up across the disciplines. Write the division down please, and share it with the person next to you.

Now let's see the results of the Inscape Art therapy Jury for Music, Drama and Dance Movement Therapy.

BETWEEN THE ARTS THERAPIES:

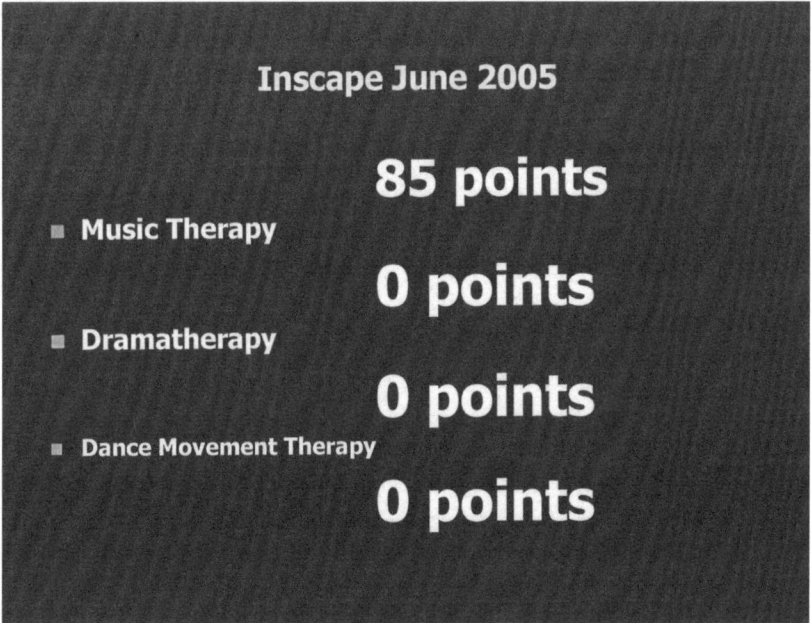

How many people came close to the result and won their bet? (Show of hands)
I did this *Ecartovision* exercise across a few Journals. You try it. You will find that, contrary to any claims, dramatherapy virtually never refers to music, dance or art; music therapy virtually never refers to art, drama or dance. With the odd exception this is the case in every edition. As with *Inscape* we do refer to other professional disciplines such as psychotherapy or psychology, but not to our 'fellow' arts therapies. . . .
Why do we think that is?
Even in collaborative arts therapies books that include chapters from different disciplines, they either never, or hardly, include references to other arts therapy disciplines in the individual chapters. Here, as an example, is an apparently interdisciplinary volume: 'Art & Music Therapy & Research' (Lee and Gilroy, 1995) Sixteen art and music therapists write very good chapters on or about research. There are 381 references in these chapters to other authors/therapist's writing and research. Now, if we see how many of these 381 refer to writing in their own discipline (art therapy chapters referring to art therapy writing and research, music therapy chapters referring to music therapy writing and research) compared to references to work from the other's discipline (music therapy referring to art therapy, art therapy referring to music therapy) . . . what do you think we see?

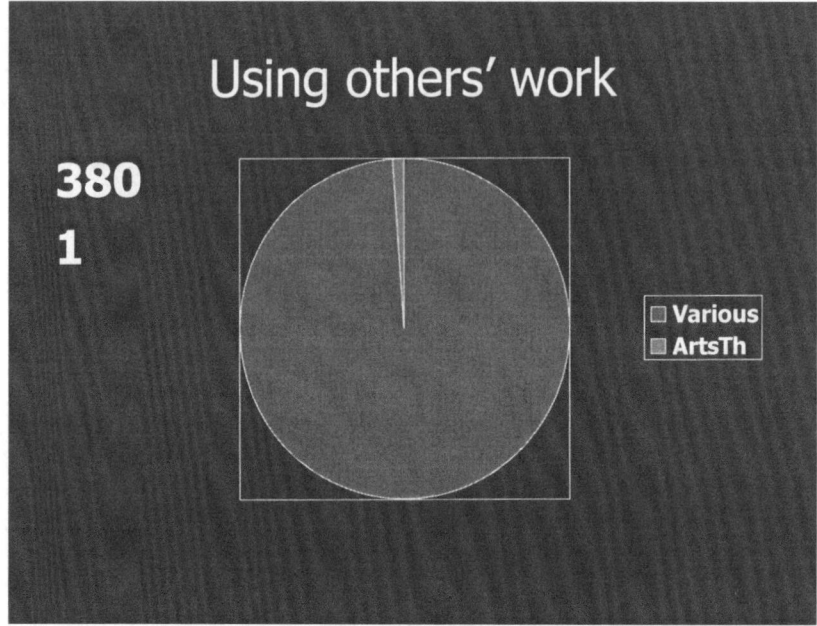

Pretty conclusive. Point made, I think.

There must be reasons for the lack of interdisciplinarity. Perhaps some of these points indicate why this might be:

- A fear of the dangers of homogeneity: of a 'one size fits all' approach to the arts therapies compared to attending to our disciplines separately as art or music therapy
- A lack of precision if concepts, ways of working become more shared or common
- That the specialisms and differences are important to benefit clients
- That general 'overviews' across the arts therapies are less able to account for, and to analyse, change, than are the specific concepts and languages of the individual arts therapies
- A lack of knowledge and/or curiosity in training and post-training
- A sense that the discipline has more in common with/to learn from/ to gain a sense of authority from an area such as psychology than with another arts therapy

The benefits of developing a greater sense of interdisciplinarity, of knowing more about each other's theory and practice for me includes:

- To benefit clients in making choices about what might suit their needs
- To gain more understanding of what is common between the arts therapies
- To learn from each other

- Research into what the arts therapies offer, the specific qualities which are distinct from other therapeutic modalities, can be made more effective by sharing information, by looking at them together rather than in isolation. There is much re-inventing of wheels across the disciplines where more open communication would focus and assist the pace of the development of knowledge.

Issues and themes – commonalities

In this keynote speech I want to argue for the latter – for an increase in interdisciplinarity, whilst showing an awareness of the issues I raised that reflect some of the reasons for the reticence in developing more relationship between the arts therapies.

To begin with, then: how can we understand difference and similarity? Well, let me start with some of the basic commonalities.

One thing we can be sure of is that in the arts therapies clients and therapists alike are engaged in an art form within the therapy session. Beyond this basic assumption, though, matters become more complex.

The entry into the arts space is a dynamic one, reflecting processes such as the relationship between therapist and client, or between clients in a group context. The initial relationship with the opportunities the arts space offers is seen as a communication between therapist and client. The decisions made at this time by the therapist, concerning issues such as being directive or non-directive in their approach, is a part of this encounter with initial meanings found in the therapy, but these are, in themselves, not differences between the arts therapies, rather they are differences of *approach* which are *not primarily located within the differences between the art forms*.

Some arts therapists, for example, might introduce, or suggest, an activity, or way of working, which would aim to support the process of the therapeutic work. This is normally following a goal to assist the client's exploration of personal material in the therapy. This idea is a *constant across the arts therapies*, that the arts experience is connected to the client's engagement with emotional material, problematic issues or areas of potential development. Any suggestion about the use of the art form made by the therapist within such an approach is informed by their perception of the psychological or emotional needs of the client, or by an attempt to assist the process of the therapy. The therapist mostly tries to follow the client's direction and needs. A music therapist, for example, says that she works without the notion of a conductor or director to the process, she never, for example, gives a beat to begin with,

> 'We usually begin with a complete silence...before the first sound is heard; then anyone can begin as they like' (Alvin, 1975 : 14).

Here, in this first moment of a therapeutic encounter in a music therapy session, we arrive at another parallel across the disciplines: that *therapeutic improvisation is a commonality*.

This is one of the key ideas about the nature of the arts within much arts therapies practice. The route into the art form and expression across all the arts therapies is one that is *based in improvisation*. It would be unusual for an art therapist to primarily give 'lessons' to the client in life drawing, for the music therapist to substantially teach scales and fingering, the dance therapist to focus on teaching in great detail a dance form, or for the dramatherapist to give direct training in a particular style of acting. This may occur in a secondary manner within the development of the language of the therapy, but, on the whole (and naturally there are exceptions which prove the rule) any introduction to methodology follows the therapeutic needs of the client. The primary encouragement is on an exploration and personal appropriation of artistic language and process to the clients' needs rather than the acquisition of an external training or precise language.

Here the emphasis is upon the immediacy of creation, and of the individual drawing on materials, processes and participation to express or to communicate, rather than to use the art form according to a prescribed tradition. There can be an element of instruction, but this is usually done indirectly, as a background or support to the client's encounter with the open space of the arts therapy, or the encounter with the arts therapy triangle of client-therapist-art form.

This does not mean to say that skill or proficiency in expression, or aesthetic considerations do not enter into the therapy. There is a difference between a belief that everyone can express themselves through the arts, and saying that the language or form does not matter. The difference, again that is common to the arts therapies, is that in the arts therapies the client can engage in a relationship with the art form and process whereby they discover, challenge themselves, and develop a relationship with the art form within the space and with the therapist, rather than being taught a proscribed notion of how to express and what to express. Skaife shows the way that choice over colour or form, over aesthetic considerations, are not seen in terms of learning or education about an art form, but rather as a part of the personal process within the therapy:

> 'The process of deciding whether to put red there or not in a picture, of taking the risk of losing the picture by restructuring the whole piece, creating a dull piece of work because of avoiding feeling, giving up on something because of feeling no good at it, all these things can be experienced and mastered with the aim of making an exciting piece of art work. Development of an aesthetic sense is part of the endeavour, without this there are no boundaries and so no precision' (Skaife, 2000 : 115).

Here Skaife neatly shows parallels between the ways in which someone's relationship with creating in an arts therapy session can be seen as part of a personal process, rather than simply as a matter of skill.

Arts therapists attempt to create a space within the therapy room which is, in many ways, similar to that appropriate for deep play. One of the best discussions of this is by Woods (2000) in her description of the art therapy studio. She stresses its role as a container, as a place which encourages absorption, and where play and mess can be tolerated. This creation of a space, whether in art, drama, music or dance, attempts to assist creativity: to create a fine balance between not seeming too controlled or contrived, whilst creating a consistent place where opportunities for spontaneity can occur. In some ways this might seem a paradox – a deliberately created place and time for spontaneity to occur! This, though, is something that every arts therapist tries to enable – a deliberate space for spontaneity. Another commonality. This spontaneity refers to artistic expression within the session, but is also central to the opportunities for therapeutic change, which are crucial to the client's use of the arts therapy

Here, then, I have shown that in very basic ways there are substantial commonalities across the arts therapies. These have included the arts' potential for expression, that the arts experience is connected to the client's engagement with emotional material, problematic issues or areas of potential development, the notion of therapeutic improvisation and the parallel with deep play.

However, I am not an 'integrationist'. I do not believe that there can be, or should be, a professional identity called 'arts therapist' where someone practises all art forms. There are substantial differences between the practice of art, music, drama and dance therapy. However, I feel it is important to understand the differences as they can shed light onto our individual disciplines. It is also useful to have a language for difference when explaining to clients, other arts therapists and to other disciplines and institutions. I will now go on to outline two key responses to these issues. The first is to propose the idea of 'foregrounding' and 'backgrounding' as a structure to understand and communicate difference and relationship between the different arts therapies. The second response is the idea is that we have, across the disciplines, core processes at work in all the arts therapies.

Differences – ways of understanding: Foregrounding and backgrounding

So, do the different art forms in the arts therapies make any difference to the client within these processes? Does the choice of dance movement compared to music make any difference? I want to contrast some examples to look at this as a way of looking at the concepts of 'foregrounding' and 'backgrounding'.

As we saw earlier the different arts therapies mostly use *specific areas* of artistic expression that are different. Gale and Matthews, in a collaborative project involving an art therapist, dramatherapist and music therapist, for example, noted areas that were *parallel or similar*. They also recorded areas of language, session structure, ways of relating to clients and the use of physical objects that were *different* (Gale and Matthews, 1998, 182-3). But what exactly are these parallels and differences, and do they make any difference to the client? I want to look briefly at the arts processes in the arts therapies in terms of what the process emphasises or *'foregrounds'*, and what it does not emphasise/involve – what it *'backgrounds'* – as a way into exploring this area. I will say more of these concepts shortly.

The creation of an image in art therapy through painting, compared to a story enacted in dramatherapy is experientially very different. The expression and encounter with the arts medium of the client varies considerably if looked at in this way. I think it is possible to say that, within the variety of practices that have been developed, clear differences can be identified between the languages and processes at work within the different disciplines. There is little extant art therapy work, for example, which consists of the client's role being primarily one of being an audience to the art therapist painting, or the dramatherapist or dance movement therapist client's experience as being primarily that of being a witness to the acting or dance of a therapist. However, one approach within music therapy involves the therapist playing an instrument whilst clients witness – their role is to be involved by listening, not making directly. As an example, this primacy of witnessing the therapist illustrates the way in which the use of one arts language and process can create a difference in the client therapist relationship. This example illustrates that there are some differences of method, tradition and experience for the client.

One way to structure and attempt to develop a language to consider difference is that of 'foregrounding' and 'backgrounding'. I have chosen this as a structure as it does not attempt to create homogeneity in the arts therapies, but rather tries to use it as a paradigm for identifying different elements within a basic assumption of relationship. By foregrounding I mean the way in which some aspects of the arts forms emphasise, or engage more significantly in, some processes, experiences and kinds of language over others in the client's participation.

By backgrounding I mean the way in which some aspects of the arts forms lessen, or reduce involvement in some processes, experiences and kinds of language for clients and therapist.

Here are some brief summaries taken from a much longer analysis in The Arts Therapies (Jones, 2005).

Dramatherapy, Music, Dance Movement and Art Therapy: 'foregrounding' and 'backgrounding'

Drama in dramatherapy emphasises physical work – the client often uses their body either through improvisation or role, movement or physical play. Dramatherapy foregrounds the therapeutic potentials of identity transformation through taking on the roles of others, fantasy characters or gives opportunities for the client to play themselves in a different time or space. In group dramatherapy a client also engages with others who have transformed their identities – for example, in a role-play where a number of people have taken on roles. The client can leave their usual identity with its attendant ways of behaving, and try out new ways to relate, or respond, to people or events. Dramatherapy foregrounds the client's opportunity to 'try not being themselves'. In addition, other people may depict the client. This might occur though someone playing them, through role play, or video playback. This foregrounds the reflective capacity of the client being outside their normal self and looking at their own life. This reflexivity and transformation is different from art therapy and music therapy, where the therapy does not emphasise pretending bodily to becoming someone else, or playing a role, or the client seeing someone else playing themselves, for example.

In music therapy, the experience of music might vary from direct involvement in improvisation, to the client and therapist listening to recorded music. A client might listen to music produced by the therapist, or work might consist of the client lying on a bed which makes use of the vibrations caused by musical sound. The Nordoff Robbins (1977) approach, for example, involves the client in making music. The therapist can make music with the client, encouraging them to improvise with musical instruments. In some work the therapist participates in the creation of music. Like art and dramatherapy, music can emphasise the ways in which objects can be used to form and hold relationships. However, music does not involve the creation of objects through mark making or manipulation in the same way as art therapy. Music foregrounds the use of objects to produce sound, or relationship, through making music, or being handled and passed, compared to the use of objects in relation to image making in art therapy.

Music backgrounds the creation of fictive states. Much music therapy stays in the here and now of the playing, rather than moving explicitly into fantasy states involving taking on other identities. Aspects of the client's identity might be foregrounded, or experimented with in creating sound, rhythm or lyrics, but they do not normally consciously play a character, or another client, for sustained periods of time. Music backgrounds the use of the body in the way dramatherapy or dance movement therapy might seek to express identities, or the development of themes through playing roles and creating stories.

Dance movement therapy, by contrast, foregrounds the physical development of relationships through dance and movement as a cultural form that allows participation and connection to a person's culture. Movement prioritises the body as communicator, and foregrounds areas such as non-verbal communication, and signals made by the body. It foregrounds the ways in which discomfort, distress or illness are reflected through the body and the ways in which movement can both reflect and release. The way the body and movement connect to identity is central to DMT. Client experiences emphasise this relationship between the body and identity, and the way in which movement reflects and allows change in this. It involves ways of working that stress how the body can experience release, transformation and new ways of experiencing the self and relationships with others through movement. It also uses the potentials of dance and movement as ways of expressing, exploring and transforming relationships

Art therapy often foregrounds the creation of static images, the creation of objects which can be kept beyond the session in which it is created, the made thing is kept over a period of time. Art therapy emphasises engagement with materials such as paper or clay which are used to reflect personal material, and to create images. The direct expressive potentials of the body of the client are not used as frequently as in dance movement therapy or dramatherapy, where the client could be engaged in physical movement, or mime, or expressing a role physically through the way they move their body.

Art foregrounds the client staying within their identity. The focus is on what they have made, they do not normally enter into different identities through role playing. When looked at within a model which looks at transference, a part of this is that the client may take on different aspects of themselves within the interaction. They may, for example, feel as a child, a parent, a rival within the therapy, but within this they stay within their own identity. There is no formal shift into taking on an identity by role playing and pretending to be themselves at age seven, or taking on the movement qualities of their mother in order to depict her. Similarly, the therapist would not actively take on a role, as in dramatherapy, where the therapist might play a role in the client's imaginary world, or in dance movement therapy where the therapist might touch or enter into physical engagement and movement work with the client.

These, then, are brief summaries to give a flavour of the ways in which the art forms can be seen to highlight certain processes or aspects of expression and the concept of *'foreground'* and *'background'* can be used to create a dialogue which engages with difference and similarity. Obviously these are very general statements, and each client and therapist's experiences will differ. However, I have attempted to provide some sense of the ways in which the arts therapies may differ for those involved.

So, does the art form matter? It's possible to see in these brief outlines areas that are parallel and that are different in terms of the ways in which the client might experience the art form and process within the arts therapy. Having reviewed the different modes and ways of expressing in this way it's important to ask does the expressive form matter? Does it make any difference to the client? If there are differences what are they?

So, can we say, for example, that the client's *experience* in music therapy is substantially different to the client in the art therapy? The answer for me is both 'yes' and 'no'. The arts forms discussed have shown the ways in which the different arts processes and languages within the arts therapies have both commonalties and difference. The way the art form affects the relationship between client and therapist also has commonalties and differences. We have seen that the arts therapies argue that they foreground the healing potentials within the arts and within the potentials of relationship, expression, communication and reflection that the arts engender. For the client the different arts therapies do offer different languages and opportunities. I would argue, though, that the above descriptions illustrate that even though the arts languages and processes within the arts therapies differ in some areas, it is possible to identify processes which are at the core of change within the arts therapies that are common. The above consideration of arts languages and processes has shown that there are differences, but I will argue that there are processes that can be identified across the arts therapies that create a common link.

Commonalities and core processes – a theoretical model across disciplines

I will now turn to the idea referred to earlier in the presentation: the proposal of a model for core processes across the arts therapies. It tries to encapsulate the specific and unique ways in which therapeutic change can occur in the arts therapies. In brief: what is special about the arts therapies? What is it that is especially useful for clients?

It's important to try to find a balance between creating a language that obscures or is over technical – and a way of describing that is precise enough, that does justice to the processes at work. 'The Arts Therapies' (Jones, 2005) includes a definition of a series of 'core processes' that tries to be precise, without creating a way of describing how something works which becomes opaque or baffling in its complexity. Nor is the idea of these 'core processes' one that is designed to be proscriptive, with fixed ideas about how they should be applied. Each therapist will use their creativity to relate to how they would be reflected in developing work with clients. As you look at the following three I invite you to look at them to see if they lie at the core of your practice. I will invite you to discuss them in relation to your own work with a partner, and then to make comments across the audience in terms of differences and parallels. If you like, to create in this hall the dialogue over commonality that needs to redress the absence I marked in the *Ecartovision* result.

The Arts Therapies Core processes

These processes are:
Artistic Projection
The Triangular Relationship
Perspective and Distance
Embodiment
Non-verbal Experience
The Playful Space and the Informed Player
The Participating Artist-therapist
The Active Witness
(Jones, 2005)

Here three of the processes are described in more detail:

the participating artist-therapist

- arts therapist can engage in the art form as a way of enhancing the client's experience of therapy

- therapist can engage in an art form with the client as a way of communicating or routes of contact and transformation through active participation

artistic projection

- For the arts therapies a vital relationship is created between inner emotional states and external forms and processes through artistic projection

- clients project aspects of themselves or their experience into arts processes and forms within the therapeutic relationship, and thereby externalise inner material

- creation of perspective, exploration and insight through the client's access to arts form, process and creativity of projected material

- art form and the relationship within the therapy can encourage the client to work with the material. This exploration can lead to a new awareness, or relationship, to the material brought

- this new position can then be integrated into the client's experience of the issue.

active witness

- being an active witness is the act of being an audience to oneself or to others, and to created work within the arts therapies

There are a series of possible witnessing interactions:

- Being witnessed by another group member or/and by the therapist
- Witnessing others or the therapist
- Clients witnessing themselves either through video, someone playing them in role or movement or music, or being represented by images or objects
- Witnessing arts work created by self or other, others witnessing art works created by self

(Pair work, discussion and questions within the conference.)

Conclusion
Many arts therapists would find Greek dramatherapist Couroucli-Robertson's position a familiar one. Areas of process and practice are common, however, each encounter has an original, fresh creative component:

> 'Through the years I have developed a personal mode of working which I try to adapt to different clients in order to meet their own individual needs' (Couroucli-Robertson, 1997 : 143).

The definitions also try to do justice to the things the arts therapies have in common, whilst not denying the differences between art, music, drama and dance movement.
In looking at the arts therapies as a whole, I would echo the position summarised by Smitskamp: their unique qualities spring from the ways in which,

> 'they can elicit specific art-related healing processes, thereby expanding the range of possibilities offered by other psychotherapies' (Smitskamp, 1995 : 182).

Many of the key opportunities that the arts therapies offer concern these potentials: of the relationship between the client, therapist and art form. I hope that this keynote has made us aware of the missed potentials of intensive dialogue and awareness between the disciplines. Through the point made in my *Ecartovision* slides, in the discussion of the reasons for avoiding and establishing more dialogue, in the concepts of 'foregrounding' and 'backgrounding', I hope to have created some ideas and structures which can be drawn on within the Conference and beyond the life of the Conference. In addition I hope that the concept and definition of 'Core processes' offers the field a structure to agree, disagree and develop in future theory, practice and research. Of course, dividing up the arts therapies in this way is an artificial construction around something that, in practice, is not separated into such categories. This was done in order to try to see more clearly the specific forces at work in creating original and exciting opportunities for client and therapist. Such descriptions of 'core processes' try to isolate *particular aspects* of the ways the arts therapies work in order to try to see the *whole* more clearly, and to identify what makes the differences and innovations in the opportunities the arts therapies offer clients.

References
Aldridge, D. (1996). *Music Therapy Research and Practice in Medicine*, London: Jessica Kingsley Publishers

Alvin, J. (1975). *The Identity of Music Therapy*, British Journal of Music Therapy, Vol 6, No 3

Andsell, G. (1995). *Music for Life: Aspects of Creative Music Therapy with Adult Clients*, London: Jessica Kingsley Publishers

Bunt, L. (1997). *Clinical and Therapeutic Uses of Music,* in Hargreaves, D.J. and North, A.C. (eds) *The Social Psychology of Music*, Oxford: Oxford University Press

Clarkson, P. and Nippoda, Y. (1998). *Cross-Cultural Issues in Counselling Psychology*

Practice: A Qualitative Study of One Multicultural Training Organisation, in Clarkson, P. (ed) *Counselling Psychology: Integrating Theory, Research and Supervised Practice*, London: Routledge

Couroucli-Robertson, K. (1997). *The Tethered Goat and the Poppy Field: Dominant Symbols in Dramatherapy,* in Jennings, S. (ed) *Dramatherapy: Theory and Practice 3*, London: Routledge

Gale, C. & Matthews, R. (1998). *Journey in Joint Working*, in Rees, M. (ed) *Drawing On Difference: Art Therapy With People Who have Learning Difficulties*, London and New York: Routledge

Helman, C. G. (1994). *Culture, Health and Illness*, Oxford: Butterworth-Heinemann

Jones, P. (2005). *The Arts Therapies: A Revolution in Healthcare*, London: Routledge

Klineberg, O. (1997). *The Social Psychology of Cross Cultural Counselling*, in Pedersen, P. (ed) *Handbook of Cross-Cultural Counselling and Therapy*, New York: Praeger

Landy, R. (1993). *Persona and Performance: the Meaning of Role in Drama, Therapy and Everyday Life,* London: Jessica Kingsley Publishers

Lanham, R. (1989). *Is it Art or Art Therapy?* Inscape, Vol 3, Spring 18-22

Li, T.C. (1999). *Who or What is Making the Music: Music Creation in a Machine Age,* in Candy, L. and Edmonds, E.A. (eds) *Introducing Creativity to Cognition*, Loughborough University, Association for Computer Machinery Press, New York Conference Proceeding

Nadirshaw, Z. (1992). *Theory and Practice: Brief Report – Therapeutic Practice in Multiracial Britain*, Counselling Psychology Quarterly, Vol 5, No 3, 257-61

Nordoff, P. and Robbins, C. (1977). *Creative Music Therapy*, London: Gollancz

Peters, D. (1994). *Sharing responsibility for patient care*, in Budd, S. and Sharma, U. (eds) *The Healing Bond*, London: Routledge

Reason, P. (1991). *Power and Conflict in Multidisciplinary Collaboration*, Journal of Complementary Medical Research, 5, (3), pp144-150

Skaife, S. (2000*). Keeping the Balance: Further Thoughts on the Dialectics of Art Therapy*, in Gilroy, A. and McNeilly, G. (eds) *The Changing Shape of Art Therapy: New Developments in Theory*, London: Jessica Kingsley Publishers

Smitskamp, H. (1995). *The Problem of Professional Diagnosis in the Arts Therapies*, The Arts in Psychotherapy, Vol 22, No 3, 181-7

Wood, C. (2000). *The Significance of Studios*, Inscape, Vol 5, No 2, 40-50

II
CONCEPTS AND DEBATES

RALF BOLLE

ON THE FLOW OF INNER IMAGES AND THE BORDERS OF CONSCIOUSNESS…

In his novels the Japanese writer Haruki Murakami is dealing with an immense variety of different spaces and energies spanned between consciousness and multiple layers of dream worlds. I am very fond of his books, since he is expressing in a modern and sometimes irritating way, what I think is the core of Analytical Psychology. I don't know whether he is acquainted with the works of C.G. Jung, but he definitely came up with metaphors of human existence that are very close to the concepts of Jungian psychology. From a specific postmodern point of view, he is in dealing with the central questions of psychotherapy. Keywords of his fascinating work are the *alternating between inner and outer landscapes, finding and valuing of metaphoric and symbolic interaction* with inner and outer realities, the *struggle for a constructive relationship to the Self and the Other* in a postmodern world and, last not least, the importance of intensive *imagination processes*.
The dynamics, that emerge from the interaction and tensions between these fields of psychic energy, affect the conscious awareness of his protagonists and their actions as well. Sometimes they are able to grasp or get an inkling of the images, fantasies and metaphors emerging from their intra- and interpsychic realities, sometimes they fail to seize them, so that they remain totally un-perceived, un-known and un-conscious.
When one of Murakami´s protagonists is faced with the inner "Other", it reads like this:

> … he 'let his body relax, switched off his mind, and let things flow through him. This was natural for him, things he'd done ever since he was a child, without a second thought. Before long the borders of his consciousness fluttered around, just like the butterflies. Beyond these borders lay a dark abyss. Occasionally his consciousness would fly over the border and hover over that dizzying, black crevasse…. That bottomless world of darkness, that weighty silence and chaos was an old friend, a part of him already… *everything* is there, but there are no *parts*….' (Murakami, 2005:90)

In my opinion this is a very appropriate description of the ambiguity of the unconscious: the fascinating, ominous and unifying, as well as its inconceivable aspects opening to the ego-consciousness, which, cast into the immensity of that space, feels small and exposed.
Of course, the implicit idea of the novel – and of life – is that of development and of activating and differentiating of the ego's latent potentialities to take up a dialogue with the unconscious. This is the underlying quest in Murakami´s novels, which always are "Entwicklungs-Romane" and it is the very aim in the developmental process of each individual and, naturally, the aim of psychotherapy.

In my work, it is a basic assumption that our experiences are continually accompanied by an underground, mostly unconscious stream of inner representations and mental images. In our fantasies and our creative activities we are relating to this stream only partly consciously. In our dreams it is flowing predominantly at an unconscious level. The patterns of human experience underlying all our actions and the mode in which we configure our social relations are a condensed resultant of both personal and collective influences.

In my professional training I was influenced rather early by H. Leuner, who developed a specific method of using daydreams in a psychotherapeutic context. I am very thankful, that he introduced me to a very interdisciplinary attitude towards psychotherapy: aspects of Drama Therapy, Art Therapy and many Jungian ideas were always the part of the approach. So later, as I completed my training as a psychiatrist and psychoanalyst, I did not loose the belief that the human psyche has to be dealt with in a multiprofessional way and that different methods can be of equal value in the healing process. Ideas of interlinkage, plurality and a resonance are very important to me.

For the context of my further reflections, I want to use a rather open definition of a symbol: all psychic realities result from very complex processes of assimilation and structuring of psychic material. These are conditioned, on the one hand, by somatic (ZNS) factors, and on the other hand by psychic factors (biographical experiences). Therefore, psychic experience is always symbolic.

In the healing processes specific symbols are used to structure and organise the therapeutic process in a goal-oriented mode, i.e. with a view to restoring health. Working with innerpsychic images and imagination has always played an important part in psychotherapeutic tradition. C.G. Jung in *Analytical Psychology* and H. Leuner in the *Guided Affective Imagery* have developed methods that promote the conscious dialogue with the inner world and emphasise the communication with intrapsychic images.

On the next pages, I want to invite you to join me on an excursion through the conceptual landscapes that are underlying the psychotherapeutic work using imagination, dreams and creative methods in general. We will start off in the territory of modern brain research and will face the main concepts about the importance and the impacts of inner images on human actions and perceptions of the world.

It is very interesting to see, that now brain researchers are referring to the ideas that have been used by psychotherapists intuitively for a long time. I believe that it is a great chance for psychotherapists to understand that central concepts of that work are now beeing re-invented by modern neuroscience. Then I will go on to a different area of reflecting the work with inner images: in the psychodynamic tradition of therapy working with symbolic expressions of inner realities has become more and more important. So we have to investigate the concept of symbols further: a symbol points beyond itself, it expresses and contains more than the conscious mind (at a given moment) can comprehend. It is a bridge spanning the (individual and collective) personal and non-personal, the phenomenal and non-phenomenal (physical and meta-physical), the conscious and the unconscious. From this point of view, a symbol always aims at new dimensions and at transformation, in other words it aims at the immanent and inherent structure of reality. At the end there I will describe a short case example showing how the ideas presented in this paper can be used in a integrative process.

Inner Images: neurophysiological backgrounds

In recent years, brain research has made remarkable progress and the results have been discussed quite frequently. The development of the so-called neuroimaging techniques has made it possible to gain new insights into the functioning of the human brain to an extent inconceivable in the past. No matter how fascinating the results are, for me it is important to bear in mind that describing the human soul on a scientific basis is still a matter of speculation.

Today's scientific insights start from the premise that neurophysiological operations responsible for inner-psychic experiences are *highly dynamic and non-linear systems*. And this basically means that very complicated and unpredictable systems are involved. It has also been asserted that unconscious processes precede conscious processes and that human conscious experiences are determined by an unconscious processing of information to a very high extent. Brain processes on the neuronal level are concerned with important human psychic activities, such as planning and decision making, the experience of emotions, the ability for empathy and sympathetic understanding and the imaginative process itself.

In his book *The Power of Inner Images – the way visions influence the brain, man and the world* ... Gerald Hüther, a well-known German biologist and brain-researcher, gives an integrative view of the actual scientific insights. I want to refer to his work, because he is summarizing brain research in a way that is very easily connected to psychotherapeutic thinking. Many of his ideas are very closely related Jungian terms and his findings can be used to understand the effects of inner images in therapy better. He uses the concept of *"inner images"* on purpose in order to emphasise that the inner structure-forming processes can not be defined accurately. As related terms he refers to: patterns, schemata or representations. These *'inner images'*, according to Hüther, *control reactions, focus attention, influence orientation, structure activities and shape inner and outer relationships*. He distinguishes between *cellular images*, connecting chemical units, *individual images*, that control the interactions between cells and functional areas, and *collective images*, which pattern communication between the individual and the community. To me it is evident, and that archetypal and personal influences can be described in this manner. He underlines also that human genetic information has been preserved almost unchanged for the last ca. 500,000 years and that changes in human behaviour are basically determined by cultural (i.e. individual and collective) processes.

The constantly ongoing flow of perceptions from the outer and inner world is continually compared with already existing emotional and cognitive memory patterns. They are adjusted and checked against one another. If the new perceptual images fit into known and pre-existent memory imprints, then no change in the individual behavioural pattern will occur. If no such memory imprints are detected at all, then the new perceptual pattern will be discharged as senseless or uninteresting and it too will leave the behavioural pattern unchanged. Significant within a therapeutic learning context are perceptual patterns, which bear a certain resemblance to those already existing. Then an active interferential process will start as well as an associative extension of the stored memory patterns into ever enlarging correlations, until the new pattern can be integrated. Again and again already existing patterns will be down-loaded, until integration into an enlarged, and thus changed, inner brain-landscape becomes possible.

Within a therapeutic context learning experiences are most important. This field also provides interesting scientific findings. In emotionally positive significant situations learning is facilitated by releasing special messenger substances of the brain (dopamine, endorphins). These substances then activate the building up of new neuronal circuits in the brain and, moreover, they change the expression of the genetic information. That is: during learning processes deep changes in the neuronal landscape take place. In this context a difficult life-situation can be looked upon as a challenge, and finding a positive solution to it can bring about interest and eagerness for other challenges. This positive feedback loop has a strong tendency to become a stable cycle of self-preservation and is referred to as "eustress" or "flow".

Unfortunately, the same cycle is called up in emotionally negative significant situations. Here, too, a vicious circle is started with the tendency of self-preservation. In this case, however, a new life-situation is experienced as a heavy burden, the lack of solutions leads to negative expectations, then fear and finally to an avoidance response and a possibly aversive behaviour. The same messenger substances are implied as in positive learning experiences, so that here too deep changes in the brain structure may occur. There is evidence, that perhaps these types of negative feedback-loops are responsible for severe depressive conditions. In my opinion, all these neurophysiological findings underline the significance of working on and with inner images. Special attention should be focused on the importance of inner images in generating new integrative behavioural patterns towards integrating and enlarging the interlinkage and communication between different memory images. I will refer to that later. Such inner images turn into healing images, when applied in the work with individuals, who have to dissolve inner blockades or rigidness. The malfunctions in the psychic processes generated by, and referring to, inner realities, are generally known as psychic disorders.

On the flow of inner images: symbol-processing and the symbol-building

It seems to me, that psychotherapeutic tradition has acknowledged both the significance of the inner landscape, with its correlations and structures, as well as its reflections in the conscious mind and its relevance to the therapeutic practice. C.G. Jung has introduced the idea of archetypal structures that form the common fundamental organization of the psychic realities. At the very basis of all healing systems a similar archetypal concept is shared: a certain specific releasing situation leads to an interruption of the dynamic flow of the natural life forces (Libido), thus causing disorders, disease and ultimately death.

As I understand it, a healing process implies the liberation of these blocked energies and their transformation into a dynamic process that then is able to support and facilitate the constructive development of body and soul. In this concept of life, energy refers to the idea of self-healing potentials. The conscious mind can approach the "aspects of meaning" of these dynamic energies in a variety of culturally determined images, rituals, narratives and myths. On the physical level the vital energy manifests itself in the biological existence, in the "just being in/ within the body", on the psychic level, it appears in its psychic representations: the symbols. The psychic experience is always symbolic, being the product of complex structuring and experience-condensing processes. On the level of physical existence, it is the nervous system which influences and affects awareness, on the psychic level, it is the integration of the biographical experience of the individual and his/her culturally determined learning.

The central focus of any therapeutic setting is to create and expand the possibilities of how to get in contact with healing oriented symbols arising from the unconscious primary life-forces and to promote a constructive communication with them (Bolle, 1998). Working with the symbolic dimensions of reality is primarily a way of working with relationships: this can mean the relationship between the inner and outer reality, of course it is also the relationship to meaningful others, who represent and resonate with inner landscapes in a "good enough way". In such a context symbols are an adequate expression of the actual situation of the individual development. Used in that manner, symbols offer the possibility of direct intervention within a symbolic intermediate space. Once we have succeeded in contacting the dynamic fields of the psyche, we can set free the formerly obstructed forces and re-establish a lively, active mutual relation with the surrounding world, with society and with the individual self. By their energetic links both to physical and psychic realities, empowered healing oriented symbols may also influence biological or somatic processes. They are able to transform the vital energy, thus ensuring stability, and create a new integration with effects on both the structure of the psyche and on the soma.

Lifted out of its ordinary "everyday" context, any object, any relationship or any action may turn into a (life-) supporting symbol. It is exclusively the *context*, i.e. the connection with the world around us, that turns these outside objects (mirrors of our innerpsychic contents) into meaningful symbols. These can be then used by the individual or community to render the basic forces of the world perceivable and accessible to experience. However, to equate a symbol with a definite psychic content would be a basic error. Symbols which can be fully translated by the mind are rather signs or metaphors.

It is a well-known tradition in Analytical Psychology to distinguish between signs, which can be explained fully in conscious concepts and symbols that can not be explained in that way. A symbol can be understood as the best possible way of communicating about a relatively unknown subject that is being perceived as something existing. In that tradition Schaverien, a British artist and analytical psychotherapist, has developed a more differentiated view on images, that develops further Jungian ideas: the concepts of diagrammatic, embodied and empowered images (Schaverien, 1969) are very useful in understanding symbolic healing processes. Basically the differentiation is made to distinguish between images that are used to illustrate a thought or a mental concept and images that open up to the experience of the material and to unconscious resonance. If the work of art has become very important for the creator it may even serve as a container of relevant emotions and can be called an empowered image and can function as a talisman.

'The *diagrammatic picture* is usually an approximation of a preconceived mental image... it is usually an attempt of a linear reproduction of this image. The intention may have been to reproduce the picture seen in the "mind's eye"... This process... is usually conscious in intent... this type of picture is controlled in its execution, and it is often figurative and specific. The diagrammatic picture may be an illustration or a description of a feeling, but it is not an embodiment... it may be an aid to communication.' (Schaverien,1969:86)

The story of the picture has to be re-told in words. It needs descriptions and further explanations by the author. Often it keeps the Art-Therapist at a distance to the creator. In an *embodied image* the physical act of painting takes precedence over the original idea that may arise from a preconceived mental image. In the picture, conscious and unconscious elements are combined and interwoven, so that the picture cannot be used as mere illustration of thoughts anymore. It has its own life, and is not immediately amenable to discourse. The process of producing the picture becomes more and more important and holds very relevant aspects of the emotional and intellectual development of the creator. The sensual experience of the materials used facilitate an intense engagement in the creating of the image itself. There is a symbolic action executed on the level of producing the image. Finally a "significant motif" or a "significant form" can arise. Embodiment can be understood as the unity of form and content.

When a "significant motif" or "significant form" appears, which is a good expression of an important inner theme of the creator that can be valued as a symbol and used in the therapeutic process. Such a significant motif could also be called an *empowered image*. It can integrate aspects of the therapeutic relationship, meaningful relationships to others as well as relationships to inner objects. It will then be an empowered talisman that can accompany the creator for a long time afterwards. In the case study that I will present at the end of the paper, I feel, that the empowerment of images is very essential here.

I believe, that the process of empowerment is a very important source of a successful therapeutic work. Let us go into details a little bit more and look on the basic structures of healing processes: in its archetypal sense, symbolic healing is not disturbed by cultural differences and can virtually affect every individual. In order to develop its full transformative potentialities however, a symbol must <u>acquire</u> the quality of *resonance*: the consciousness of the individual and the community must enter a state of resonance with the archetypal space of experience.

'Lacking inner resonance, symbols are dead – mere pictures or monotonous, grinding litanies. Only in the presence of resonance new sources of psychic energy can be made accessible. The image of a plug introduced into the socket arises. Suddenly the symbol lights up and energy is released for actions that would otherwise be impossible to perform.' (Sandner,1994:286, translation R.B)

According to Sandner (1994) the basic archetypal thematic fields of a symbolic healing process are:

- returning to the origin
- banishing the evil
- the dynamic relationship between death and resurrection and finally
- the re-establishing of a stable universe

It seems to me, that only those symbols resonating with profound archetypal and biographic experience have deep healing potentialities. The potential for healing is not in the symbol beforehand, but has to be transferred to it by a long process of establishing various kinds of relationships to collective and individual values. In this way they are charged up energetically and will finally execute a healing effect. The condition of *being related* (*being in resonance*) is of central significance. – This all shows clearly in the relationship between healer and patient. – The very substance of symbols must be *interactional* and *transactional*.(Quekelberghe, 1993) A symbol is situated at the intersection between healer and patient, the collective myth and the individual experience, between matter and psyche.

One of the archetypal aims of symbolic healing is that the individual is enabled to relate to his personal or the collective myth of creation so that he can recreate himself and find new orientation. The established relationship with the healer and with the symbol permits the patient to find a comfortable distance towards the emotional impact he experiences during the process of re-orientation. He can so gain an *aesthetic distance* from the very strong and sometimes overwhelming emotions that accompany transformative processes. In this way, even the most extreme situations can be integrated. It is not the variety of different and specific methods applied, but rather the interactive field that enhances the healing effect (Best, 2003; Bolle, 1996). Artistic or musical creation alone is not a healing experience by itself. It only unfolds its healing potentialities, when the activated interactional space is able to exert a structuring influence and so permits a meaningful expression.

It appears to me, as if, in a certain, curious way, the origins of the world and the origins of the psyche have become interwoven. From the view of depth-psychology they are certainly not to be separated: earliest pre-personal experiences during pregnancy, birth and infancy determine the way we perceive the world we live in, whether as a home, or as place, where we are just tolerated or even feel threatened. Pre- and perinatal engrams (Grof, 1978; Janus, 1991) colour our very perception of reality. For the adult, the contact with these engrams can acquire the qualities of a mystical experience.

> 'It is this foetal consciousness at the very basis of our soul, that we always ominously relate to and from which we can again and again (re-)define ourselves.' (Janus 1991:230, translation R.B)

Basically, all psychic activities which contact the unconscious, are suitable to process healing-relevant symbols. Human psychic structure can evolve only in a relational context. Relatedness and the experience of relationship are both premises and functions of the human psyche (Stern, 1992).

visions
new perspectives
transcendence

resources
competences
abilities

**resonance
crosslinkage
communication
relationships
plurality**

context
integration

stability
harmony

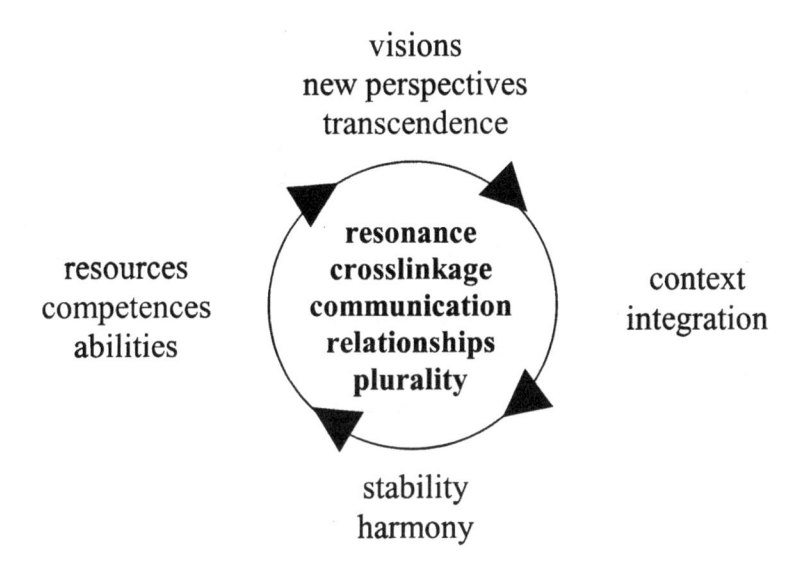

Fig. 1: Dynamics of healing images

In my opinion, during an enduring therapeutic process individual symbols will emerge and be received by the conscious mind. Within the therapeutic relationship these symbols will be empowered and thus become effective. In order to integrate these psychic contents which can reflect broader and larger contexts, individual symbols must be charged energetically by also relating them to the personal biographic realities. Effective symbols of the soul condense individual and collective realities. This means that symbols must, to a certain degree, reflect the actual objective consciousness, i.e. they must have enough realistic objective reference to what the majority regard as reality.

Integration	comprehensibility, world view, reality
Transcendence	unfolding new perspectives, the experience of openness
Finality	sense, meaning, content
Action	gestalting / creation, expression, representation
Resonance	reciprocity / interaction / correlation and contact
Communication	inner dialogue, personal reference, social context
Competence	capacity to act, to control, quality of management
Resources	sources of power and energy
Context	inner landscape, outer relationships
Stability	order, harmonious relations

Fig. 2: Basic themes of healing images

Since in western culture we are lacking an unbroken tradition, that would permit us to address the underlying energetic processes of our actual reality as gods, angels or demons, I think it is necessary to come up with modern terms to express these themes. The unconscious has become the predominant gate that opens into transcendental dimensions, and expressions of the unconscious, whether in dreams, images or representations or in forms that involve the body (e.g. dance, drama, or music), have now become the only possibility to relate to the collective structures of the soul. The moment we enter such a space something very impressive happens: whenever consistent symbols of complex psychic processes emerge, they are a deep experience of beauty, and in this understanding, an aesthetic experience. This immanent beauty, this *radiance* as Trungpa (1989) calls it, is a central aspect of the healing process.

On the banks of consciousness: methods of imagination

In his essay "The Transcendental Function" (written in 1916, but published four decades later in 1958), C.G. Jung analyses the different ways to concentrate on fantasies and work with them. In his early work he describes the process in rather general terms. He suggests that:

> 'inner images and/ or words are:
> expected
> perceived
> documented
> expressed and enacted
> with hands and/or with the whole body' (Jung, 1958:79, translation R.B).

I really value this early definition on the nature of Active Imagination, because it displays the whole range of possibilities of the unconscious processes to express themselves: besides modelling and artistic formulation in pictures, images, stories and sculptures, Jung showed great interest in drama, music and imaginations. His 'extended concept of imagination' represents a rather modern viewpoint that includes a wide range of therapeutic methods and still opens a route to integration of different levels of expression.

Jung used the term Active Imagination for a large variety of imaginative and creative methods, in particular active "doing". His approach seems relevant for today's psychotherapeutic controversies about the *work in the third space*. As mentioned above, Jung reduced the all-importance of the classical method of interpretation by adding non-verbal processes to the frame of his approach to Analytic Psychology. Non-verbal procedures became a natural part of Analytical Psychology: imagination, sandplay, painting, sculpturing, music and dance. These have become self-evident methods as important as the (verbal) reflections on dreams, imaginations and fantasies.

For C. G. Jung the two poles of therapy were given on the one side by the process of *creative formulation*, and, on the other side by the process of *understanding*. He wrote:

'The ideal approach would be a constant or rhythmic alternation of both methods. One seems impossible without the other one, though it occurs in practice: the will to express grips the object at the expense of the senses, or the need to understand, ignores prematurely the process of expressing. The unconscious contents want to appear clearly first, and this is possible only, when they are expressed, and only afterwards analysed, when all their statements have been made visible and tangible. Vague discerned contents require visible expression in order to become more definite. This is only possible by drawing, painting and modelling. Hands often unveil the secrets that the mind is trying to uncover in vain. During the Gestalting / shaping process the dream continues to unfold more detailed in a waking state, and the initially unperceivable, isolated contingency is integrated into the whole personality, though the individual may be unaware of this.' (Jung, 1958:103, translation R.B)

It is this latter aspect, which Jung considered very significant. Again and again he emphasised the necessity for integration of the imaginative realm and its symbolic meaning into everyday life, considering this a matter of high moral responsibility. Moreover, he maintained, this was the only way to dilate and further the conscious mind. This idea he largely exposed in his concept of individuation. It is necessary, he insisted, that the psychic contents should be considered both in a collective (i.e. social) as well as in an individual (i.e. personal) context, if we want them to unfold fully their therapeutic effects. This view led him to his explicit concern with both the *collective meaningful* as reflected in myths and in the personal history of the individual. This basic idea of Jung has been included and has gained great actuality in modern self-concepts like that of the "narrative self", to name but one of them.

'No one would have had the slightest idea, what to do with Gorgo´s head, had he not been acquainted with the mythological act. Individual images work similarly: they need to be embedded in a context, which is not only a myth, but individual history as well.'(Jung, 1940:263, translation R.B)

H. Leuner, a Jungian psychoanalyst, has devised a differentiated concept and method of working with images: the Guided Affective Imagery. Within this day-dreaming-technique, the imaginative process is accompanied by an active dialogue with the therapist. The imaginative work may be initiated by motifs or it may unfold freely, rising from the inner underground imagery. Interpretation of the imagery is of secondary importance. The direct perception by the senses, the phenomenological perception of the imaginative experience is primary and leads to the differentiation and promotion of the conscious ego functions. In this context the creative expression requires due attention and is part of the method. The imagery mirrors the dynamic configuration of the psyche at that moment, its complex-fields, archetypal themes and energetic aspects. The produced and verbalised images can be interpreted both on the subject level, i.e. as a symbolic expression of intrapsychic processes and on the object level, as aspects of outer relational patterns. Within the imaginative process diverse fields of experience can be inter-connected and cross-linked. The perception of inner images turns into emotional and sensual experiences that are to be understood as reflections of the individual's actual life situation. Moreover they open the door to archetypal or resource-oriented experiences as well as to important relational patterns of the personal present and past. The unconscious psyche reveals its need for meaning and outlines the paths to this goal. Thus, Guided Affektive Imagery (Leuner, 2004) offers a valuable possibility for direct work with the symbolic expressions of the energetic primary forces of life.

On the stream of inner imagery and the banks of consciousness

In my therapeutic practice different levels of working with conscious, half-conscious and unconscious material interweave. It is always important to connect the different experiences into a meaningful whole. This process, that can develop parallel to an artistic or to an art-therapeutic process, weaves dreams, imaginations fantasies, reflections, emotions, actions and life-forming impulses into one interrelated and interconnected unity. It may well happen that the place, where all these life-threads meet, is perceived only indistinctly and intuitively. Yet sometimes a concrete image, a representation or some certainty may form. At other times this inner place of integrity exerts its influences out of that which is dark and undefined and can be grasped only by the observed changes in the outer life situations. The implicit objective of each therapy is to raise the quality of outer life, to enlarge the ability to establish relationships and to widen the work-capacities. That, what has been obtained in the imaginative world, must be put into effect in daily life, in order to own it.

I will illustrate the interrelations mentioned above by exposing an extract of a case study from within my practice:

After many years of marriage, the patient was left by his wife. He felt depressed, lost and saw no way out of his situation. He was leading a retired life, was reading a lot and had almost no contact with other people. He was a very responsible, rational, reality-orientated person, but hardly able to open up to his creative and vivid impulses. On the contrary he used to feel cut off from others and was suffering from inner emptiness and severe loneliness.

After we had managed to establish a positive therapeutic relationship, he related the following dream:

"I am at the railway station in Crailsheim. I feel lost. The rails are deserted and empty. I do not know where to go."

As we worked on this dream, which he felt did not make any sense, we concentrated on the question: to what extent was the dream reflecting his own life-situation. He lacked any biographical references to this town. For him it was an unattractive, unimportant, uninteresting place. It was, he said, only a *transit* railway station. He wouldn't know, he said, where one could travel to from there. The dream image, the railway station, soon became a starting place for fantasies and ideas concerning other "life"-journeys. He confessed, he would like to go to St. Petersburg or Paris. But he doubted whether there was a way to get there with Crailsheim as a starting point. More and more he came to see this transit station as a symbol of his own life-situation, in which he felt lost, aimless and lonely. All interesting trains of his life had already left. With due respect for his inner world, we linked and related this image to his outside reality. It got more and more charged emotionally and transformed into a symbol, which he fostered carefully. He went to Crailsheim by train to take photos there. A tour through the city confirmed, that there was nothing *really worth seeing*. His first trip there missed its aim, because there had been no filmroll in his camera, that had been long out of use. He made another trip to Crailsheim and shot photos over hours; he took great interest in details and large survey perspectives and thus transformed his inner journey into an external, enacted experience, accompanied by manifold emotions and inner dialogues. Due to a ray of light getting into the negatives the developed photos were marked with a strip of intensive red, like a high-energy band.

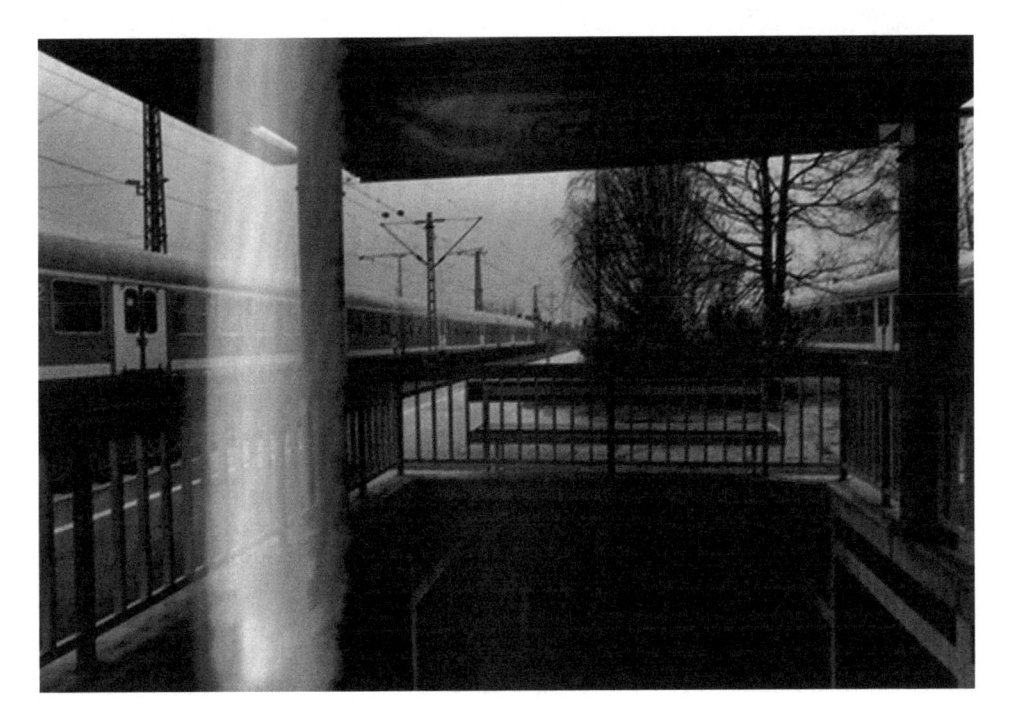

Fig. 3: The trainstation and the intruding high-energy band

This accidental strip required, we agreed, more attention: the trip to Crailshaim had provided pictures, which could be interpreted as expressions of hopelessness and inner emptiness and at the same time they made visible the latent forces of an un-lived liveliness. Within the therapeutic relationship and by the close attention which the patient was paying to his own creative process, he soon managed to re-establish a relation to his creative and lively potentials. It was a remarkable moment for both of us, when we realised that one of the photos he took, whilst sitting on the train, revealed two opposing aspects: initially a wasteland photo, but when turned upside down, it changed into a hopeland and/or homeland scenery.

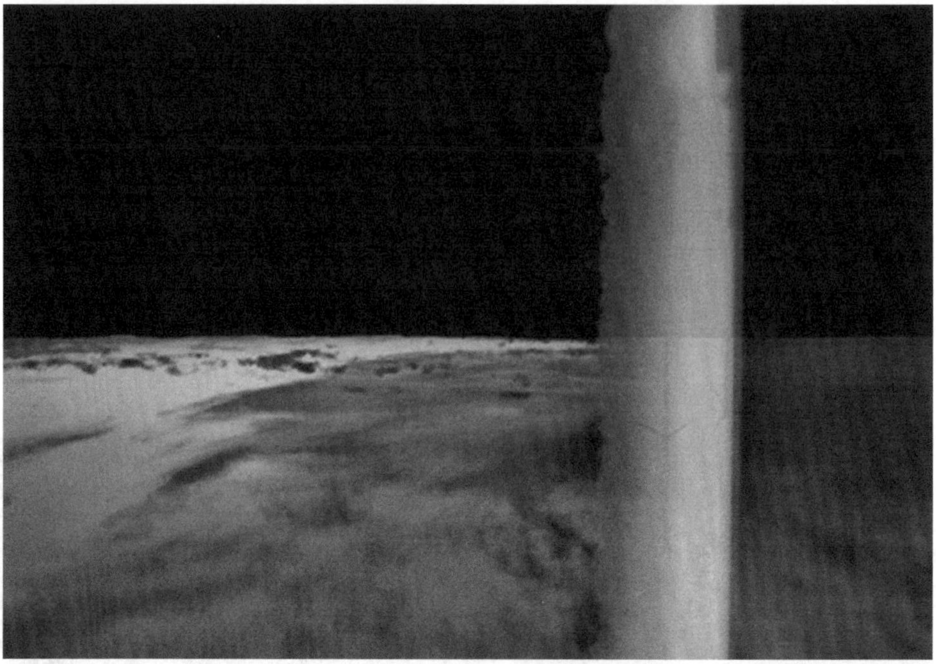

Fig. 4: Approaching earth

It looked like a spaceship approaching the earth. This photo opened a totally new perspective, created through the discussions about the seemingly real picture of the station: out of a rather objective, emotionless and isolated life, a world of palpable reality, a vision of return and landing on the earth was born. The fantasy about the possibilities of landing on almost every spot offered an unexpected enlargement of life-perspectives. It suddenly revealed its symbolic potentials for creating a new way of life.
Certainly, the therapeutic work is not accomplished and has not come to an end after images like that come up. Its aim is to include these symbols into a lively context of inner and outer controversies. If we succeed in binding together imaginations, actions and every-day reality, constructive changes and transformations in life may occur.

References
Best, P. (2003). *Interactional Shaping within therapeutic encounters: Three dimensional dialogues*, USA: Body Psychotherapy Journal, Vol 2.1, pp 26-44
Bolle, R. (1996). *Am Ursprung der seelischen Welt – Initiationsmuster und interaktives Feld*, International Journal of Prenatal and Perinatal Psychology and Medicine Vol 8.2, pp 479-502
Bolle, R. (1998). *Symbol und Heilung – zu den archetypischen Strukturen des symbolischen Heilens*, In: Gottschalk-Batschkus, C., Rätsch, C. (Hrsg) Ethnotherapien-Therapeutische Konzepte im Kulturvergleich, Verlag für Wissenschaft und Bildung, Berlin, pp 204-209

Elger, C. et al.(2004). *Das Manifest – elf führende Neurowissenschaftler über Gegenwart und Zukunft der Hirnforschung*, Gehirn und Geist, 6/2004: 30-32, Heidelberg

Grof, S. (1978). *Topographie des Unbewußten -LSD im Dienst der tiefenpsychologischen Forschung,* Klett-Cotta, Stuttgart

Hüther, G. (2004). *Die Macht der inneren Bilder – wie Visionen das Gehirn, den Menschen und die Welt verändern*, Vandenhoeck & Ruprecht, Göttingen

Leuner, H. (2004). *Katathym-imaginative-Psychotherapie, (KiP,)* Springer-Verlag, Stuttgart-New York

Janus, L. (1991).*Wie die Seele entsteht – Unser psychisches Leben vor und nach der Geburt,* Springer-Verlag, Stuttgart-New York

Jung C.G. (1940). *Psychologie und Religion*, GW 11, 1979, Walter-Verlag, Olten

Jung C.G. (1958). *Die transzendente Funktion*, 1916/, GW 8, 1982, Walter-Verlag, Olten

Quekelberghe, R van(1993)*Grundzüge symbolischen Heilens im Kulturvergleich,* Ethnopsychologische Mitteilungen, 2, No 1: 3-17

Murakami, H. (2005). *Kafka on the shore,* – novel, The Harvill Press, London

Schaverien, J. (1992). *The Revealing Image – Analytical Art Psychotherapy in Theory and Practice*, Kingsley Publishers, London

Sandner, D. (1994). *So möge mich das Böse in Scharen verlassen Eine psychologische Studie über Navajo-Heilrituale*, Walter-Verlag, Solothurn/Düsseldorf

Stern, D. (1992). *Die Lebenserfahrung des Säuglings* Klett-Cotta, Stuttgart

Trungpa, C. (1989). *Feuer trinken, Erde atmen – Die Magie des Tantra,* dtv München

MICHAEL BARHAM

LEAD PIPE IN THE LIBRARY: ART, CREATIVITY AND CONSCIOUSNESS

SO WHAT?
(with apologies to Miles Davis)

One
This paper concerns how we create narrative in order to construct meaning. You, the reader, will notice that it is divided into thirteen sections. Before reading, cut out thirteen small pieces of paper and write the numbers, from one to thirteen, one on each piece. Place in a hat or bag and draw one out at random, then another, and another, and so on until you have them all. This will dictate a possible order to read this paper. As you read observe how you make sense of it, how you construct your own narrative.

There is only one reference to the arts therapies in this paper, hence the subtitle, 'So What'. As you read keep in mind 'so what?'. Keep asking yourself, what does this mean for me? How is it relevant?

Finally, this paper is dedicated to Sir Arthur Evans, the British archaeologist who claimed that he had discovered the labyrinth constructed by Daedalus at Knossos – the lair of the Minotaur. Attending the conference allowed me the opportunity to visit Knossos and see at first hand the fiction that Evans had created. As arts therapists we could be described as archaeologists of the psyche, what fictions do we create....?

This paper attempts to provide some explanations for the way we construct our meanings and our selves including the creative shaping effect on the mind of social narratives i.e. our experiences in, knowledge about, and creative transactions with the fictional and real social worlds. Chomsky (2000) forefronts what he takes to be the permanently intractable identity of consciousness in relation to creativity. His wish to insist on its 'mystery' poses a problematic perspective that I here wish to challenge with my hypothesis; a particular interpretation of the idea that the mind and the neurological system match social narratives. This is based upon the idea that in order to understand how life imitates art, we must appreciate the relationship between our participation in the symbolic systems of fiction, film, drama and so on, art, and our social narratives.

If the organising principle of the mind is narrative rather than conceptual, it is important to understand the nature of narrative, how it is built around established social expectations and our reaction to deviations from such expectations. According to Bruner, (1986) narratives organize our experiences by imposing patterns inherent in their symbolic systems, language employed, discourse modes, and the forms of narrative explication. These phenomenological, meaning-framing social narratives depend upon shared meanings and cultural narratives as well as upon shared modes of discourse for negotiating differences in meaning and interpretation. One of the aims of literary interpretation and translation seems to reflect Paz's (1992) idea that we wish to capture the signs freed into space by a text in order to re-codify them into another language. The codification of cultural narratives gives us insight into the creativity of the human mind.

Two

The phenomenological approach to narrative mental organization and 'meaning-making' has been proliferating these last several years in social anthropology, linguistics, literary and film theory, and philosophy. Jakobson and de Saussure were influenced by Nietzsche, and Foucault, Searle and Derida by Husserl to name a few. Phenomenology has an all out effort to establish meaning as the central concept of philosophy as well as psychology rather than observable behaviour, or the input-output of information technology. Its aim is to discover and to describe formally the meanings that we create out of our encounters with the world, real and fictional, and then to propose hypotheses about narrative processes.

The phenomenological reduction is an attempt to generate a description of the contents of consciousness that excludes all reference to the natural standpoint. Husserl describes the attitude of the natural standpoint in terms of an empiricist view of mind, which finds that when we look upon an object, what we actually perceive are fragmented, discrete, partial, perspective views of the object. We associate one sense datum with the next and thereby infer, by induction, the existence of the object. To avoid this fragmentation, the phenomenological reduction constructs meaning with the symbolic systems embedded in language and images. Social narratives, including both linguistic and pictorial components, organize our experiences by utilising schemata, the philosophical constructs of a worldview. These schemata are the characteristics of the narrative flow, the sequential knowledge components in the narratization and interpretation of social experiences. The central concepts of a social narrative are meaning and the philosophical processes involved in the construction of meaning.

Three

Parallel to Husserl's idea that the mind's task is to extract the constant, invariant features and meaning of objects from the perpetually changing flood of information it receives from objects is the neurological task of the brain. If the brain is structured by language, then neuro-narrative strategy derives from a theory of the brain as a highly connected or programmed mechanism in which basically the narrative competencies are different neurological dimensions of the brain. Calvin (1997) has demonstrated the importance of narrative explication on the physiological development of the brain. Yet another dimension must be considered: plasticity of the brain, the tendency of synapses and neuronal circuits to change as a result of mental activity. Plasticity weaves the tapestry on which the continuity of mental life depends. Action potentials not only encode information; but also their metabolic after-effects alter the circuits over which they are transmitted. We develop new neural pathways from new social narratives. Mind with its pattern of meaning is the personalization of the brain. The schematic scripts of a neuro-narrative strategy support a phenomenological framework.

Meaning and schematic scripts, which are the sequential segments of the social narrative, are critical to the physiological development of the brain. Although the brain's architecture takes shape in the foetus, it can only assume its final form with the ability to interpret reality through stimuli including textual and pictorial images. The world we see is literally the creation of our brain: we are most definitely neither computers nor cameras. Bruner (1983) thought that even new-borns have a rudimentary way of representing their environment, with his contention that many cognitive abilities are innate. Schematic scripts work either primarily pictorially, in an auditory manner or kinaesthetically (somatically) in discourse comprehension. This is confirmed by recent research in neurolinguistics. What implications do these findings hold for readers-viewers? Robinson (1991) sees the sensory orientations as shortcuts to the body, to the somatic response to words. Visualisation makes the words come alive. Images and words alike 'make sense,' 'feel real,' only when they reach down to the body.

Four
According to Gass (1970) when a reader forms an image of a breakfast scene, for example, a table with butter and marmalade on it (which the reader inferred, because they were not mentioned in the text), then the reader is not treating the text as literature, because it is a 'conceptual breakfast'. Do we react emotionally mainly to the sensory scripts in the text, film, drama or the thoughts in our heads? And if we react mainly to our own thoughts, is it irrelevant whether the novel, film or drama is interpretative or formulaic, *i.e.* being only one dimensionally plot-driven, and following a simplistic linguistic formula?

However, interpretative novels because of their complexity require slower reading and thus provide the opportunity for elaborate images to develop, which also stimulate more imaginative powers. One may recall at this point Chekhov's famous observation that if a story tells us there is a gun on the wall, later it will certainly fire. It is plausible to assume that proficient readers have acquired this conventional wisdom during incidental learning and have converted it into a specific reading strategy. In general, more mature readers will have more developed strategies including more elaborate schemata. Therefore, one may predict, for instance, that more mature readers of literature will construct a stronger surface-representation than less mature readers, and that they will be more aware of the parameters, which determine, besides textual factors, the comprehension process. In the comprehension process, the relation of words or expressions to other words or expressions and the relation of images to other images constitute, along with reference, the sphere of meaning.

Specific experiences will enhance the connectivity in highly specific neuronal circuits. The key factor is stimulation of the brain. Our brains are physiologically changing constantly (Greenfield, 1997). We cannot establish as yet a causal relation between the physical and the phenomenological in the human brain; however, it is sufficient to be aware of the correlation between these two levels of operation. Different modes of thinking and social narratives encapsulate our inner resources for interpreting, in our exquisitely unique fashion, the world around us. In the narratization and interpretation of our personal experiences, framing or schematising provides a means of constructing a worldview, characterising the flow, and the sequencing of events. The special, persistent feature of a narrative is the schematic bias of what we will observe in our environment (real or imagined) and what we will connect from our past life. Providing a framework of interest, excitement, and emotion, this schema favours the development of specific images, thoughts, or feelings, and provides a persistent description of the social world and its psychological patterns. The very process of experience is formed by schemata steeped in socio-philosophical conceptions of our world – the constituent beliefs and the larger scale narratives holding them in the temporal configurations of plots.

Five

Our exposure to social narratives begins with the cultural tales that we are exposed to as children. Bettleheim (1969) argued that fairy tales (the first social narratives) teach us how to think in social situations. Neurological story patterns, beginning at an early age, have organising effects on our mental processes similar to the scenarios of our external reality. Stories can engage our attention and can have a surprising capacity to develop our minds and move our emotions as imaginings stimulate belief. Our minds pay attention to story patterns, the symbolic systems of narration, and cultural codifications (cf. Von Franz, 1977).

Good dramas or narratives, such as, for example, Eco's (1995) *The Name of the Rose*, offer different levels, alternate or multiple readings of its story. Linguists have always insisted that no story can be understood or have meaning at a single level unless it is simply formulaic. Jakobson (1960) urged that all meaning is a form of translation, and that multiple translation, polysemy, is the rule rather than the exception: an utterance can be conceived of as referential, expressive, poetic, contact preserving, and as metalinguistic. So, we can interpret *The Name of the Rose* in various ways, indeed in various ways simultaneously.

Six

We experience the larger scale narratives of novels, films and dramas because we hope they will engage us, that their plots will snare us, and that we will be concerned for the fictional characters, their actions and fate (Bazin, 1997). Although we may disagree about the impact of any particular novel or film, we sometimes do not become psychologically involved with the characters of a 'formulaic work' with its predictive structure and a lack of didactic purpose and complexity of language, plot, and character. On the contrary, we do report empathic responses to a protagonist in an 'interpretative work,' marked by a didactic purpose and a complexity of language, plot and character (Kermode, 2000). Interpretative works have different symbolic systems than formulaic works. The subtlety and complexity of syntactic rules lead us to believe that such rules are learned instrumentally by reading and viewing experiences.

Story type seems to be a way of both organising the structure of events and organising the telling of them. Something in the actual narrative triggers an interpretation of story type in the participant, an interpretation that then dominates the participant's own creation of what Iser (1978) calls a "virtual text." What then are "triggers" and what are the subjective forms of story-type that come to dominate the participant's mind? Are story-types merely subjective or are the triggers objective literary or semiotic signs telling the participant what story type it is and what stance to take toward the story? Stories are, in Ricoeur's (1983) view, models for the redescription of the world, however, the story is not by itself the model, but a representation of one of the possible models we carry in our own minds.

The philosophical dimension is conditioned by sociological and psychological factors, and based upon particular background framing, or experience, conditioned by individual cultures and by people's individual make-ups: 'what is perceived depends on the observer's perceptual frame of reference' (Hohulin quoted in Tabakowska, 1993: 59). 'That the world is my world, shows itself in the fact that the limits of that language (the language I understand) mean the limits of my world (Wittgenstein, 1973, also cf., Katan, 1999: 74). Thus, social and cultural narratives are always present to filter our reality. Williams (1978) alerts us to that what he calls the emergence of 'structures of feeling' depend upon the cultural forms available for use. This is the same pattern of the translator who moves himself within, and among a variety of languages, from his native language and culture and beyond. Phillips (2000: 128) wrote:

'Without translation in its familiar sense of transferring from one language into another, and in its more metaphorical sense of moving across, or removing to another place, there can be no sense of history, of alternatives, of aspirations, or of possibilities. And contemporary so-called multi-cultural societies depend for their viability on their members' enthusiasm, however ambivalent, for translation. Our relationship to translation has become a virtual synonym for our relationship to ourselves.'

When attempting to understand our relationship to ourselves, we often need therapists. It could be said that we are in need of translation, to be moved from one place to another through language. We see therapists when we have reached the limits of our language, using our available descriptions of what is happening. We don't start therapy because we want to learn another language as Italian or Swedish. We don't say that we are unhappy in English and we would be better off in Italian. If we are in English, we want a different English, a more interpretive narrative vocabulary to enhance our understanding of the world.

Seven

For Goodman (1978) who speaks of possible worlds, the major aim of art's themes and plots is to contribute to and enlarge upon our understanding of the world. The linear incidents that make the plot, versus the timeless, motionless, underlying theme create the power of great stories in the dialectical interaction they establish between themselves (Kermode, 1983). So using such approaches, the participant begins by placing a story in one genre, which may have powerful effects on their reading or viewing, and they may change their view as they participate. The actual text or drama is unchanged, however, the virtual artwork changes often in the act of participation. When we study the participant's conception of what kind of story they are encountering or recreating – we are in fact asking not only about the actual narrative, but also the relation of words and images, the schematic scripts in the interpretative process.

To experience a story is to participate and get engaged in an internalised experience of make-believe, where our personal schemata match the schematic qualities of the fictional narrative. Bartlett's (1932) research demonstrated that when participants were given stories inconsistent with their schemata and their expectations, recall was usually distorted in the direction of personal schemata. Where we encounter a story that is different from our usual understanding, we have difficulty fitting it into our existing schema, and subsequently tend to alter it until it is congruent with our existing narrative. I argue that different readers and viewers probably utilize diverse schemata during encoding of fictional material, which might produce different impressions of the same material (cf. Gersie, 1997).

Eight

Ricoeur (1981, 1983) argued that the meaning of make-believe in narrative is built upon concern for the human condition: stories reach sad, comic or absurd resolution, which must be simultaneously constructed on two landscapes, action and consciousness. As Anscombe (1981) argued, action includes agency, intention, and situation, whereas consciousness includes what those involved in the action do or don't know, think, or feel. If the intentions and actions of a story's character are to achieve verisimilitude, the story must have internal consistency, however, it can use violations of such consistency as a basis of drama – as in the changed character identities in the dramas of Pirandello.

Some modern writers like Joyce and D.M. Thomas create a world made up entirely of the psychic realities of the protagonists, leaving knowledge of the objective world in the realm of the implicit. Joyce leaves objective reality at the horizon of the story as matters of supposition. Even Manet, in the often-quoted scholarly folklore, argued against objective representationalism as the only way to depict reality in painting by exclaiming, "Nature is only an hypothesis." With respect to narrative, Iser (1978: 61) agrees with Manet's phenomenological idea that the participant composes reality.

> 'Fictional texts constitute their own objects and do not copy something already in existence. For this reason they cannot have the full determinacy of real objects, and indeed, it is the element of indeterminacy that evokes the text to "communicate', with the reader, in the sense that they induce him to participate both in the production and the comprehension of this work's intention.'

It is this relative indeterminacy of a text, which allows a wide spectrum of possible worlds. Instead of formulating meanings themselves, stories initiate possibilities of meaning. The form of the narrative, the story type, actualises performance of meaning in Iser's sense. Several discourse properties of stories are critical for interpretation of meaning. The first property I wish to highlight here is *presupposition,* construed as the creation of implicit rather than explicit meanings. With the explicitness of formulaic stories, is interpretation an option? A second property is a *subjective perspective:* the depiction of reality through the filter of the consciousness of protagonists in the novel. A third property is a *multiple perspective.* (Barthes (1977) argues that without multiple codes of meaning a story is merely "readerly," not "writerly.") A fourth property relates to a variety of *senses of metaphor*, which keeps meaning open to interpretation in its progressive revision of senses.

Nine
How does discourse portray a subjunctive reality, which is the key to the issue of discourse in great drama? One of the more systematic ways in which this is accomplished is by a text's violating the formulas that regulate much of popular writing. One way is expressing a meaning beyond the literal words we write, or for meaning something other than what we write as in irony, or for meaning less than the literal words we write. Instead of using a formulaic style, meaning is created with gaps and the recruitment of presuppositions to fill them. Good novels, films, and dramas have implicatures to increase narrative tension by forcing meaning-performance upon the participant. I here adopt a general use of 'good' as in Kermode's (1975) sense. Interpretative stories have dialogue that offers more than pure information, which is a feature of formulaic narrative forms with its minimisation of presupposition, restricting the participant from understanding anything about the story or the writer's mind beyond the information presented.

It has often been assumed that a deeper appreciation of a writer's mind is made available through the pedagogical powers of interpretative narratives. By participation in the interpretative images and texts of fiction we can possibly sense the writer's intentions as well as develop a larger-scale map for life and our social transactions. Vygotsky (1978) pioneered an idea about a larger scale map for life, the now famous Zone of Proximal Development. This is an account of how the more competent artists assist the young and the less competent to reach that higher ground, from which to reflect more abstractly about the nature of things. Vygotsky challenges us to find a way of understanding humans as a product of culture as well as a product of nature.

For Vygotsky, language was the agent for altering the powers of thought – giving thought a means for explicating the world. In turn, language became the memory-bank for new thoughts once achieved. It was that connection that helped create, for example, not only the writers Joyce, Proust and Green, or the film-maker Bergman and dramatist Ibsen, but also the readers and viewers whose virtual texts could be shaped by the novels, dramas or films they were experiencing. Accordingly, we are part of culture that we participate in and then recreate. The power to recreate reality, to reinvent culture is why this is so important for therapists to understand.

Ten
As Allen (1995) argues, even though stories as instruments of imagination and reason do not cause us to believe in the reality of the narrative, they can engage us to the extent of creating within us the sometimes pleasant and unpleasant states we experience when moved by real life events. Why do we become so involved with characters in works whose existence is merely imagined? Emotional contact with people, real or fictional, involves imagination, assumptions, and inferences including attributions. Through this process of imagination we make an interpretation of the story, constrained and guided by considerations similar to

those we utilize when interpreting behaviour in the real world. The interpretation of fictional or real behaviour is achieved by explaining intentions, using attributions, either situational (external) or dispositional (internal), as in the example of explaining why some people read and view primarily formulaic works and others primarily interpretative ones.

The foregoing perspectives can be used to generate a range of questions. Is there a correlation between the ascription of either situational or dispositional attributions to explain a fictional character's behaviour and the schematic qualities of different types of fiction, film and drama? Furthermore, is the possibility of finding the works philosophically elucidative related to interpretative and formulaic schematic qualities? On the assumption that engagement with a fictional character and retrieval of the deeper textual meanings are related to schemata which guide our experience of a story, do different types of discourse modes possibly compel a certain schema upon us?

Do all participants of the different media assign multiple meanings to stories? And do all stories elicit these multiple meanings? What kinds of story categories evoke this 'meaning attribution' process? Is interpretation affected by story type, and what does story type mean philosophically? And how are multiple meanings triggered? What is there in the text, film or drama that produces this multiple effect, and how can one characterize the susceptibility of participants to polysemy?

Language structures are arbitrary with respect to how they fulfill particular functions, however, interpretative thinking has a priority, in communicative needs – a priority that reflects higher-level social dimensions including identification and empathy. Interpretative forms, as metaphors are not mastered either for their own sake or merely in the interest of more efficient communication. One of the most powerful discourse forms in human communication is narrative. Bruner (1990) found that narrative structure is even inherent in the praxis of social interaction before it achieves linguistic expression. Narrative requires crucial interpretative constituents if it is to be effectively carried out. Narratives with interpretative linguistic structures could possibly contribute to situational attributions, and show our need to appreciate the relationship between our participation in the symbolic systems of fiction and film and our social narratives.

Eleven

Imagination is important for interpretation; fictional interpretation is largely a matter of understanding the meaning of the story where words and images often have to be taken nonliterally, and often can be hinting at events beyond the literal structures of the narrative. Sometimes, figuring out the events of the story is a matter of understanding the intended pictorial and linguistic representations. I wish to maintain that since the language of fiction functions symbolically, interpretations are to some degree a matter of calculating intentions and meaning. This view is disrupted by the impact of de Saussure's effect on interpretation of a cinematic narration by indeterminacy being an internal property of this medium's concern with, for example, montage (See Metz, 1999). Clearly, there are interference factors of the pervasive roles of intentionality, (Anscombe, 1959, and Gibson, 1998) and indeterminacy (Kermode, 1975, 2000).

A central point of my claim is that if we don't use our capacity for imagination, for a richer experience of a narrative by simulation, our cognitive style is formulaic. The formulaic schemata probably do not allow us to simulate the mental states of fictional characters. Similar to the autistic person, the individual with formulaic schemata probably has difficulty understanding that other people have different beliefs, knowledge, desires, and generally a different mental map of the world from themselves. If imagining is simulation, we have possibly an explanation to the puzzling phenomenon of why some individuals can't empathise with others and their situations. The basic manner, by which we make emotional contact with other people, real or fictional, involves – and could be said to be dependent on – imagination.

This is comparable to the presupposed principle of a hypnotherapist, like Erickson (1987) who used words in a narrative form to encourage the subject to focus selectively on their experience and if the words are not open to interpretation, the words will probably jar the subject's experience and prevent them entering a trance. Similarly, Klein (1989) began inquiring whether the object of analysis was not so much archaeologically to reconstruct a life as it was to help the patient construct a more contradiction-free and generative narrative of it (cf., Phillips, 2000). In which case, what constitutes a narrative, or better, a good narrative? A good hypnotherapist is similar to a good writer because they assist the creation of a virtual reality. Bruner (1986: 37) said about a virtual reality that:

> 'The virtual text becomes a story of its own, its very strangeness only a contrast with the reader's sense of the ordinary. The fictional landscape, finally, must be given a "reality" of its own – the ontological step. It is then that the reader asks that crucial interpretative question, "What's it all about?" But what "it" is, of course, is not the actual text – however great its literary power – but the text that the reader has constructed under its sway. And that is why the actual text needs the subjunctivity that makes it possible for a reader to create a world of his own. Like Barthes, I believe that the writer's greatest gift to a reader is to help him become a writer…Beyond Barthes, I believe that the *Great* writer's gift to a reader is to make him a *better* writer.'

Bruner's subjunctivity here (i.e., subjunctive conditionals) of interpretative narrative art, as our subjunctive connections in the real world, places the action in the characters rather than only in the plot. This subjunctive ability for connection between others and ourselves may be provided by the forms of narrative that the culture offers us. As Bruner (1986) argued, life could be said to imitate art. We account for our own actions and for the human events that occur around us principally in terms of narrative, story, or drama. What makes Schaffer's drama a powerful virtual and subjunctive world for us is not only events, but also his characters. Aristotle in the *Poetics* conveniently distinguishes between "agent" *(pratton)* and "character" *(ethos),* the former being a figure in a drama whose actions merely fit the requirements of the plot, and no more, while the latter has traits beyond those required. Ricoeur (1983) reminds us that Aristotle's idea of *mimesis* includes the notion that drama reflects "character in action" and action surely involves plot and its setting.

Twelve
Asch (1946) demonstrated that character is not a fabrication of autonomous traits but an organised entity. Asch made this clear by demonstrating how differently the trait *intelligent* was interpreted depending on whether the character to whom it was attributed was also described as *cold* or as *warm*. In the first case, intelligent meant "crafty," while in the second it was taken to mean "wise." Apparent character is perceived as a *Gestalt,* not as a list of traits that account for particular actions. And the Gestalt seems to be constructed according to some sort of theory about how people are. For example, a character can have some sort of core characteristic that directs their behaviour from within. But if the character behaves in a way that violates that core characteristic, we easily explain it away by invoking circumstantial evidence. In an estimation of another person, real or fictional, we can, for example, describe a *poor person* dispositionally by stating they are lazy and have no ambition, or we can describe them situationally by stating they have the disadvantages of particular social economic circumstances. Do we need to be categorical like many politicians or is there a possible interaction between internal and external variables? We need to know how others look out upon their world, their social narratives.

Similarly, this research is interested in the phenomenological windows we use through which we look out upon the world. Some individuals experience a wounding marital conflict on the stage or in a film or novel and feel the psychological pains, as others just feel barrenly informed about the facts. Each drama, film or novel we encounter comes wrapped in thought-markings, which are illocutionary invitations to the use of reflection, elaboration, fantasy and possibly even trance. Searle (1969) argued that it is the illocutionary force and not the locution that signifies the writer's intent. To the extent that the scenes are chosen for their power to transform imagination, and are presented in a manner inviting speculation, to that extent the art form becomes a part of culture making. The audience, in effect, becomes a party to the interpretative process. How the playwright, scriptwriter or novelist writes comes eventually to be how she or he represents what she or he writes about, and how the participants interpret the art form, represents the richness of their social narratives.

Thirteen
Research on the relation between symbolic systems of fiction and our social narratives can contribute to the important reorientation that is taking place between social/cognitive philosophy, the neuro-sciences, and literary and film theory. I also believe that this dialogue can assist the arts therapists to understand more about the process of our way of working and playing together and the importance of the imagination to wellbeing. This research on the characteristics of social narratives provides us with a greater understanding of the nature of the mind and is particularly relevant in our world today, since the social shaping of information technology is not on 'meaning' but information, not the construction of meaning but the processing of information. Tendencies within areas of

functionalist positivist thought (Dennet, 1987, 1998) with its current fixation on mind as information processor has led philosophy away from the objective of understanding mind as a creator of meanings and social narratives. On the other hand, the phenomenologists have focused upon the symbolic activities that we employ in constructing and in making sense not only of our world, but also of ourselves. They believe that language, syntax, and literary and pictorial dimensions in our narrative modes, more than the positivistic laws of information technology, affects our behaviour.

References

Allen, R. (1995). *Projecting Illusion: Film Spectatorship and the Impression of Reality*, Cambridge: Cambridge University Press
Anscombe, G.E.M. (1959). *Intention*, Oxford: Blackwell
Anscombe, G.E.M. (1981). 'The Intentionality of Sensation', in *Collected Works*, Oxford
Asch, S., (1946).'Forming Impressions of Personality', *Journal of Abnormal and Social Psychology*, no. 41, 258-290
Bartlett, F.C. (1932). *Remembering: An Experimental and Social Study*, Cambridge: Cambridge University Press
Barthes, R. (1977). *Image, Music, Text,* New York.: Hill and Wang
Bazin, A. (1997). *Bazin at Work: Major Essays and Reviews from the Forties and Fifties*, tr. A. Piette and B. Cardullo, ed. B. Cardullo, New York and London: Routledge
Bell, D.S. (1999). *Husserl: Arguments of the Philosophers*, London: Routledge
Bettleheim, B. (1969). *The empty fortress: Infantile autism and the birth of self*. New York: The free press.
Bruner, J. (1983). *Child's Talk; Learning to Use Language* New York: W.W. Norton
Bruner, J. (1986). *Actual Minds, Possible Worlds*, Cambridge, Mass.: Harvard University Press
Bruner, J. (1990). *Acts of Meaning*, Cambridge Mass: Harvard University Press
Camus, A. (1965). *Essais* / Introd. par R. Quilliot. Textes établis et annotés, par R. Quilliot et L. Faucon Series: Bibliothèque de la Pléiade ; 183 Paris : Gallimard,.
Calvin, W. H. (1997). *How Brains Think: Evolving Intelligence, Then and Now*, London: Weidenfeld & Nicolson
Chomsky, N. (2000). *New Horizons in the Study of Language and Mind*. Cambridge : CUP
Dennet, D.C. (1987). *The Intentional Stance*, Cambridge, Mass.: MIT Press
Derrida, J. (1973). *Speech and Phenomenon and Other Essays on Husserl's Theory of Signs*, tr. D.B. Allison, Evanston, Ill.: Northwestern University Press
Derrida, J. (1978). *The Truth in Painting*, Chicago: University of Chicago Press
Derrida, J. (1992). *Acts of Literature*. Derek Attridge, ed. Publisher: London: Routledge.
Eco, U. (1994).*The Name of the Rose*, New York: Harvest Books
Erickson, M.H. (1987). Central themes and principles of Ericksonian therapy. edited by Stephen R. Lankton Series: Ericksonian monographs; no. 2 Publisher: New York: Brunner/Mazel.
Foucault, M. (1965). *Madness and Civilization: A History of Insanity in the Age of Reason*, trans. R. Howard, London: Routledge.
Gass, W. (1970). *Fiction and the Figures of Life*, New York: Alfred A. Knopf
Gersie, A. (1997). *Reflections on therapeutic storymaking : the use of stories in groups*, London: Jessica Kingsley Publishers
Gianakaris, C. J. (1992). *Peter Shaffer*, Basingstoke : Macmillan
Goodman, N. (1978). *Ways of Worldmaking,* Hassocks, Sussex: Harvester Press

Goodman, N. (1984). *Of Mind and Other Matters,* Cambridge, Mass.: Harvard University Press
Greenfield, S. (1997). *The Human Brain,* London: Harper Collins
Iser, W. (1978). *The Act of Reading,* Baltimore: Johns Hopkins University Press
Jakobson, R. (1960). '*Closing Statement*: Linguistics and Poetics', 350-377
Katan, D. (1999). *Translating Cultures*, Manchester: St. Jerome Publishing
Kermode, J.F. (1975). *The Classic*, London: Faber
Kermode, J.F. (1983). *Forms of Attention: Essays on Fiction*, Chicago: Chicago University Press
Kermode, J.F. (2000). *Shakespeare's Language*, London: Penguin
Klein, M. (1989). *Developments in Psychonalysis*, ed. by J. Riviere with a preface by Ernest Jones, London: Karnac
MacGillivray, J. Alexander, (2001). *Minotaur*, London: Pimlico
Metz, C. (1999). *Some Points in the Semiotics of the Cinema*, in Braudy, L. and Marshall Cohen, eds. Film Theory and Criticism: Introductory Readings, Oxford: OUP
Nietzsche, F.,(1969). *Thus Spoke Zarathustra*, trans. R.J. Hollingdale, Harmondsworth: Penguin
Paz, O.'Translation: Literature and Letters', tr. I. del Corral, in Schulte, R. and J. Biguenet, eds. (1992) *Theories of Translation: An Anthology of Essays from Dryden to Derrida*, Chicago: University of Chicago Press
Phillips, A. (2000). *Promises, Promises*, London: Faber and Faber
Ricoeur, P. (1981). 'The Narrative Function', in *Hermeneutics and the Human Sciences,* ed. and tr. J.B.Thompson, Cambridge: CUP, 277
Ricoeur, P. (1983). *Time and Narrative,* Chicago: University of Chicago Press
Robinson, D. (1991). *The Translator's Turn*, Baltimore: The Johns Hopkins University Press
Sartre, J.P. (1957). *Being and Nothingness*, tr. H.E. Barnes, London: Methuen
Shaffer, P. (1977). *Equus*, London: Penguin
Searle, J. (1969). *Speech Acts,* Cambridge: CUP
Searle, J. (1998. *The Mystery of Consciousness*, London: Granta Books
Tabakowska, E. (1993). *Cognitive Linguistics and Poetics of Translation*, Tübingen: Gunter Narr Verlag
Taylor, C. (1989). *Sources of the Self*, Cambridge Mass.: Harvard University Press
Von Franz, M. L. (1977). *Individuation in fairy tales*, Zurich: Spring Publications.
Vygotsky, L.S. (1978). *Mind in Society: The Development of Higher Psychological Processes,* ed. M. Cole, S.
Scribner, V. John-Steiner, and Souderman, E. , Cambridge, Mass.: Harvard University Press
Williams, B. (1978). *Descartes,* Harmondsworth: Penguin
Wittgenstein, L. (1973). *Philosophical Investigations*, tr. G.E.M. Anscombe, eds. G.E.M. Anscombe and R. Rhees, Oxford: Blackwell

PAULINE MOTTRAM

BREAKING NEW GROUND – EXPANDING OUR VISION

In the initial theorising of British Art Therapy there was acknowledgement of diverse roots ranging from art theory, art history, philosophy, sociology, social anthropology, psychology and psychiatry. Subsequently British Art Therapists have long identified an uneasy tension between words and images (Skaife 1995). Debate has been endemic within the profession. The pioneers of art therapy disagreed over the significance, role and function of the "art" and the "therapy" in clinical practice. (Hill. A (1945), Naumberg, M. (1958), Kramer (Wadeson 1980), Adamson E (1984), Lyddiatt (Thompson 1989)). The art process and the image were regarded by some as the primary curative factor, and an opposing view was held by others who asserted the primacy of psychotherapeutic interventions as the major factor. A core theoretical formulation of the art therapeutic triangular relationship evolved in the early 1990s and this currently underpins most British Art Therapy theorising. (Wood, 1990, Case 1990, Schaverien, 1990) This model looks to psychoanalytic understandings to conceptualise intra- and inter-personal dynamics in art therapy clinical practice (Dalley 1984, Thompson 1989, Case and Dalley 1992, Schaverein 1994).

Grounding artwork solely in psychoanalytic (or any particular) understanding can result in artistic re-presentation and symbology being reduced merely to signs that indicate those particular tenets and principles (Pereira 2002). How we frame our work imposes tacit epistemological assumptions, which in turn frame our practice and understanding and reinforce our conceptualisations. My research into British art therapists' practice shows that solipsistic matching of psychoanalytic theory to dynamics observed in art therapy can obstruct the recognition and development of our discipline specific tacit knowledge (Mottram 1992, 1999, 2002).

To engage in the debates of our post-modern world in this paper I venture outside the traditional UK academic art therapy framed debates and explore some of the current debates that circulate in critical art theory, social psychology and cultural studies.

I do not wish to suggest that psychoanalytic understanding is not useful in art therapy theoretical explication. For example, I find the work of Anton Ehrensweig (1967) particularly helpful in considering the intra-psychic processes of creativity. He employs a Kleinian framework to articulate his observations that in the processes of painting an inability to tolerate fragmentation and an excessive desire to control inhibits creativity. He identifies a need initially to loosen ego rigidity and to surrender creatively to a state of manic oceanic fusion or a de-differentiated unity. Ehrensweig suggests that through maintaining a state of passive watchfulness and half-conscious scanning, a hidden order that operates below a level of conscious scrutiny is apperceived and new symbols emerge in the resultant creative integration of fragmented aspects. He suggests that the subsequent phases of critical scrutiny and completion of an artwork engender similar dynamics to the paranoid schizoid and depressive positions described by

Klein. I regard that Ehrensweig's conceptualisation, due to his focus on process and Kleinian psychoanalytic understandings, does not give sufficient import to artistic prospective meaning making processes that arise out of consideration or confrontation with the unknown.

With regard to the creative process, Arthur Koestler echoes ideas similar yet different to Ehrensweig's notion of a 'hidden order': for example, he identifies what he calls a less conscious 'matrix' that operates below conscious rational thought (Koestler 1975). He suggests that a creative act consists of a new synthesis of previously unconnected matrices of thought. He calls this process 'bi-sociation' and he describes it as "...forging new combinations out of seemingly incompatible contexts". (1975:182). He states that "...the creative person's mind seems to regress from disciplined thinking to less specialised more fluid ways of mentation." (Koestler 1978:149) This type of mentation may present as images, mental pictures and dreamlike sequences.

In similar vein, through his work with groups, psychoanalyst Wilfred Bion (1962) regards processes of fragmentation and integration to be interdependent and intrinsic to the creative process. He does not regard 'fragmentation' to be regressive or pathological, nor does he confine this to an early developmental stage, instead he regards there to be alternating processes of fragmentation and integration throughout life. He names the fragmented unassimilated raw, unprocessed sensory data 'beta' elements. These are transformed by an 'alpha' function in the creation of meaning. He conceptualises a notion of 'container' and 'contained'. A sufficiently strong ego is able to 'contain' processes of fragmentation or disintegration until the chaotic fragments (beta elements) can "link" (through alpha function) in new constellations and a new meaning and coherent order emerges.

Ehrensweig's concept of 'hidden order', Koestler's concept of 'bi-sociation' and Bion's concept of 'alpha-function linking' seem to point towards somewhat similar conceptualisations of intra-psychic creative processes. All three also notice that creative processes require a relinquishing of conscious rational control, a phase of fragmentation, chaos, and a-logicality that is accompanied by an attitude of passive waiting and less conscious apprehending, a position of unknowing, and ultimately a new constellation integrates/emerges. The danger to creative resolution is a reactive fear of fragmentation, premature closure and imposition of order.

Martin Jay (2002) explores the dichotomy that images 'show', (they are tied to what they resemble and they can transcend a specific culture) whereas words 'tell', (they re-present conventions and signs that are culturally determined.) Art Therapists professionally are usually placed in clinical cultures where staff inter-act by 'telling'. Communication is based upon succinct verbal expression of a clinical culture of agreed conventions and signs. Yet our work is with artistic processes of 'showing'. Our clients show us, and we see what they show. In its very nature art is subversive. I believe that part of the on-going debate about words and images in art therapy arises out of the incompatible paradigms that we endeavour to straddle in our work.

Art Therapy it not only concerned with creative processes. The concreteness of the visual image opens up many other areas for consideration. Intra-psychic dialogical processes as well as inter-personal dialogic webs are engaged in the making and viewing of art and in the construction of meaning. I find that Hermans (2004, 2001,a,b, 1996) notion of a dialogical self enables me to address more adequately the inter-personal, cultural, collective and social processes that I find are intrinsic to art therapy practice. Hermans fluid theory proposes that neither 'self' nor 'culture' are reified but are viewed as co-created within a historical and cultural context. Hermans develops Bakhtin's (Holquist 1990) understanding that dialogue is not dyadic but at its minimum is triadic (comprising self-relation-other). 'Self' and 'other' are viewed as co-existing in a dynamic plurality of multi-voiced positions (Hermans 2004).

This post-modern de-centering of a unitary concept of self produces an array of micro-narratives rather than an overarching meta-narrative.

Art is one of the many communicative cultural products of a society. I am increasingly fascinated that Art Therapy theory is developing to the exclusion of insights and debates emerging in relation to images and visual culture in social and cultural studies and in critical art theory. Surely as ART Therapists we should have much to contribute? Why is our voice absent?

Rose articulates a criticism of the psychoanalytic perspective, which 'concentrates on the psychic and visual construction of difference at the expense of considering the social construction and consequences of difference' (Rose 2001:135). Visual images can be regarded as being made within a context of competing operational discourses. Visual images can work on both a level of psyche formation and also on a level of social construction. They can contain, represent and reflect inner and outer dynamics, psyche and social. They present a dialectic: how social processes are subjectively articulated and how subjectivity is socially articulated. I believe this fertile dialectic has been occluded in British Art Therapy theory through the current psychoanalytic hegemony. Art re-presents a particular construction of subjectivity within a society and concurrently art is also a spontaneous response of a community to its experience of existence. Art can be regarded as both a container for and a site of creation of meaning (Pacey, 1977). This meaning is both individual and subjective, as well as collective and social.

How and where images are seen and where, why and how images are made, determine their social meaning and influence. They are an aspect of social and subjective practice. Rose (2001: 137) states:

> 'It is possible to think of visuality as a sort of discourse too. A specific visuality will make certain things visible in particular ways, and other things unseeable, for example, and subjects will be produced and act within that field of vision.'

I find it of interest that in standard British art therapy practice we do not interrogate the visuality of images. Whether the seer is the maker or the viewer, the seer constructs meaning, or brings frames of meanings, in response to the visual phenomena. In extending Rose's understandings to art therapy I prefer to expand this understanding of visuality to include the communicative negotiations inherent in art therapeutic viewing of images ie: the maker operates within his/her own particular discursive practices and produces an image, which reflects his/her discursive formation. When the therapist as viewer sees the image, active participation is required to begin to see the maker's discursive formation, and to co-create a mutual understanding through careful dialogue. The therapist does not merely view from his/her perspective of habitual or preferred constructs and discourses.

Rose (2001) suggests that images can be analysed in terms of Production (how the image is made); Image itself (what it looks like); Audience (how it is seen). I believe that this construction artificially separates aspects and does not take sufficiently into account social and personal dynamics engendered by images. The relationships between artist and medium, and between artwork and audience are inter-active and dialogic. Levine (1992:72) considers Ricoeur's notions of 'hermeneutics of generosity' and the 'hermeneutics of suspicion': he believes that to see an image's transcendent dimension we need to take on an attitude of generosity and give ourselves feely to image with awe and respect, and allow it to overflow our preconceptions. The image reveals. But Levine asserts that just as the image is always more than it is, it is also always less. With an attitude of suspicion we can regard there to be something hidden from us and we wrestle with the image to reveal it. 'Only in the to and fro of suspicion and generosity does the double nature of the image stand revealed.' (ibid:74)

McNiff (1998:186) explores his reaction to viewing an image:

'Although the arts offer researchers a wealth of perceptible phenomena, the subtleties of the creative process cannot be encapsulated within isolated frames of observable behaviour which are seen as parts of an overall pattern of linear causes and effects. In my experience, the impact of artworks on viewers is more environmental. When I perceive an artwork, I enter its environment which is composed of a complex interplay of forces.'

Post Colonial theorist Hall (1999:310) regards viewer and viewed as mutually constitutive and he holds that the articulation between viewer and viewed is an internal relation:

'The subject is, in part, formed subjectively through what and how it 'sees', how its 'field of vision' is constructed. In the same way, what is seen – the image and its meaning – is understood as not externally fixed, but relative to and implicated in the positions and schemas of interpretation which are brought to bear upon it.'

Hall (1999:311) states that the impact of image

'is immediate and powerful even when its precise meaning remains, as it were, vague, suspended – numinous." And he describes "the image's capacity to connote on a much broader social field, to touch levels of experience which seem remote or 'archaic', beyond the purely rational level of awareness, and which disturb by the very way in which they exceed meaning.' (ibid).

An image can point to that which has not as yet been articulated verbally. It operates within and beyond constructed discourse – in the border zones of the verbal and preverbal. Numinous art can operate as an agent for social change and is in contrast to mannered art that is in the service of the known/dominant discourse. The numinous art work is produced by an artist who operates in the margins of society and social understandings. The numinous art work and its artist are subversive of dominant discourses. They present the audience with 'knowing unknowing'. The discourse of this type of image is hybrid: there is sufficient of the recognisable and known for the image to be partially intelligible/acceptable to the viewer, but it also presents something not known, something new, a mystery awaiting exploration, which gives it its numinosity.

Considerations through art go beyond existing discourses to the sites of creativity where meaning is made, where dominant discourses are subverted, and the new emerges. This necessitates a concept of human agency: of creating and concurrently being created. Pacey (1977) regards that:

> 'The work of art embodies, and re-enacts, a moment of vision which is a moment of *recognition*. The potter recognises, in a lump of clay, his capacity to transform it...the capacity for transformation...is in both maker and material.'

Art, as a container for and a site of creation of meaning, continually offers a possibility of making, and re-making connections and understandings. Henzell (1995:193-196) states that an image shows rather than says. It can be looked at in a multitude of directions, and several elements can be apprehended simultaneously. In this engagement images and words enhance each other in a dialogical co-construction of meaning.

From a broader global and social perspective, Freedland (2001:84) suggests that in these times of globalisation, mass migration and loss of territorialized notions of homeland, the maintaining of cultural traditions can hold a community together but hybridized or hyphenated diasporic identities also emerge and these are expressed through various art forms. She identifies (2001:86-87) the current context of internally diverse and evolving communities, of political turmoil and complex negotiations of personal identity. She holds that art is crucial for addressing the personal and collective questions raised by this "ever-new, and often precarious, world situation."

Instead of espousing the traditional paradigm wherein art process and objects are the raw material for psychological research, McNiff (1998:24) suggests that artistic inquiry is a research method in its own right.

> 'Imagination is an intelligence which is highly underrated in our approaches to research. It is the basic tool that all people use to approach and understand new areas of experience and to revise what they already know.' (ibid:184).

I suggest that art presents a particular ambiguity in that it is able to function as a container for inter-personal social meaning and also to point concurrently beyond what may be constructed to other levels of experience and constructions of understandings that may be negotiated through dialogical encounters around and through the art work.

In regard to inter-personal construction of social meaning, Barthes (2000:109) states that '...every object in the world can pass from a closed, silent existence to an oral state open to appropriation by society.' Once appropriated it is given significance and meaning, and it becomes a sign. (ibid: 111). Holquist (1990:81) in a similar vein identifies how words name, direct and connect the "dark chaos of inner sensation" to the outer world in a constant exchange and creation of meaning. Hall (2000) draws attention to how images can point beyond the known. He recognises (ibid 2000: 311)

> '...the image's capacity to connote on a much broader social field, to touch levels of experience which seem remote or 'archaic', beyond the purely rational level of awareness, and which disturb by the very way in which they exceed meaning.'

I would like to expand on these insights by suggesting that images may 'connote' in a multi-layered manner i.e. they may evoke primitive and/or archaic infantile dynamics such as those conceptualised by Kleinian and British Object Relations theoretical formulations (Glover 2004). They may address the current hegemonic discourse and constructed meanings that operate on 'purely rational levels of experience' i.e. the contemporary known, agreed and collectively accepted social understandings. In a Bakhtinian (Holquist 1990) sense they also present opportunity for hetereoglossia: multiple and divergent constructions and negotiations of meaning. As divergent meanings are constructed and become attached to the art work, resultant centripetal processes can disrupt and disperse collectively accepted social understandings opening spaces for new and hither to unknown constructions and constellations of meaning attribution.

Jay (2002) discusses the notions that no culture is distinct, integrated, coherent and boundaried. Instead culture can be regarded to be a 'porous container'. (ibid:273) What is inside and what is outside interact and this results in 'hybrids' and 'quasi-subjects' and 'quasi-objects' that both include and exclude. Jay (ibid:274) cites Merleau-Ponty's notion of 'flesh of the world': He suggests that figurality cannot be entirely reduced to discursivity; images cannot be entirely reduced to words through discursive cultural mediation. Images remain in excess of cultural filters and they resist total subsumation by a particular culture.

Debray (1996:153) talks of the 'corporeality of images' that '.....disrupts the smooth symbolic order of surfaces – like the flesh before and behind the word.'.
Jay (2002:276) presents a notion of 'a stubborn residue of what culture thought it had left behind....' He identifies a 'persistent disruption' of culture by 'visual experience' and he proposes that we live with the dialectic of culture and nature, as neither is sufficient without the other. Jay (ibid:274) cites Latour's argument that '...it is impossible to reduce natural visual experience to its cultural mediations as it is to disentangle it entirely from them.'

I find in my art therapy work with patients and students that I remain fascinated, because I have never found closure in my understanding. I know that I can never fully understand. I believe that the rare times when I think I may understand are the potentially most damaging to my understanding, to myself and to others. It may be that in time a hidden order may emerge from the not-knowing and a more articulated encompassing meta-narrative may be articulated. But I also wonder if art therapy theory does require a totalising myth? We work in very complex terrains that may be resistant to definitive mapping.

I think of paint, the basic stuff of our work, and I think of Elkins' (2000:5) superb description of paint as 'liquid thought' and how in the act of painting, thoughts are 'embedded in paint'. Elkins uses the term 'hypostasis' to indicate what he identifies as a 'general infusion of spirit into something' (ibid:44). He explores the concrete and symbolic aspects that are juxtaposed and which interpenetrate in an artwork:

> 'Hypostasis is the feeling that something as dead as paint might also be deeply alive, full of thought and expressive meaning... paint is a window onto something else, a transparent thing that shimmers in our awareness as we look through it to see what the painter has depicted: but it is also a sludge, a hard scab clinging to the canvas.' (Elkins 2000:44)

He points to the fundamentally unsettled and unsettling qualities that, in remaining unresolved, compel and fascinate us:

> '...and when it is merely paint, it begins to speak in an uncanny way, telling us things we do not quite understand – in the language of alchemy and religion – with soul, spirit and formal life...paint seems irresistibly to mean. It never speaks clearly because as any sober scientist or humanist will tell you – every meaning is a projection of the viewer's inarticulate moods. Substances are like mirrors that let us see things about ourselves that we cannot quite understand.' (Elkins 2000:45)

He articulates the inter-relationship of maker (viewer) and artwork and he highlights the continual dialogical processes elicited in making and in viewing Paint

> '.... is always speaking but never saying anything rational, always playing at being abstract but never leaving the clotted body. Painting is something that is worked out in the making and the work and its maker exchange ideas and change one another.' (Elkins 2000:78)

He succinctly identifies the movement of meaning in an artwork, through various levels or forms: physical sensory, concrete reality and constructed perception.

> 'The meaning seems to travel like an electric current, sparking from the artist's body to the chemicals and from there to the eye of the viewer.' (Elkins 2000:98).

Conclusion

Post Colonial theorist Hall (2000) expresses understanding that meaning can be regarded as always in process and that it is continually involved in an inter-weaving and inter-playing of similarity and difference. I find that the experience of art can present rifts and openings in both intra- and inter-personal meanings. In rifts and openings 'I' positions may be challenged and unsettled and meaning may be re-negotiated. I increasingly use this as a central understanding, as well as my point of departure in my art therapy practice and theorising.

Within art therapy practice and theorising, the post modern challenge is to integrate creatively seemingly disparate and/or fragmented intra-personal perceptions and inter-personal exchanges. Understanding of 'dialogical space' constellates client and therapist within poly-vocal positions in a flattened hierarchy. 'I' positions may be made, and re-made. Attributions of meaning may be challenged and re-negotiated and meaning may be re-created or transformed, as the dialogical self is constructed and re-constructed in and through negotiation around the artwork. 'I' positions, subjectivity and meaning may be intra- and inter-personally contested, re-negotiated and re-created.

Dialogical reflection and revelation around the unfurling immediacy of the art therapy image enable co-development of understanding, and co-creation of meaning, within the particular historical and cultural situatedness of the art therapy sessions. The challenge is to contain multiplicity and not-knowing in order to be able to integrate and/or synthesise meaning. This indicates a continual dialogical process of re-negotiation of and between self and other.

I believe that a reactive fear of fragmentation, premature closure and imposition of order can endanger the creative progression of art therapy theorising. Chambers (1994:133) states:

> 'The world is marked by language, not engulfed by it. While continually translated into the texts we read, watch, listen to, write, interpret and live by, the world stubbornly resists closure. The alchemy of language is not so powerful. It is through this rift, this opening, that our bodies, our gestures and our language are constantly renewed: drawn on by the desire for the promise of the impossible.'

In my current theorising of art therapy practice, I find most useful understandings that provide insight into social and intra-personal creative processes that operate within and beyond constructed discourse in the border zones of the verbal and preverbal: a 'knowing unknowing'. Vital processes and dynamics in our practice can be occluded by rigid espousal of any particular perspective. By breaking new ground and expanding our vision, multiple perspectives can be both discovered and uncovered, and our theorising and explication of practice can be consequently widened and enriched.

References

Adamson, E. (1984). *Art as Healing.* Coventure
Barthes, R. (2000). *Mythologies.* London: Vintage Classics
Bion, W.R. (1962). *Learning from experience.* London: Tavistock

Case, C. (1990). *Triangular Relationship 3* Inscape Winter 1990 p20-25
Case and Dalley (1992). *Handbook of Art Therapy*. London: Routledge.
Chambers, I. (1994). *Migrancy culture identity*. London: Routledge
Champernowe, I. (1971). *Art and Therapy: an Uneasy Partnership*. American Journal of Art Therapy: 10(3) Apr pp131-143.
Dalley, T. (ed.) (1984). *Art as Therapy*. London: Tavistock Publications
Debray, R. (1996). *Media Manifestos: On the technological transmission of cultural forms* (translated Rauth, E) London: Verso
Ehrensweig, A. (1967 ed1993). *The hidden order of art. A study in the psychology of artistic imagination*. London: Weidenfeld
Elkins, J. (2000). *What painting is"* London: Routledge.
Freeland, C. (2001). *But is it art? An introduction to Art Theory*. Oxford: Oxford University Press
Glover, N. (2004). *Psychoanalytic Aesthetics: the British School.* accessed 05.08.2004 http://human-nature.com/free-associations/glover/index.html
Hall, S. (1999). 'Looking for Subjectivity: Introduction' pp 309-314 in Evans, J & Hall ,S *Visual Culture: the reader*. London: Sage
Hall, S. (2000). Conclusion: the multi-cultural question. pp209-240 in Hesse B (ed) *Un/Settled multiculturalisms: diasporas, entanglements, 'transruptions'* London. New York: Zed Books
Henzell, J. (1995). "Research and the particular" p185-205 in *Art and Music Therapyand Research* ed Gilroy,A &Lee,C. London: Routledge
Hermans , H.J.M. (2004). *Introduction: The Dialogical Self in a Global and Digital Age*. Identity: an International Journal of Theory and Research 4(4) 297-320
Hermans, H.J.M. (2001a). The dialogical self: towards a theory of personal and cultural positioning. *Jn: Culture and Psychology* 7:3:243-281
Hermans, H.J.M. (2001b). Mixing and moving cultures require a dialogical self. *Jn: Human Development* 44:24-28
Hermans, H.J.M. (1996). Voicing the self: from information processing to dialogical interchange *Jn: Psychological Bulletin* 119:1:31-50
Hill, A. (1945). *Art vs Illness*. London, Allen & Unwin
Holquist, M. (1990). *Dialogism. Bakhtin and his world*. London, New York: Routledge
Jay, M. (2002). Cultural Relativism and the visual turn. *Jn Visual Culture* vol 1 (3) 267-278
Koestler, A. (1975). *The act of creation*. London: Picador
Koestler, A. (1978, '83ed). *Janus: a summing up*. London: Pan Books
Levine, S. (1992, 1997ed). *Poiesis: the language of psychology and the speech of the Soul*. London: Jessica Kingsley
McEvilley, T. (1995, 1999ed). *Art and Otherness*. Documentext McPherson &co
McNiff, S. (1998). *Art-Based Research*. London: Jessica Kingsley Publishers
Mottram, P. (1992). *Relational Dynamics in Art Therapy*. unpublished paper 'Praxis & Visions' Conference Copenhagen
Mottram, P. (1999). *Art Therapists' accounts of the skills and interventions used in working clinically with individual clients' images*. Unpublished MA by Res thesis University of Hertfordshire
Mottram, P. (2002). *Art therapists' accounts of working with images*. Arts Therapies Virtual Journal (University of Derby UK)
Naumberg, M. (1958). 'Art Therapy: It's scope and Function', in E.F. Hammer (ed) *'Clinical Applications of Projective Drawings'* Springfield, Ill.: C.C.Thomas
Pacey, P. (1977). *A sense of what is real*. London: Brentham Press
Pereira, F. (2002). Fairburn, dreaming and the aesthetic experience. Chpt 7 p111-125 in *Fairburn and Relational Theory* Pereira and Scharf, Eds London: Karnac

Rose, G. (2001). *Visual Methodologies* London: Sage
Schaverien, J. (1990). *Triangular Relationship 2* Inscape Winter 1990 p14-19
Schaverien, J. (1994). *Analytical Art Therapy: further reflections on theory and practice.* Inscape vol. 2 pp41-48.
Skaife, S. (1995). *The Dialectics of Art Therapy.* Inscape vol. 1 pp2-7.
Thompson, M. (1989). *On Art and Therapy: an Exploration.* Reading, Berks: Cox & Wyman Ltd
Wadeson, H. (1980). *Art Psychotherapy.* John Wiley and Sons, Inc.
Wood, C. (1990). *Triangular Relationship 1.* Inscape Winter 1990 p7-13

PETER SINAPIUS

ART AS THE CENTRE OF ART THERAPIES EDUCATION

1. Introduction

Art has to be the centre of art therapies education. However, the piece of art is not the purpose of art therapy. The process of creating is the decisive moment.
Art therapy is the science of relationship. If I stand here looking to a painting I have to relate to it to enable myself to express my feelings, my images, my visions and my passions. I have to get a sensitive feeling about it. Art therapies education is dealing with how we can relate to a piece of art by creating it.
There is no way to explain, what a painting is about (Boehm 1995). Mark Rothko said:

> 'No possible set of notes can explain our paintings. Their explanation must come out of a consummated experience between picture and onlooker. The appreciation of art is a true marriage of minds. And in art, as in marriage, lack of consummation is ground for annulment.' (Mark Rothko 2001)

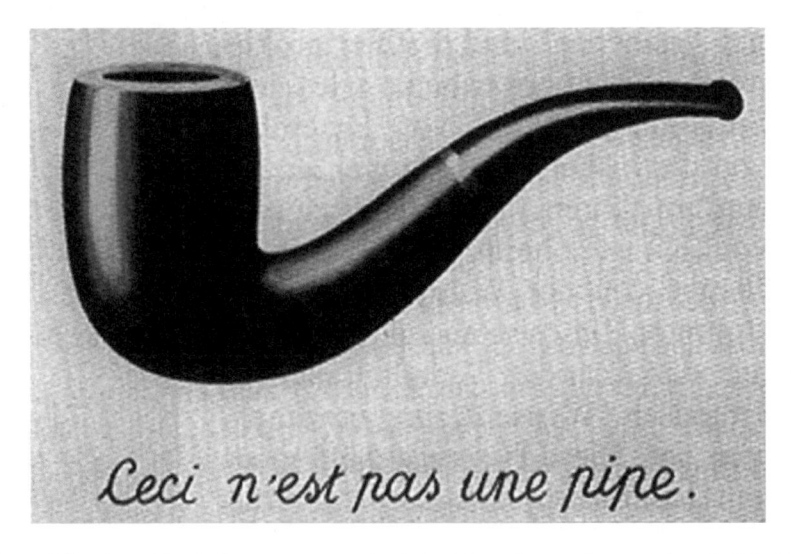

Rene Magritte: 'Ceci n'est pas unce pipe', in: Kunstforum International, Bd. 173, 2004, Ruppichteroth, p 72.

Art is not about *what* we see on a painting, it is about *how* we could look at it (Sontag 1967). If we recognize a pipe in a painting, we can relate to it with the term "pipe". The word "pipe" is not especially concerning this painting, it means everything that is looking similar to a pipe. The word "pipe" is only a reference to the painted or real pipe. There is no doubt our relation to this individual painting is different having a sensitive feeling about what this painting looks like. And, indeed, this feeling is much different from our relation to a real pipe that we are smoking. Obviously we are able to relate to a painting like this in different ways.

2. Three ways forming a relationship

Before I speak about pictures, that have been painted in art therapy, I use a simple object like an apple to find out how we get into a relationship to it and how the apple can become part of our history.

The first level of a relationship between me and this apple is the physical one. If I look at an apple, I recognize that this apple is different from me. I am not this apple and the apple is not me. On the level of its physical appearance there is no doubt that I am not an apple and the apple is not me. I have nothing to do with it.

The second level of a relationship between me and an apple is an emotional one. If I get interested in an apple, I have to go into a certain relationship to it. The question is: What do I have to do with this apple? To find out something about it, I bite into the apple. I don't let it be as it is. I eat this apple and I annex it. The result is not that I by myself become similar to an apple. Something different happens. I like the taste or I don't like it. With a sensitive feeling, I try to find out what I have to do with this apple. I get into a relationship with it. I respond to it with a feeling, that tells me, how it tastes: sweet, sour, juicy. I don't get this feeling if I only look at this apple. I have to bite into it to get to a perception. Having this experience, I make this apple into a part of my own history.

The third level of a relationship between me and an apple is the spiritual one. If I speak about "apple" in general, without seeing it and without eating it, I don't speak about a special apple, but I get an idea of an apple. If I imagine an apple in my mind, I have transformed an apple in an image of it. This transformation of the physical appearance to an idea is the way art happens. In my mind I relate the term "apple" to the essence, to the character of an apple. The apple I speak about cannot be understood as a physical thing. It is a spiritual matter. It has nothing to do with a real apple in its physical appearance. I create this apple in my mind. The question is not what I have to do with this apple, when I bite into it to get a sensitive feeling. The matter is what the species "apple" is about. If I get an idea of that, I have understood something about an apple.

By this, I have described three levels that determine our relationship to our surroundings: the physical, the mental and the spiritual level.

3. The painting and its context

Assume that I go by night into my neighbor's garden to steal an apple from his tree. In this case this apple is different from all the other apples. It has its meaning through this story, which distinguishes it from each other apple. This apple is connected with my personal story. It gets its meaning because I went into my neighbor's garden to steal an apple from his tree. Only if I tell you this story, this apple gets the same meaning for you as for me: the apple taken out of my neighbor's garden.

If we look at a water-color painting without any object like a pipe, an apple or anything else on it, we have to find another way to describe what we see. At first we may describe its physical conditions: Its ground, the paint, and its proportions. We see what it looks like physically. But on this level, we get no more an idea of its image than we get an idea of the taste of an apple by only looking at it. At first, this painting is a strange object for us with its own history, with which we have nothing to do.

Usually emotion is our reaction looking at a painting: We like it or not, it looks strange or familiar. We judge it. So far it is a matter of taste that determines our relationship to this painting. Looking at its colors we get a feeling of grief or happiness, of warm or cold, of calm or movement. Our feeling is more about what the physical conditions of this painting. The colors are causing something like a sound we don't hear with our ears; we hear it with our soul. This sound only gets real between the painting and the onlooker (Bockemühl 1985). In order to get this feeling we have to create a personal experience like biting into an apple. We are producing its image.

Beyond that an art therapist might pose the questions: What does this painting mean, what is its image and what has it to do with the person, who painted it? As soon as I have this question, I go over the personal emotions I got looking at it the first time. The question aims now at the circumstances with which the painting was connected. The context of this painting might disclose its real meaning, which let us know something about its author.

In this case, a painting is similar to an apple that I have stolen from my neighbor's garden. I have to know something about its history to understand its meaning. We don't get its meaning by only looking at it. Its appearance has no evidence about what has happened in therapy. But if I tell you the story about it, we are able to see it with other eyes.

4. Forming a relationship through painting

The painting, I am thinking about is connected with the following situation:

Nadine was 14 years old, when she came to art therapy. She was suffering from acute asthma. She liked to draw and to paint. At first she was doing what she liked most. Having put a shell in front of her, she drew it very carefully and with her own accuracy by using a pencil and a small piece of paper. I did the same and so we both were absorbed in our work. At the end of our meeting, we compared what we had done and spoke about it.

After some more meetings, I had the desire to paint a common painting with Nadine like a conversation piece. We took a large piece of paper between us, choose painting in water-colors and decided not to speak before we had finished the painting. The colors on the paper were our words and the basis for our conversation. About half a year, we painted common pieces every week. Through this process we developed something that was speaking through the relationships of colors.

As a result of art therapy, the relationship between Nadine and her surroundings was directly affected: the asthma-attacks which had lead her to art therapy, disappeared after half a year (Sinapius 2005).

In therapy with Nadine we can see two different processes of creating:

- At first we drew a shell. Each of us was absorbed in his/her own work. Tracing something we saw in front of us and looking for a good result, we tried to get into a relationship to an object by drawing this object. Like biting into an apple we tried to get a feeling of the shell by drawing.
- Then we painted a common piece. There was no image beyond the painting itself. We didn't relate to an object, we related to what the partner was doing. The image was developed by painting: The relations between the colors. The image that the painting was about was arising between Nadine and me.

In this example, we relate in different ways to the painting as an object of art. The painting may tell something about a shell. In this case it is something like a document of history. Beyond that, a painting could be part of history. It gets its meaning during the process of doing (Aldridge 2002). Art may open a space between you and me. In this case art therapy is acquiring a social significance. The image that determines art therapy is the process of getting new access to our surroundings.

5. Art and therapy

This understanding of art, of including the creative process, already determines contemporary art. Looking at art of the 20th Century, we see its theme is the discrepancy between the painting as a closed document, about something that happened in the past, and the context with which it was connected. In the art of our days, the process of creating gets more and more important. The production and setting of art is getting more important than the piece of art itself.

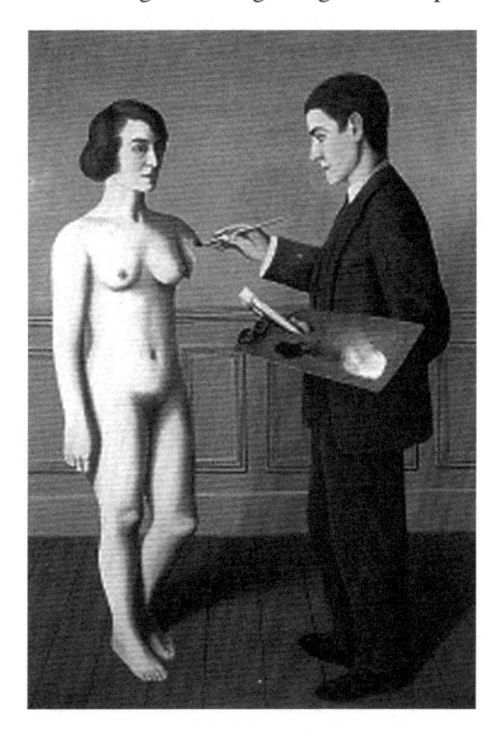

Rene Magritte: 'Impossible',
in: Gombrich, E.H. (2002). Die Geschichte der Kunst. Berlin, Phaidon Verlag, p 591.

Two short examples might illustrate that:

- In 1928 Magritte painted the "Impossible": He painted himself while he was painting a model he is creating at the very moment we look at it. He is not depicting reality. The painting is not a document of the past. It is creating a reality that is present. It happens at that moment, we are looking at it.
- Contemporary art is going one step further. In 1952 John Cage composed a work the contents of which is only the noise of the listeners: The listeners are the musicians. Almost at the same time, the shadows of the onlookers are part of Rauschenberg's "white paintings" (Rolling / Sturm 2002). And in the sixties Joseph Beuys transformed the traditional understanding of art. His images get real in a social and political context (Mennekes / van der Grinten 1984 / Harlan 1986).

The decisive moment is not the analysis of the piece of art; it is the way we are taking part, the way we are looking at it. Art is the science of relationship. From this point of view, art in therapy is more than a document of the past. It is something that gets its meaning in the moment we are participating: Each action, movement, shape or color in the therapeutic process is part of our way to communicate through art. The art therapist needs the artistic skills to create this process.
This is the reason that art has to be the centre of art therapies education.

References
Aldridge, D. (2002). *Forschungsmethoden Künstlerischer Therapien* / Grundlagen Projekte – Vorschläge: Musiktherapieforschung – eine Erzählperspektive. Stuttgart, Maier

Bockemühl, M. (1985). *Die Wirklichkeit des Bildes / Bildrezeption als Bildproduktion*: Rothko, Newman, Rembrandt, Raphael. Stuttgart, Verlag Freies Geistesleben

Boehm, G. (ed.) (1995). *Beschreibungskunst – Kunstbeschreibung:* Ekphrasis von der Antike bis zur Gegenwart: Bildbeschreibung. Über die Grenzen von Bild und Sprache. München: Wilhelm Fink Verlag

Harlan, V. (1986). *Was ist Kunst? Werkstattgespräch mit Beuys*. Stuttgart: Urachhaus.

Mennekes, F. / van der Grinten F J (1984). *Menschenbild – Christusbild*. Stuttgart: Katholisches Bibelwerk

Rolling, S. / Sturm, E. (ed) (2002). *Dürfen die das? Kunst als sozialer Raum: Zwischen Agitation und Animation.* Aktivismus und Partizipation in der Kunst des 20. Jahrhunderts. Wien, Turia & Kant

Rothko, M. (2001). Mark Rothko: Foundation Beyeler, Ostfildern-Ruit: Hatje Cantz Verlag.

Sinapius, P. (2005). *Therapie als Bild – Das Bild als Therapie: Grundlagen einer künstlerischen Therapie.* Frankfurt a.M.: Peter Lang

Sontag, S. (1967). *Against Interpretation*. New York: Straus & Giroux

Picture references
Rene Magritte: 'Ceci n'est pas unce pipe', in: Kunstforum International, Bd. 173, 2004, Ruppichteroth, p 72.

Rene Magritte: 'Impossible', in: Gombrich, E.H. (2002). Die Geschichte der Kunst. Berlin, Phaidon Verlag, p 591.

PETER RECH

ON THE SYMPTOMATOLOGY OF THE IMAGE

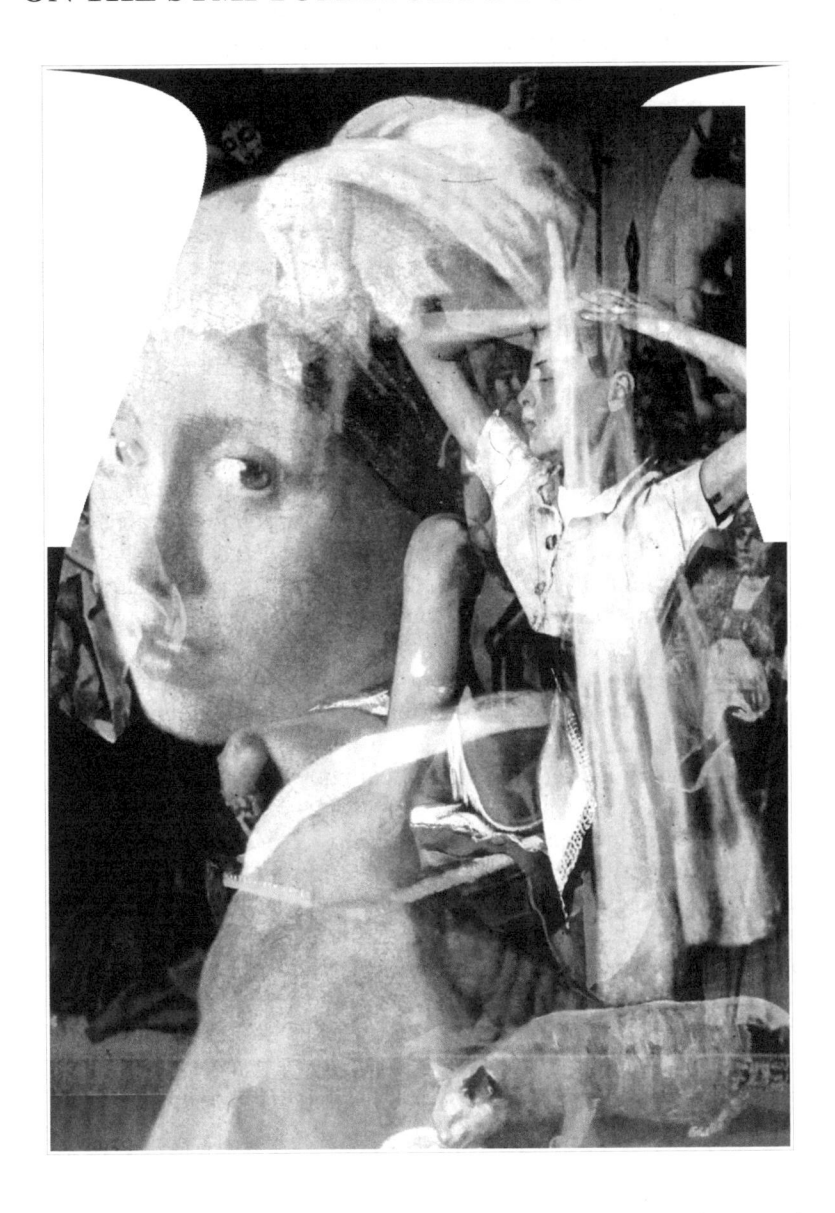

Image and imagination are related. They both communicate objects and events independent of reality. Both are *the* media in that they are also mediums of and for the creative visual therapies. They are the centre of all arts therapies.
The deceptive appearances of images work on us like drugs. They stem from a former satiation through the body of the mother. Images are places of consolation in remembrance of a former "1-ness".

Originally, therapy meant helping the ill person to view his illness – which aims at nothing other than a process of self-healing – as a myth, and ultimately to realise and accept it: this manner of speaking embraces notions which the ill person narrates about himself, and which his environment uses to regard his illness. On both sides, inner images begin to develop that take a sparing view of both the diagnosis and the progression of the illness. This view underlies the contradictory processes of transference. Therein ensue desires that augur the "1-ness" with the mother.

The therapeutic dyad, the "2-ness", appears as a conversation, which is specifically what a therapy should not be. Intense resistances against the therapist abruptly occur. The therapeutic procedure begins to halt. In reality everything is urging to break up the whitewashing of the illusions. In order to realise that *one* single truth which is relevant to each particular, individual patient – a truth which in the case of therapeutic interactions is never actually nice – one needs the *di-version,* via the spellbinding beauty of the images, which are for the main part deceptive. That which is beautified in the images has to do with illusions that are fixed between birth and death "in mother **tongue**".

Thus arts therapy could be said to constitute no more than an attempt at making visible whatever individual universes lie hidden behind the metaphors of a given illness. What order does an image possess underneath its proposed mysteriousness? The demystification of an image proceeds symbolically, and is at the same time undermined symbolically, in the process of talking about it, which is babbling. Babbling makes audible an image beyond what is visible in/on the surface (Kandinsky, 1912, 1952: 45-52).

A patient is subject to the wishes for healing. A therapist is subject to the phantasmagorias of science. Both are connected in their individually significant misjudging of the truth of a given illness. In any case, to realise the truth of an illness does not always necessarily lead to healing.

Visual arts-therapeutic perception should go over and beyond the pictorial in the images, since both patient and therapist are led by the nose, by mirror-inverted and snugly fitting self-deceptions, which represent the nature of counter transference (which itself comes close to complete folly). In the overlapping of inner images their I's become so alike, that the deconstruction of the exchange between both unconsciousnesses involved presents the only therapeutically sensible *way out*. A therapist can only cure or heal to the extent which "his own complexes and inner resistances allow him to" (Freud). Affects and obsessions (particularly the therapists') are caged in *presentable* self-images. How may the truth of the illness still unfold for the patient in images that are not beautifying?

The painting of images still activates most obviously the contradiction between the veiling and the unravelling nature of images as the echo *and* the resounding of one unconscious towards/with another.

Man is thrown back and forth between images and perceptions; this way therapy corrupts us most temptingly with exterior images. One simply loses sight of the symptomatology of the life story. Furthermore, that which is relived in the process of painting is confused with the memories in the images.

Images fascinate, captivate, although they are only surfaces with height and width.

The effect of images between whatever is visible on/in them on the one hand and what shifts in the lives of those who paint, and henceforth view them, on the other is solely situational. Reproduced algorithmically, images behave like results of numerators and denominators. Written on the one side is 'what counts'; it counts how often a thing occurs that stays '*mute*' in the denominator. '*Fact is*' what is imperceptible. An illness appears like an 'eerie feeling' (Freud), as if it had a pictorial interiority. Right from the beginning of our lives we need to overcome "loneliness, silence and darkness (...) as those true moments (...) of child's fear that never quite ceases" (Freud). The fact that no *narrative* level of an illness can fully conform to this un*demonstrative* level of an illness makes the "dream" of arts therapy so "hard". Therapeutically, an image is never sufficient. "An image *is* (in fact) more than a thousand words".

Man is a 'confidant.' The *unconscious*, which is '*respons*-ible' for the production of the images, is *not visible*. To the same extent to which there are images, we feel liberated from having to wise up to ourselves. Without it being decodeable, something does return in the images that exists *outside* of that whose 'con-ception' it effectuates. It is something at once forever lost and unforgettable, which must have once acted like a prohibition. The therapeutic aspect of images is the fact that/the manner in which they rile their recipients into a continually repetitious talk about something that seems to oppose the inner images with such impressive force, as if they were concentrating on just this forbidden material. *Thanks to* the razzle-dazzle of the images the unconscious is strongly perceived internally (Jung). Thus the creative visual arts therapies are inclined to present themselves as fantastical "imaginative journeys."

That which could be affected by said prohibition is deleted in its possible truthfulness from memory for all time. Thereby the verifiability of the fact that every first forbiddance aims at the desiring of the mother is falsified.

Arts therapy *draws* – structurally as well as with respect to contents – from many mistakes. It wastes its time with creative activities. As if artistic practice alone is what characterises arts therapy! It ignores the reasons behind the images. In its early stages at least, anthroposophical art therapy was honest enough to rejoice in understanding art therapy to be a covering (as opposed to an un- or dis-covering) medical procedure; perhaps even in the sense of *the* most pictorial ode to the images:

"*A cornucopia of blossoms,/Another of fruits,/how I'd like to linger and/arrange them for celebration!/But a flurry sweeps/through the airs so wild;/Where all congeals,/Rejoice in the image!/Hail the images!/They went ahead,/And others follow -/Thusly and henceforth!* " (Goethe to Zelter on the 11.12.1831, in Werke, 1998:285).

Art therapy is not conceived as 'a flurry sweeping through the airs so wild'. Therapeutic activity is meant to pictorially overcome all that is congealed. In his worlds of images, the patient is made self-conscious, is tangled, caught, but also (all the same): held.

In this, most of all, the directly imaginative therapeutic methods are to date debunked. In the jargon they are called, as already mentioned, quite bluntly "imaginative journeys". Here arts therapy reaffirms most obstinately that it is useful to avail oneself of the deceptive appearances of images. Arts therapy as a perfecting of the fact that the deceptive appearances of the images act like drugs (see above). Is this ab-*use* now fateful or fruitful?

The images which illustrate these words are computer printer digital collages of artworks, in combination with six important quotations and with three theses. The collages follow the principle: "Not to claim possession of the image, but rather to let oneself be possessed by the image: allowing one's knowledge about the image to be snatched away. The risk is high, of course." (Didi-Huberman, 2000:147-149, 196.)

The question 'what do images stand for?', seen art historically, is the question also for the arts therapies. As well qualified in the field of Byzantine studies, Hans Belting (2001:14,17,126,130,146.) speaks, with regard to Antiquity, of the "era of the image" which was replaced by the "era of art" of the Italian and Dutch renaissance.

Slogan 1: *"The longer I observe the less I see".* (Didi-Huberman, 2000:231)
Thesis I:
IN CLASSICAL ANTIQUITY THE IMAGE PERTAINED TO THE CONDITION OF DEATH

Slogan 2: *"The motivation behind human image-making is death"*
(Belting, 2001:17, 143, 146)
Just visualize – what every educated European has in mind – the oldest cemetery of Athens. There the statues depict the dead, the spentness of their lives. The Roman steles will keep up the careful description of the dead. But don't forget that the old Egyptian statues have revealed themselves in the expectation of otherworldly animation (Panofsky, 1980). Let us think of the late medieval times and their old books of hours. Are we to blot out the old perceptions? As a reminder, the lid of sarcophagus (Greek: 'carnivore') should always stay before one's eye.
And then after all, in the artworks, we see 'more and more' the birth of Christ.

Slogan 3: *"Uterus Mariae – I am the place which you inhabit" (=every picture is held by the virgin)* (Didi-Huberman, 2000:234)
Thesis II:
IN ART, THE MERGING – AS BECOMING (ONE) FLESH WITH THE MOTHER – BECOMES A THEME ("...THE WORD HAS BECOME FLESH...")

Slogan 4: *"In all works of art death is concealed by the woman "* (Didi-Huberman, 2000:234)
You might say the first metaphorical use of imagery takes place within the subject of the birth of Christ. A lesson for all of us is the painting by the Master of Hohenfurth, who was active in Prague around 1350; mother and child fondle and cradle each other like woman and man.
Thesis III:
THE CHILD IS INCREASINGLY OMITTED IN ART. THE 'BECOMING FLESH' ITSELF EMERGES.

Courbet's "L'origine du monde", despite the fact that it was painted in 1866, still shocks viewers today. From 1963 through to 1995, Tracey Emin spends the night In a tent (which has now been burnt in a gallery) with friends that come to visit her and which stay the night, with relatives, with her mother, with her lovers. Their names are appliqued to the inside of the tent. The tent presents itself as a uterine image folded inside-out. Tracey Emin's coffin from 1997 is a textually lidded image that pre-empts her own death. This art-*work* stays very close to the underlying motivation of every image, which is death.

Slogan 5:*"The images themselves are not reason enough to destroy them [...] but you must preach [...]. that the images are nothing: God does not ask for them"* (The thinking of Martin Luther, in Belting, 1990:519

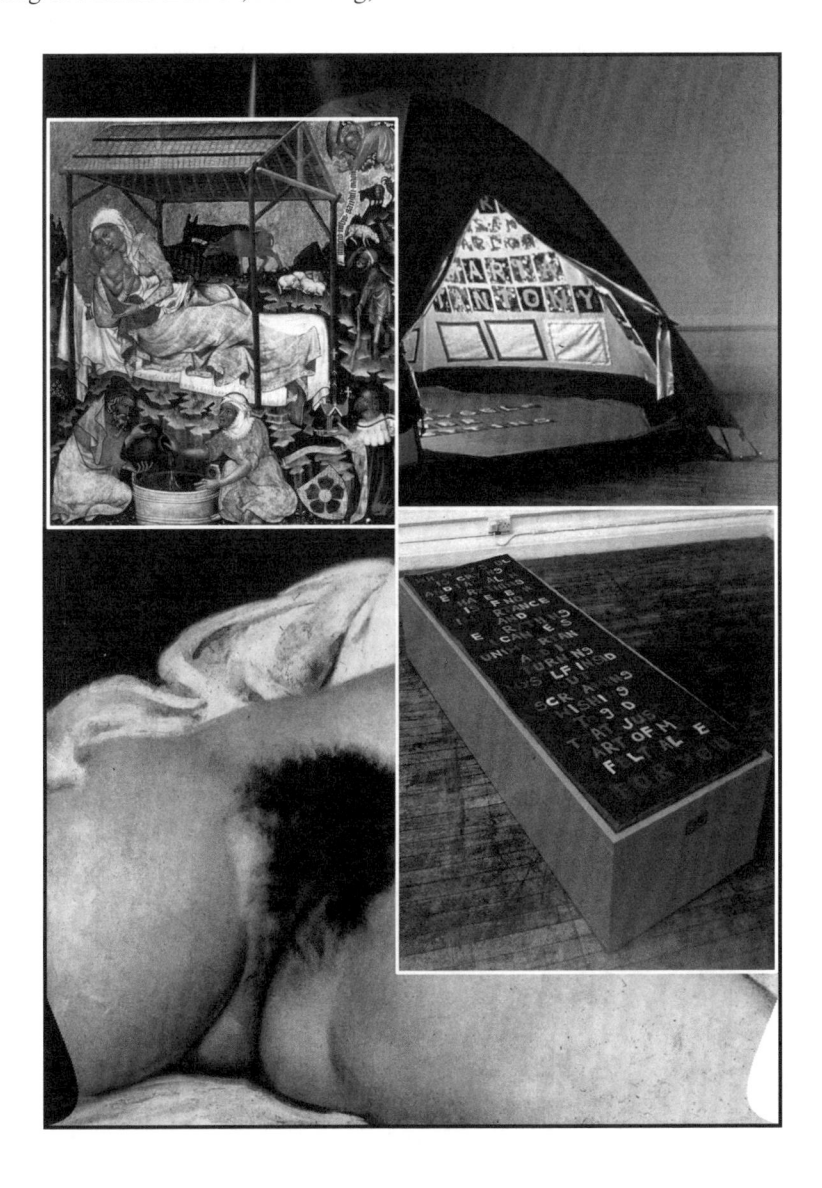

The "Girl with a pearl earring" (around 1665) – almost every single person in Western Europe knows this masterpiece by Jan Vermeer. Balthus' "Dreaming Therèse" (1938) is the alternative of our time. The crucifixion is more and more hardly visible. Death 'gets lost' in the image – an excuse. The image is accusation and wrathful claim.

Slogan 6: "... *the aim of the image is to kill the image*" (Didi-Huberman, 2000:229)
And the art therapeutic results? Unwillingly / unknowingly / *unconsciously* they recreate the change between the two 'eras'. The "era of art" could only unfold through the "killing of the image" (Didi-Hubermann, 2000).
What is given away within mysterious or enigmatic 'picture puzzles' still remains with the images, until finally 'painting a pretty picture' becomes a useless exercise. The 'cross'-ing out of the image is initially prevented by art. Does being ill not actually deserve the 'demythologising' of the comforting images?
Art therapy is moving between faking as changing that which underlies any appearance so that it looks like being real *and* hiding the narcissistic parts in how

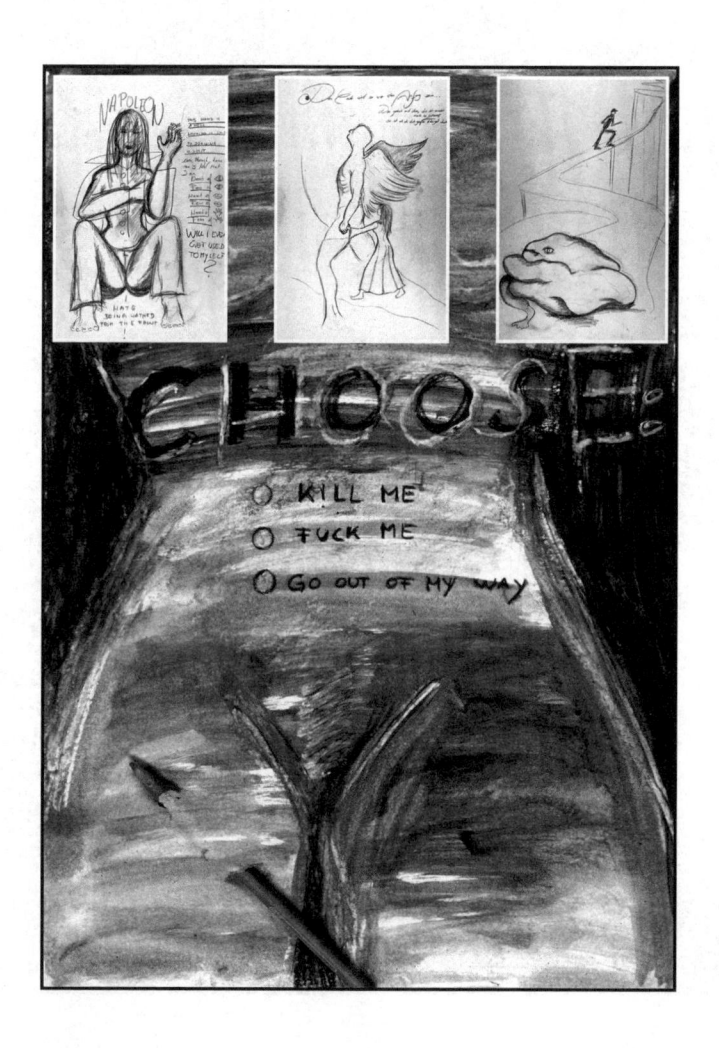

the corresponding artwork has become into being. In so far the nature of art therapy is symptomatic for itself. The problem is that symptoms can neither be hidden nor be seen. Art therapy is suggesting hypnotically as if symptoms could be recognized within pictures. One cannot see anything through pictures. You never see more as a picture; you see objects within a picture, but the object you see is not the object. (You can see it in every picture of Rene Magritte.)

What this article wants to contribute to the problems of art therapy – namely more in the light of the collages and less on the basis of scientific words (therefore the play with the slogans and the pictures) – , is to show that art therapy would have the wrong idea of itself were it to give the impression as if painting and looking at pictures would be simply salutary. The circumstances are more difficult to understand. The complexity can be partially cleared up – in addition to the psycho-analytic answers going through the matters which need thinking about the image, about that what can be imagined, about imagery, about the power of imagination – by the latest results of art history which have a lot in common with art therapy. The names which stand out in this connection – as Hans Belting (2001) and Georges Didi-Huberman (2000) were saying.

In their beginnings, pictures were attempting to be in agreement with death. They had to bring the dead to life in a metaphoric sense. Later on, the salvation of the dead has brought out the 'picture maker' as an artist. On the whole, he replaced the subject of the dead with the subject of the mother of God as the *Immaculata*. The subject of death has been exchanged for the subject of the woman. The point is whether this symptomatologogy of the picture within its mechanisms has remained the impetus of making pictures. That iconoclastic moment will be the sticking point of art therapy. As far as suffering and diseases go, art therapeutic experience has to take the picture's veil off.

References:

Belting, H. (1990). *Bild und Kunst*. München: Beck Verlag
Belting, H. (2001). *Bild-Anthropologie*. München: Wilhelm Fink
Didi-Huberman, G. (2000). *Vor einem Bild*. München, Wien: Carl Hanser
Kandinsky: (1912) (1952). *The Inner Sound*, In Ueber das Geistige in der Kunst. Bern: Benteli
Mayr, D.F. (1999). *Der Riß der Geschlechter. Madonna. Der Diskurs. Die Hysterie. Und Hölderlin.* Wien: Passagen
Panofsky, E. (1980). *Studien zur Ikonologie*. Köln: DuMont
Rech, P. (1997). *umgekehrt. Bilder und Unbewußtes*. Wien: Passagen
Werke Goethes, I, (1998). *Goethe to Zelter on the 11.12.1831*, Darmstadt: Wissenschaftliche Buchgesellschaft

layout of the collages: Niklas Zimmer
translation into English: Niklas Zimmer

III

PRACTITIONER RESEARCH AND ASSESSMENT OF PRACTICE

MARTIN D. COPE

INTRODUCING A NEW METHOD OF ARTS-BASED THERAPEUTIC RESEARCH: NARRATIVE PHENOMENOLOGICAL ANALYSIS

This paper summarises the research conducted by the author as part of his MA 'Upgrade' in Dramatherapy at the University of Plymouth, U.K. (Cope, 2005).

The Research Setting
The research was conducted within a residential Therapeutic Community. It housed twenty-four young people, aged 10-16 years, with general emotional and behavioural difficulties. These young people manifested elements of dysfunction such as learning difficulties, developmental delay, attention deficit hyperactivity disorder, autism spectrum disorders, post-traumatic stress and personality disorder. Often their histories involved aspects of dysfunctional families and abuse: emotional, physical, sexual and neglect. Issues of separation, abandonment and loss predominated. The author, and therapist/researcher of the study, had pioneered and developed weekly individual and group dramatherapy within the community for a number of years. The dramatherapy approach had similarities to the non-directive play therapy of Axline (1947). Dramatherapy sessions were voluntary and client-centred (Rogers, 1951). This placed the onus of personal change and development on the individual's latent internal power to heal him/herself (Bannister, 1997: 9-12).

Aim
The research aim was to empower clients thereby enabling them to provide their own perspectives on their experiences of individual dramatherapy to date.

Focus
There has been much debate concerning the efficacy in studying the creative arts therapies. Brenda Meldrum stated:

> "The notion that therapy is an art form whose creativity is lost if too closely examined has in the past led to the resistance of clinicians to empirical study." (Meldrum, 1999: 179).

Cope (2005) drew dramatherapy practice and research together. The author became a reflexive researcher. Thus, he placed his professional self in his research, just as he would do in his dramatherapy practice (Etherington, 2004). The study adopted a client-centred perspective to research. It followed suggestions (Aigen, 1993; Grainger, 1999; Meldrum, 1999; Ansdell & Pavlicevic, 2001; Wilkins, 2001) and presented an 'arts-based' research methodology that embraced the creative process of dramatherapy.

Philosophical Background

The artistic, creative and client-centred approach to research favoured an underlying narrative philosophy. This developed as the study progressed. In recent years, there have been many therapeutic disciplines that have adopted a narrative approach to their practice and theory. Most have been influenced by the pioneering work of Michael White and David Epston (1990). They conceptualised therapy as a process of storying or re-storying one's existence when the predominant story frame denied lived experience.

Unfortunately, narrative approaches to therapy have either used the terms 'narrative' and 'story' synonymously, or have lacked clear definitions. Martin McQuillan (2000: 2) implied that narratives are potentially everywhere and in everything. However, McQuillan also stated that, "the definition of the term 'narrative' is unstable and still 'up for grabs' (2000: 323)." The following are 'working definitions' that were developed by the author through the course of the research:

Narrative: *"The basic symbolic units of existential meaning."*

Narrativisation: *"The construction or reformulation of symbolic categories of narrative meaning."*

Story: *"An amalgamation of numerous narrativised symbols into a containing, yet fluid, structure."*

Dramatherapy: *"A client-led dramatic, creative and reflective exploration of personal and social narrative-symbolic structure to promote insight and integration."*

Identity: *"One's internal subjective sense of self."*

Personality: *"One's external embodiment of self."*

These definitions have been influenced by symbolic interactionist and social constructionist ideology (Mead, 1934; McNamee & Gergen, 1992; Burr, 1995; Denzin, 1995). Symbolic Interactionism in its simplest form, describes humanity as a 'dynamic interaction' via a vast array of human-made symbols and their related meanings. It is argued within this paper that 'narrative' symbolism and meaning dominates social existence, be it reality or fantasy. Furthermore, narrative symbols, meanings and categories are socially constructed in the very act of living as social beings. This leads to the construction of narrative realities, identities and personalities.

Narrative is universal. We may chose to construct ourselves from any of the narrative stimuli we receive everyday; for example, money, television, billboards, house size, role models, language, conversation, fashion, transport or commercial goods like perfume and make-up. All have a potential to shape and re-shape our lives, personalities, identities and cultures: a potential for narrativisation.

Donald Spence (1982) differentiated between historical truth and narrative truth.

Historical truth may refer to experience in the moment whereas narrative truth is the representation of the historical truth in one's recollections, stories, re-enactments, identity and personality. Narrative truth manifests a transformed version of the historical truth, a reduction, categorisation, elaboration and/or fabrication. It may be achieved via the process of narrativisation. Experiential meaning must always enter the realm of narrative truth as soon as the moment has passed.

A narrative approach to individual dramatherapy could be conceptualised as a client-led narrative-symbolic exploration within the 'potential space' of client and therapist (Winnicott, 1971; Bannister, 2003). Clients offer narrative-symbolic aspects of themselves and their lives through the context of their play and creativity. Clients reconnect to themselves by narrativising, or re-storying, their existence. They develop narrative truth that does not deny lived experience but also offers appropriate distance to move on from traumatic events.

The narrative approach to the author's arts-based dramatherapy research may be conceptualised in the same way. The only difference is that participants were creatively re-storying their experience of individual dramatherapy to closer approximate lived experience. This added a therapeutic element to the research which was particularly relevant given the study's setting within a therapeutic community.

Methodology

There are many approaches to narrative analysis within the research literature (Reissman, 1993; Josselson, Lieblich & McAdams, 2003; Angus & McLeod, 2004). Unfortunately, most methods have concentrated on participant verbal narration and have missed the equally important symbolic representations of narratives within non-verbal communications, gestures, facial expressions, emotional tone and imagery etc.

The new method of arts-based therapeutic research introduced in this paper is called Narrative Phenomenological Analysis. The approach adds a narrative conceptualisation and methodology to the rigour and prescription of Clark Moustakas' (1994) procedure for Transcendental Phenomenological Analysis. Moustakas' philosophy reflects qualitative, constructivist, postmodernist thought (Creswell, 1998). He mirrors concepts of 'content' and 'process' (Yalom, 1995: 129-188) which are frequently used in creative arts therapies, and the concepts of 'symbol' and 'meaning' inherent to symbolic interactionism. Moustakas (1994) described noematic and noetic dimensions of phenomena. For Moustakas, noematic referred to the texture of existence, the 'what', 'when' and 'where'. Noetic encompassed the structure, the 'how' and 'why'. Thus, the following can be seen as potentially synonymous with each other:

1. Noematic – texture – symbol – content and;
2. Noetic – structure – meaning – process.

Moustakas' analytical procedure effectively reduces the content and process of statements provided within participant interviews. Similar inter-subject themes are formed into an 'essential structure' that describes the essence of the experience of a phenomenon. Narrative adaptations frame research within narrative-symbolic interaction and permit the inclusion of non-verbal, contextual data for analysis. Furthermore, the phenomenological 'essence' of participant experience, or historical truth, may be re-conceptualised as a form of narrative truth.

Procedure

The study adopted detailed ethical procedures and sensitive recruitment. Informed consent was required from the participant, their legal guardian and from the principal of the therapeutic community. All ten individual dramatherapy clients volunteered to take part in the study. This 'purposeful' sample (Creswell, 1998: 62) comprised seven boys and three girls aged eleven to sixteen. The respective gender ratio within the therapeutic community was three boys to one girl. Participants were at different chronological stages of dramatherapy and manifested different needs and developmental levels. Consequently, they were all using the dramatherapy space in very different ways. The mixed group was deemed supportive to the research given the phenomenological aim to identify experiences common to all participants.

Participants chose when to conduct the research. This was termed the 'study session'. Pre-established boundaries were maintained by the behavioural contracts that were drafted by each client in their first dramatherapy session. The study session lasted up to 45 minutes for each participant. The location was the drama studio. This was where the majority of dramatherapy took place and there was a tremendous choice of creative materials for clients to choose from. These spanned the disciplines of drama, music, movement, art, play and circus skills. Maximisation of client choice, especially in the form of expression, is one of the first steps to client self-empowerment and regeneration (Bannister, 2003).

At the time of research all dramatherapy sessions were video recorded for the safety of client and therapist. The study sessions were also video recorded with the secondary purpose of providing contextual, non-verbal data. Stringent policies and procedures surrounded this additional use of the videotapes within the study.

When the participant felt ready to engage in the study session, both parties were fitted with discrete radio microphones with a cordless link to a four-track recording system. This system maximised audio-recording quality, was sensitive to subtle verbalisations, permitted freedom of movement, and playback speed could be varied.

The study session was conducted as an unstructured 'open' narrative interview (Robson, 1993: 231; Moustakas, 1994: 114-115; Mattingley & Lawlor, 2000). The interview schedule contained one overarching question posed by the therapist/ researcher: "What have been your experiences so far of the dramatherapy sessions?" Simple language was used for some participants depending on individual needs and development level in order for them to fully understand the task. All participants were given the opportunity to respond creatively, artistically and/or verbally.

Therapeutic practice and research were drawn together. The only difference between the study session and a typical dramatherapy session lay in the focus.

Participants were exploring their specific experience of individual dramatherapy within the study session. They did this in the same creative and reflective way as they would explore their life experiences during dramatherapy sessions.

The interviewing technique used within the study session mirrored the author's professional client-centred approach to dramatherapy. Anderson and Goolishian (1992) succinctly described the approach. Clients are the experts of their own lives and experiences and the therapist consequently comes from a place of 'not-knowing'. The therapist adopts a Socratic style of interaction and questioning. This follows the philosophy of Socrates and person-centred therapy. A position of ignorance is assumed from the therapist in order to empower clients to explore and display self-generated knowledge. This is opposed to the pedagogic style of 'teaching', or the 'rhetorical' style of persuading or impressing, from the therapist's point of view (Anderson and Goolishian, 1992).

Research participants 'directed' their artistic, creative and verbal responses. However, it is acknowledged that the therapist/researcher's own narrative person situated within an established relationship with the participants will shape his clients' constructions. The interactive phenomenon of the therapeutic space has thus been described by some as a process of co-construction of experience and meaning (McNamee & Gergen, 1992; Cattanach, 1999, 2001). However, within a client-centred, Socratic perspective, clients are encouraged to **lead** the construction. Therefore, the experiential creative aspect of the study session symbolised client search for, and representation of, meaning. The reflective aspect enhanced cognitive structuring of meaning into knowledge.

Central to this art of interviewing is the preservation of dramatic and metaphoric parameters forged by participants within the study sessions. This ensured that the participant and the researcher maintained appropriate distance from material with the potential for client re-traumatisation (Bannister, 2003).

The client-centred, Socratic form of interviewing is a style based upon years of experiential training and professional practice in facilitating the generation of client insight and re-connection to self. In this respect, creative arts therapists need not be 'trainee' researchers. They have trained for years and are experts in this style of reflexive interviewing.

Prior to de-briefing, respondents also had an opportunity to critically reflect upon the study session itself. Dramatherapy clients were therefore significantly empowered to express their own perspective on the dramatherapeutic process and on the research methods used to approach their experiences of that process. Participants reported positive experiences of the study sessions. However, some said that it was not an easy process to think, reflect or feel.

Assumptions

As is tradition within phenomenological analysis, the therapist/researcher created his 'epoche' prior to conducting the study sessions. This was in order to suspend therapist preconceptions that may impose an 'a priori' hypothesis upon client expression of experience (Moustakas, 1994: 85-90; Creswell, 1998: 52). It was assumed that, despite individual differences, there is an 'essential structure' to the narrative truth of client experience of individual dramatherapy. Pre-judgements and previous interpretations were set aside in order to assume a position of ignorance of this structure. A client-centred, Socratic style of interviewing was adopted in order to maintain the 'bracketing' of the research aim.

Data Analysis
Audio and visual data were recorded onto A3 'landscape' data templates (Figure 1).

Participant:

CONTENT (data)			PROCESS (interpretation)		
No.	Trancscription	Context	Tone	Imagery	Theme

Figure 1: A3 'landscape' data template (reduced size).

These templates produced a formula of texture and structure, of symbol and meaning, of content and process. 'Content' is split into 'transcription' (audio data) and 'context' (corresponding video data). All expressions from both participant and researcher were recorded in this way. This data was augmented with reference to memos and field notes written during and after the study session by the therapist/researcher. The 'process' or interpretation section is in three parts: tone, imagery and themes. Narrative personality psychologist Dan P. McAdams (1993) suggested these three categories to direct lines of interpretation when analysing personal narratives. McAdams related the terms to one's developmental socialisation. Crossley (2000) directly illustrated a narrative analysis method using these terms for one's personal narrative.

Cope (2005) further extended McAdams' technique. The 'tone' represented the feel or emotional content portrayed by the participant within the study session. The 'imagery' referred to images represented, spoken or embodied within the dramatherapy space. Imagery also referred to the images and pictures that spontaneously arose in the therapist/researcher's mind when interacting with the participants. The 'themes' represented the initial strands of meaning that developed from the transcript, contextual data, tone and imagery. This was prior to the formation of more overarching intra-client and inter-client themes. Attention to tone, imagery and themes at this stage, facilitated a deeper analysis of narrative-symbolic interaction. Also, the therapist/researcher has consistently worked with these aspects during dramatherapy practice and in reflection.

Moustakas' (1994) procedure of transcendental phenomenological reduction was applied to the data templates for each participant. This procedure was expanded to include all relevant client expressions rather than focusing purely on significant participant statements. Every expression relevant to the experience was listed (Horizonalisation) and formulated into non-repetitive, non-overlapping expressions (Invariant Constituents). Invariant Constituents were clustered and thematised. Invariant constituents and themes were referred back to the data templates to check for explicit expression or compatibility. This process validated the invariant constituents and themes. Only valid invariant constituents and themes were retained.

Validated invariant constituents and themes were used to construct individual textural and structural, content and process, descriptions. Verbatim and contextual examples from the templates were included. A variety of structural interpretations were formed by what Moustakas termed 'imaginative variation'. Dominant interpretations were then thematised. Every thematic paragraph of content was followed by an indented paragraph of process. The reader was consequently encouraged to judge for themselves the relationship between content and process for each theme and for each participant within the study.

The ten individual textural-structural descriptions illustrated the diversity between clients and their deeper search for meaning as the study session progressed. All individual descriptions were then reduced to form a composite textural and structural description which blended content and process. Individual invariant constituents and themes were included in this composite description. This retained the narrative-symbolic foundation of the study sessions and preserved respondent idiosyncrasy. It also displayed the interpretative steps taken. Finally, the composite description was reduced to form the 'essential structure' to the narrative truth of client experience of individual dramatherapy.

Trustworthiness

A complete set of verification procedures specific to the subjective nature of the qualitative piece of research were built into the design (Lincoln and Guba, 1985; Krefting, 1991; Creswell, 1998). The therapist/researcher included an autobiographical account and an anonymous description of the setting and mixed sample. Description of the research conditions informed the 'transferability' of the findings to other therapeutic contexts.

The therapist / researcher engaged in on-going external professional supervision and tutorship throughout the research process. These peers maintained honesty in his approach. They critiqued potential sources of researcher bias: method, interpretation, preconception and hidden motivation. Creswell terms this 'peer review or debriefing' or 'devil's advocate' (1998: 202). This adds 'credibility' to reflexive research, and indeed practice.

Further credibility came from the researcher's professional use, and documentation, of the Socratic interviewing technique. Similarly, the arts-approach to research, consistent with the artistic process of therapy, may have added 'dependability' verification. Wilkins has stated that research has intrinsic validity when "it is concerned with people's perceptions, the knowledge they create through doing, not with 'objective' reality (2001: 47).

Participants checked their individual textural-structural descriptions for credibility and accuracy and the descriptions were adjusted accordingly. Creswell termed this 'member-checking' (1998: 202). The clear 'audit trail' (Robson, 1993: 406) permitted an independent auditor to assess methodology, interpretation and product. Only similar interpretations between researcher and auditor were retained. This ensured interrater consistency and reliability. These procedures added objectivity, or 'confirmability', to the reflexive research (Creswell, 1998: 193-218).

Participants may have expressed what they thought the therapist/researcher wanted from them: a response to social pressure (Krefting, 1991; Robson, 1993). Procedures from dramatherapy practice were built into the design of the study to counter this possibility. Most have already been outlined such as the intrinsic validity of creative action, a Socratic interviewing technique and 'peer review or debriefing'. The therapist/researcher was mindful of client and personal process. He encouraged participants to qualify their expressions and strived for a balanced respondent critique. Therefore, consistent with dramatherapy practice, research clients were encouraged to lead the co-construction of meaning.

Results

All ten participants expressed different levels of creative, artistic, metaphoric and verbal symbolism within the study sessions. The variety of client explorations spanned: drama, character and role, costume, dance, sword-fighting, sand tray, modelling clay, literature, music, singing, rhythm, imagery, feelings and cognitions (Cope, 2005). Most participants used a similar artistic medium to that favoured within their past dramatherapy sessions. Some examples are cited here.

In response to the study session question, Tanya reflected upon on-going dramatherapy work. She had spent a number of sessions building an image with modelling clay to represent her life and feelings. Tanya said, "It was hard to like focus on how my anger was like working and that ... it has helped me loads like dealing with emotions and that." Tanya created a flower out of modelling clay to symbolise her experiences of dramatherapy. This is how she described her creation:

> "The colour red represents anger (petals), purple is emotions (stamen), pink happiness (stalk), green is the meadow (base) ... well it's like all step-by-step ... well you have to have grass first, and then the stalk ... and then you have to have the middle bit and then the petals ... yeh step-by-step ... actually, I've actually made the red as ... as if it was on the ground ... it would actually look like fire probably."

The flower appeared to represent Tanya's difficult dramatherapy journey into her internal emotional state. There is a sense of growth, of understanding layers of feeling. There is also a twist. If the petals, "like fire", were on the ground a powerful and destructive inverted image materialised. Tanya's anger (petals, fire) had engulfed her emotions (stamen) and begun to destroy her happiness (stalk), with a potential to even burn her foundations (meadow).

John also communicated his experience of dramatherapy as an emotional voyage.

He used the love of his life, music, as his study session medium. John directed the session. He narrated his experiences through song and rhythm accompanied by the therapist/researcher on the keyboard mirroring style and tone. This musical interaction was typical of John's dramatherapy to date. John sang about his initial dramatherapy sessions:

> "Number one, number one, number one, number one would be like, would be like, the feelings that you can't really give out ... you have to think, you have to look, you have to look at yourself and think ... number one wouldn't be very feelings, number two would just be getting in the feelings ..."

John reported the remainder of the dramatherapy sessions to be "definitely in the feelings." John went on to sing about the range of emotions, "bad feelings, good feelings, exciting feelings, hyper feelings, all types of feelings," that he had felt, represented and understood through music during dramatherapy.

Tim used his study session as a typical dramatherapy session for him. He spontaneously directed a powerful dramatic interaction. Vivid gruesome images materialised e.g. Tim's character hurled the severed heads of children towards his attackers. Tim hummed the pop song, 'Left Outside Alone' by Anastasia. The drama provided a window into, or demonstration of, Tim's dramatherapy experience. He used metaphor to explore, with safety and containment, his abandoned 'severed' identity and personality.

Alternatively, Carl used less distance and designed a piece of drama to precisely reflect the quality of his experience of dramatherapy as "helpful." The therapist / researcher was placed in the role of a victim of violence, Frederick. Carl stated that this character represented him when he "goes downhill". Carl played a doctor to represent his experiences of his therapist. Thus Carl maximised the scene's potential to generate empathy. Carl also played characters to symbolise significant people in his life. None of the characters could save Frederick from a lonely, desperate and painful place. However, the doctor knelt down on a level with Frederick. He offered comfort and support during the bearing of pain, listened and called the ambulance. The doctor's attention was enough to ensure Frederick's survival.

Carl verbalised his appreciation of his therapist's undivided attention. Carl had experienced dramatherapy as sacrosanct and helpful. He discovered ways of coping with and learning about self, others and relationships. Carl was learning to be active in his own survival.

Kate however, had not experienced dramatherapy as sacrosanct. At the time the drama studio was used for more than dramatherapy by the community. Unbeknown to the therapist, Kate's favourite dress, used regularly in dramatherapy, had been destroyed by one of her peers. During her study session she bravely communicated her anger and sense of injustice. This needed to be acknowledged. Kate then instigated a pretend but forceful sword-fight with the therapist/researcher. This powerful interaction symbolised her anger and inferential 'en garde' attitude.

Many clients identified dramatherapy as a place to transform their social-emotional functioning. They discovered that their destructive, anti-social or dysfunctional behaviours were often related to experiencing difficult feelings. Dramatherapy offered an opportunity to contain difficult feelings and discover more creative, constructive, functional and pro-social forms of expression. Clients developed their identities and personalities in this way. John and Phillip both constructed an image of their development within their study sessions.

John moved from music into character. He created a sinister, dark and frightening role called the 'Lonely Ghost'. He said in a haunting voice:

"You don't know I'm here Martin ... you can't see me 'cos I'm invisible ... now you look around, I'd run, I am the ghost of the lonely, to come and KILL YOU."

John delicately described how the Lonely Ghost represented his isolation and loneliness within the therapeutic community. John said the following about his experience of dramatherapy: "It helps me communicate with people but it doesn't help me like have conversations." John had used dramatherapy to re-connect to the self and to life. His search for the truth led to an understanding of his position within a desperate place. It was hard but real for John and he wanted to move on. Phillip had often used modelling clay to symbolically craft his world around the dramatherapy space. He used a large part of his study session to verbally reflect upon how dramatherapy had allowed him to actively overcome many personal and social fears. Throughout his discussion, Phillip inadvertently crafted his 'Mega Man' out of modelling clay. He presented Mega Man as an image to represent how his identity and personality had developed. Phillip said:

"Yeh! This, is Mega Man ... I wanna keep it ... it's got a bit of X (Tai-kwon-do instructor) ... it's got a bit of confusion ... it's got a bit of, bright colour, like stands out ... it's got a round body, like sphere body, perfect ... a bit of, not sure what, you know like hanging about, like you know not happening much ... nice big bold head and collar thing, stands out strong ... it's got a bit of coolness, it's brilliant, and then bright pink, reminds me of my girlfriend ... that darker like purpley-red – Christmas ... the bright yellow standing out like 'look at me' ... bold colour on head, tough, and side ... like knows what to expect, getting hit by a thousand waves at the same time ... body, sphere, perfect, round ... just perfect, that thing on the back is confusion, not really knowing where to go ... he can fly."

Phillip explained how he had used dramatherapy to transform a debilitating fear of crowds. He had explored and contained difficult feelings, built self-confidence and become much less marginalised. Mega-Man symbolised Phillip's personal and social development as an integrative transformation of identity and personality.

These examples give a flavour of the diversity of narrative expression within the study sessions. They contributed towards the following 'essential structure' to the narrative truth of client experience of individual dramatherapy. Clients have experienced the growth of a largely positive and communicative therapeutic relationship. They have felt heard, important, validated, supported, empowered, confident, safe, secure, comforted, equal and the expert on themselves. However, clients experienced dissatisfaction, anger and a lack of trust when dramatherapy was not sacrosanct in time and space. Clients experienced positive 'time-out' from everyday life, a space for catharsis and feeling. Clients have explored the symbolic world through creative art and language. They have used this symbolism to express themselves (externalisation), especially emotions, and to represent the context of their lives (sociograms). Clients developed insight into self, others and relationships. Their introspective, reflective and social skills evolved and began to transform dysfunctional ways of being. Consequently, clients experienced dramatherapy as a method to move towards integration, to develop social-emotional functioning, identity and personality.

Discussion

These specific clients have worked within a predominately containing, supportive and safe therapeutic relationship. They led an often difficult process of being and reflecting and of coming to terms with abandonment and loss. Clients began to integrate feelings, thoughts and behaviours within the context of their lives. This added support to Robert Landy's drama of engagement and separation (1992) and theory of distancing (1983). Some participants, e.g. John, have reported a cognitive process of understanding their feelings and related behaviours within individual dramatherapy. Consequently they may have reconnected to the self and gained a form of control, of thought over being. Thus beginning a process of transformation from a previously under-distanced, 'unintegrated personality' (Winnicott, 1971). Conversely, certain clients, e.g. Phillip, appear to have experienced individual dramatherapy as a safe validating place to 'be' and to feel. This again shows a reconnection to self. These clients began to transform potential processes of repression or dissociation and a related over-distanced, unintegrated state. It is possible that individual dramatherapy allowed clients to work towards an optimum balance, or integration, of feelings, thoughts and behaviours, of social-emotional functioning, of identity and personality.

The author's dramatherapy practice and arts-based research could both be described in narrative philosophical terms. Clients/participants led a creative and reflective exploration of the narrative-symbolic units and categories of personal and social meaning. This process empowered the clients/participants to construct or reformulate symbolic categories of narrative meaning: a process of narrativisation, of re-storying their experiences. Clients/participants had begun to construct a form of narrative truth that was closer to lived experience, yet sufficiently distanced to allow them to move on from traumatic events. Clients/participants were integrating their narrative personalities and identities.

There were a number of limitations to the study. Findings were temporally, spatially and inter-personally specific. Some researcher bias was accepted as an aspect of subjectivity. This rendered the 'epoche' process only partially pure. However it was argued that bias was reduced, as in dramatherapy practice, by the measures adopted to address trustworthiness.

The main limitations to this study are housed within the dualism of qualitative and quantitative philosophical debate. One can only be quantitative and qualitative as the diversity and balance of nature dictates. Landy's drama of engagement and separation illuminates the subjective versus objective battleground that has arisen over the years. 'To be or not to be', 'fantasy or reality', neotic versus noematic', identity and personality, to be reflexive, to hold ambivalence of feeling. Extremities epitomise the need for balance in life between the subjective-qualitative and objective-quantitative aspects of narrative-symbolic existence. Clients search for balance between the subjective and objective nature to their lives on their journeys towards integration. Creative arts therapists seek balance between subjectivity and objectivity within their reflexive practice. Arts-based therapeutic person-centred research strives for the same equilibrium in order to build insight into, and evaluate, therapeutic practice.

It would be interesting to follow-up this research with a longitudinal study. The same subjects could be approached at various intervals after termination of individual dramatherapy. The author could then investigate chronological narrativisation: whether client narrative truth of individual dramatherapy changed over time? Would the 'essential structure' of reflective perception survive chronologically?

This paper has introduced a method, and shown the benefits, of drawing together dramatherapy practice and research. There are also important implications for dramatherapy theory, education and communication. The philosophical and methodological underpinnings to this research may direct further academic pursuit which could build understanding of the creative arts therapies. – An understanding that, when grounded within person-centred research, is **largely based upon client perspective**.

References

Aigen, K. (1993). *The Music Therapist as Qualitative Researcher.* Music Therapy, 12, 16-39

Anderson, H. & Goolishian, H. (1992). 'The Client is the Expert', in S. McNamee and J. Gergen (eds), *Therapy as Social Construction.* London: Sage

Andsell, G & Pavlicevic (2001). *Beginning Research in the Arts Therapies.* London: Jessica Kingsley

Angus, L.E. & McCleod, J. (2004).*The Handbook of Narrative and Psychotherapy: Practice, Theory and Research.* London: Sage.

Axline, V.M. (1947). *Play Therapy.* New York: Ballantine Books

Bannister, A. (1997). *The Healing Drama.* London: Free Association Books

Bannister, A. (2003). *Creative Therapies with Traumatized Children.* London: Jessica Kingsley

Burr, V. (1995. *An Introduction to Social Constructionism.* London: Routledge

Cattanach, A. (1999). 'Co-construction in Play Therapy', in A. Cattacnach (ed), *Process in the Arts Therapies.* London: Jessica Kingsley

Cattanach, A. (2001). 'Practitioners as Researchers', in L. Kossolapow, S. Scoble & D. Waller (eds), *Arts – Therapies – Communication.* London: Transaction Publishers

Cope, M. D. (2005). *Approaching Client Experience of Individual Dramatherapy: A Narrative Phenomenological Analysis.* Submitted to the University of Plymouth (UK) as a dissertation towards the degree of Master of Arts by advanced study in Dramatherapy. Plymouth University Library, Unpublished

Creswell, J.W. (1998). *Qualitative Enquiry and Research Design.* London: Sage

Crossley, M.L. (2000). *Introducing Narrative Psychology.* Buckingham: Open University Press.

Denzin, N. (1995). "Symbolic Interactionism', in J.A. Smith, R. Harre and L.Van Langenhove (eds), *Rethinking Psychology.* London: Sage

Etherington, K. (2004). *Becoming a Reflexive Researcher.* London: Jessica Kingsley

Grainger, R (1999). *Researching the Arts Therapies.* London: Jessica Kingsley.

Josselson, R. Lieblich, D. and McAdams, D.P. (2003). *Up Close and Personal: The Teaching and Learning of Narrative Research.* Washington: American Psychological Association

Krefting, L. (1991). *Rigour in Qualitative Research: The Assessment of Trustworthiness.* American Journal of Occupational Therapy, 45 (3), 214-222

Landy, R.J. (1983). *The use of Distancing in Dramatherapy.* The Arts in Psychotherapy, 10, 175-185.

Landy, R.J. (1992). *The Dramatherapy Role Method.* Journal of the British Association of Dramatherapists, 14.

Lincoln, Y.S. & Guba, E.G. (1985). *Naturalistic Inquiry.* Beverly Hills, CA: Sage.

McAdams, D. (1993). *The Stories We Live By: Personal Myths and the making of the self.* New York: Morrow

McNamee, S. & Gergen, K.J. (1992). *Therapy as Social Construction.* London: Sage

McQuillan, M. (2000). *The Narrative Reader.* London: Routledge

Mattingley, C. & Lawlor, M. (2000). *Learning from Stories: Narrative Interviewing in Cross-Cultural Research.* Scandinavian Journal of Occupational Therapy, 7, 4-14.

Mead, G.H. (1934). *Mind, Self, and Society.* Chicago: University of Chicago Press.

Meldrum, B. (1999). 'Research in the Arts Therapies', in A. Cattanach (ed), *Process in the Arts Therapies.* London: Jessica Kingsley.

Moustakas, C. (1994). *Phenomenological Research Methods.* London: Sage

Riessman, C.K. (1993). *Narrative Analysis.* London: Sage

Robson, C. (1993). *Real World Research.* Oxford: Blackwell

Rogers, C. R. (1951). *Client-Centered Therapy.* London: Constable & Co.

Spence, D. (1982). *Narrative Truth and Historical Truth.* London: WW Norton & Co.

White, M. & Epston, D. (1990). *Narrative Means to Therapeutic Ends.* Adelaide: Dulwich Centre

Wilkins, P (2001). 'Creative Approaches to Research', in L. Kossolapow, S. Scoble & D. Waller (eds), *Arts – Therapies – Communication.* London: Transaction Publishers

Winnicott, D.W. (1971). *Playing and Reality.* London: Tavistock.

Yalom, I.D. (1995). *The Theory and Practice of Group Psychotherapy*. New York: Basic Books.

LAMBROS YOTIS

ARISTOTLE'S POETICS IN DRAMATHERAPY ASSESSMENT AND EVALUATION

Introduction

Different cultural frameworks in Drama and in Theatre have assigned various meanings to the notion of "performance", both as an individual experience and as a group phenomenon, within dramatherapy theory. Contemporary Dramatherapy is usually concerned with the process of change in each client's individual performance within a closed group therapy framework (Jennings, 1994). Furthermore, individual one-to-one Dramatherapy for both adults and children has also been developed by a number of practitioners (Jenkyns 1996, Cattanach 1999). In addition to the above models of work, a performance created by a dramatherapy group for an invited audience has often been used as a therapeutic tool, its aim being to include within the dramatherapy outcomes the benefits of a public theatre performance, thus forming a particular method of work within dramatherapy practice (Johnson 1980, Emunah 1994).

Inasmuch as the performance itself is created through a dramatherapy process, this therapeutic practice becomes both a special form of theatre performance and of therapeutic intervention. In reference to this specific therapeutic intervention within the spectrum of psychotherapies, the term "Dramatherapy Performance" has to be defined. Such a therapeutic use of performance may vary each time according to the aims, process and practice of work in relation to the specific client group. However, there are certain common processes for this therapeutic approach, regardless of the clients' particular psychopathology.

Within a maturation process of a dramatherapy group, the therapist often confronts the demand of the group members for a performance. This usually occurs when the cohesion of the group, the clients' ego strength and the overall creativity within the group have reached a point which allows for further transformation of the therapeutic practice into a social event. The formulation of a therapeutic project that includes a performance in front of an invited audience can be proposed either by the Dramatherapist or by the group members. This event aims at confirming the clients' individual changes and achievements through sharing with and gratification of non-group members.

I would define **"Dramatherapy Performance"** as a performance event which is created by and contained within a therapeutic process and which is based on the group members' personal material that is evoked, worked through, reconstructed, combined and projected into a dramatic form in order to be presented to an invited audience.

The above definition implies that a "Dramatherapy Performance":

- Has a healing intention;
- Includes therapeutic work towards a final product to be witnessed by an audience of invited non-group members;

- Contains only those parts of the group members' personal material that are worked through therapeutically and are ready to be exposed;
- Connects both the process and the final product to the group members' lives;
- Is differentiated from theatrical and "para-theatrical" performances, the intrinsic healing quality of which is not subject to validation.

This model of therapeutic work has been particularly used with clients with schizophrenia, even if at first it was not defined as a model of Dramatherapy. Eljine and Evreinov, whose early work on therapeutic performance with patients in asylums in the Soviet Union at the beginning of the 20th century, can be considered as pioneers in this field (Jones, 1996). Another model of therapeutic performances via the production of ancient Greek Tragedies in psychiatric hospitals was practised in Greece in the 1960's (Lyketsos, 1980). These were stage-directed by psychiatrists with a psychoanalytic orientation who valued the "catharsis" produced by the ancient Greek Tragedies as a therapeutic factor for the patients. Further work concerning therapeutic performance in Dramatherapy has been described by a number of practitioners via theatrical, para-theatrical and ritual perspectives (Bielanska et al, 1991, Grainger, 1999, Landy, 1995, Mitchell, 1992). Most of these practitioners have stressed the importance of the factor of structure and containment to clients with fragile boundaries, such as the ones suffering from schizophrenia (Johnson, 1993, Langley, 1983).

Theoretical context
In order to evaluate "Dramatherapy Performances" both as dramatic constructs, as well as the performance of the participating individuals within them, one has to employ a theoretical model. Although this therapeutic practice can bring to light obvious benefits for the participating clients, no system or instrument of evaluation has been created until now in order to accredit-quantitatively or qualitatively – its outcomes within the field of health care. In order to develop such an evaluation instrument it is important, first of all, to conceive "performance" – a term mainly used in the performing arts – within the field of health care. Then, one could accept, metaphorically, the schizophrenic condition as a "performance" within mental health care in general, as well as in dramatherapy practice. In this case, the schizophrenic condition could be observed as behavioral patterns, communication and expressive skills apparent during the clients' everyday life in social, clinical or rehabilitation settings. Furthermore, one could focus on the performance of an individual with schizophrenia within a dramatherapy project and the process of change in the schizophrenic symptoms occurring during this project throughout the sessions and during the presentation on stage.

This process could be viewed as the client's adventure in his or her personal Tragedy. The reason for the latter is that, according to the theorists of the Tragedian form, tragedy exists in situations of conflicting rights. My argument here is that any performance of a client within a psychiatric institution in general, as well as within a therapeutic session such as in Dramatherapy, can be seen as a contemporary tragedy, despite its dramatic, comic, or satiric style.

Living in times in which the major value is individuality, an inability to have self-boundaries can be seen as a major tragic phenomenon. If we consider Tragedy as resulting out of **two conflicting human or civil rights**, then individuals with schizophrenia become contemporary tragic figures, struggling between **a biological disposition** they did not choose for themselves and **a psychosocial need for adaptation**. The use of the ancient term "Tragedy" in the contemporary world can be related to situations involving conflicting values and the possibility of revolution: "The tragic action in its deeper sense is not the confirmation of the disorder, but its experience, its comprehension and its resolution. In our time, this action is general, and its common name is revolution. We have to see the evil and the suffering, in the factual disorder that makes revolution necessary, and in the disordered struggle against the disorder" (Williams in Drakakis & Liebler, 1998: 178). The context of these "Dramatherapy Performances" also defines the process of change in the stigmatising attitudes towards people with mental illness. Because these performances show the clients' struggle to overcome their biological nature in order to communicate social meanings, they can be seen, despite their context, **as contemporary tragedies**.

Within this theoretical framework, the need for assessment and evaluation of such therapeutic practice needs to be based on the semiotics of the tragic form. Contemporary semioticians consider the tragic mode as first defined by Aristotle in his work ***Poetics***, originating in Ancient Greece in 330 B.C., as the first "sign-system" in Theatre (Elam, 1980: 5). Aristotle first described the quantitative and qualitative elements of a tragic structure able to produce a cathartic outcome. Aristotle's Poetics describe the fundamental elements of the Tragedian form and distinguish "quantitative" from "qualitative" elements.

The quantitative elements are the sequential parts of the tragedy. According to Aristotle's Poetics the quantitative structure of a tragedy consists of an introduction (prologos), the chorus' entrance (parodus), the dialogues (episodes) and the chorus parts (stasima), and the exit (exodus). An ideal tragedy consists of three episodes, where all action between the tragic characters takes place, each followed by a chorus part, which expresses the public opinion and the people's feelings about these actions. The qualitative elements are the fundamental intrinsic processes of a tragedy. The qualitative elements consist of the Plot (Mythos), the Characters (Ethos), the Ideology (Dianoia), the Diction (Lexis), the Music (Melos) and the Design (Opsis) (Table 1). Each one of these processes will be further described hereby.

Quantitative Poetic Elements	*Qualitative Poetic Elements*
• Prologos (Introduction)	• Mythos (Plot)
• Parodus (Chorus' entrance)	• Ethos (Character)
• Episodes (Dialogues)	• Dianoia (Ideology)
• Stasima (Chorus parts)	• Lexis (Diction)
• Exodus (Exit)	• Melos (Music)
	• Opsis (Design)

Table 1. Aristotles' Poetic Elements

As Butcher explains in his study on Aristotle (1920 : 334):

> "Of the six elements into which Aristotle analyses a tragedy, plot holds the first place. **Plot** in the drama, in its fullest sense, is the artistic equivalence of "action" in Real life. [...] "Action" in Aristotle is not a purely external act, but an inward process, which works outward, the expression of a man's rational personality. [...] It must include outward fortune and misfortune, processes of the mental life".

Considering the above as a metaphor for the creation of a "myth" within the dramatherapy group's process, one can regard the development of the group's plot within the stages of a "Dramatherapy Performance" process.

As described in Aristotle's Poetics, Ethos and Dianoia are the two sides of character:

> "They are two distinct factors which unite to constitute the concrete and living person. [...] **Ethos** is the moral element in character. It reveals a certain state or direction of the will. It is an expression of moral purpose, of the permanent disposition and tendencies, the tone and sentiment of the individual. **Dianoia** is the thought, the intellectual element, which is implied in all rational conduct, through which alone ethos can find outward expression, and which is separable from Ethos only by a process of abstraction. [...]
>
> Ethos reveals itself both in the speech and in the actions of the dramatic characters. Therefore, it is more apparent in the dialogic parts of the drama (episodes). "Wherever moral choice or a determination of the will is manifested there ethos appears" (Aristotle Poet. Vi 5, in Butcher, 1920 : 340-343).

According to Aristotle,

> "Dramatic Dianoia is embodied only in speech not in action. [...] Under Dianoia are included the intellectual reflections of a speaker; the proof of his own statements, the disproof of those of his opponents, his general maxims concerning life and conduct, as elicited by the action and forming part of a train of Reasoning" (Butcher, 1920 : 343).

Lexis is the diction; it refers to the verbal expression. Concerning the clients of a dramatherapy performance process, Lexis can refer to all verbalisation processes including work through body "sculpts" expressing inner feelings and thoughts which are named, given titles and turned into words, but also to the words characters use in role-playing, singing, narrating, as well as the words clients use to relate to each other during the session. In this procedure Lexis provides an assessment of the clients' potential to express their inner world through words, to capture and express meaning in language. The lack of verbal use was already noted as part of the clients' negative symptoms, especially "alogia", which often produces muteness within the group.

Aristotle addressed the role of Music in his work "Politics":

"In rhythms and melodies we have the most realistic imitations of anger and mildness as well as of courage, temperance and all their opposites" (Butcher, 1920 : 131).

In his work "Poetics", **Melos** (music) expressed the image and reflection of a moral character. According to Aristotle's theory of the unique imitative capacity of music, the external movements of rhythmical sound bear a close resemblance to the movements of the soul.

Aristotle conceived the **Design** as the least important element of the Tragedy, however much it might contribute to the overall impression. However Butcher, interpreting Aristotle, reminds us:

"Color and form too have a similar capacity though in an inferior degree. The instinctive movements of the limbs, the changes of color produced on the surface of the body, are something more than arbitrary symbols; they imply that the body is of itself responsive to the animating soul, which leaves its trace on the visible organism" (Butcher, 1920 : 135).

Considering Design from a dramatherapy angle, I include not only the set and costumes, but also the real and symbolic use of props and objects, the position and status of the persons in space, their use and transformation of space, and the light they transmit or absorb as energetic presences. Thus, Design appears indispensable for the dramatic evolution.

All the aforementioned quantitative and qualitative elements of a tragic play confirm and promote the phenomenon of catharsis within and throughout a tragedy. Since Aristotle's Poetics, a number of interpretations have been given to the term "catharsis" (Chronopoulos, 2000), which are grouped into four basic views: the medical (physiological) view of catharsis as a physical cleansing function of the spectator, the moral view of purification, the intellectual view of clarification and pedagogic development, and the aesthetic view which refers to the intrinsic structure of a tragic action. Else (1967), in his work 'The Argument', expresses the latter aesthetic interpretation and views catharsis in relevance to a fatal or painful action, **the tragic passion**. According to the aesthetic view of catharsis, this phenomenon lies within the play itself and, mostly, within its plot. Catharsis is enacted on stage through 'mimesis', through the actors' performance, and its essential element is the moment of 'anagnorisis' (recognition), where the characters are confronted with the truth. Else argues that the spectator or reader does not perform the purification, but it lies within the structure of the play itself. For Else, catharsis is a functional and transitional component of the **tragic structure**; catharsis is not limited to the end of a Tragedy, but it is followed by the dissolving of pity and by a sense of pleasure.

Based on the above theoretical framework, I created an instrument which combines the poetic elements of the tragic form in relation to the symptoms of the clients' disorder (as can be noted in their performance within dramatherapy practice). Because the population I worked with suffered from schizophrenia, I focused on schizophrenic symptoms, and especially those of "affecting flattening", although this conceptual framework can be useful for any client group. This instrument can be applied for the assessment of dramatherapy sessions, as well as for the evaluation of a period of therapeutic work via performance-making which is described above as "Dramatherapy Performance". The name of this instrument is "Dramatherapy Performance Evaluation". It examines the different areas of performance-making according to Aristotle's Poetics and observes within each element of the Poetics the clients' symptoms and their change. I shall now explain further the qualitative elements on which "Dramatherapy Performance Evaluation" is based.

Besides, it is noteworthy that contemporary diagnostic criteria in Psychiatry are also based on a medical "sign system", which is constructed and organised in a rational way according to the presence or absence of particular psychiatric signs and symptoms. Psychiatric diagnoses are defined according to behavioural observation and registration and not to subjective experience. For example, the fourth edition of the Diagnostic and Statistical Manual of Mental Disorders' (American Psychiatric Association, 1994) outline a psychopathologic taxonomy as a subject for critical analysis, representing thus a fundamentally Aristotelian conception of the phenomena of mental disorders (Carson, 1996). The schizophrenic symptoms are classified as positive symptoms (delusions and hallucinations) and negative symptoms (related to state of interpersonal and social functioning). According to Andreasen' s taxonomy (1982) the negative schizophrenic symptoms are grouped in clusters, one of which is the cluster of "affective flattening". This cluster of symptoms consist of the following: unchanging facial expression, paucity of expressive gestures, decreased spontaneous movements lack of vocal inflections, poor eye contact, affective non-responsivity, inappropriate affect, global affective flattening. Since previous pilot studies (Yotis, 2002) and observation throughout the whole of the dramatherapy process with individuals with schizophrenia indicated a significant change on the clients' affective flattening, this cluster of symptoms was selected to be used in the formation of the instrument "Dramatherapy Performance Evaluation".

Construction of a new instrument

I will now show how the schizophrenic negative symptoms were connected to the dramatherapy performance elements in order to create a new instrument (a questionnaire) for the evaluation of a dramatherapy performance for a group of clients with schizophrenia, namely "Dramatherapy Performance Evaluation". As Table 2 shows, the Poetic elements are connected to one of the clusters of schizophrenic symptoms: "affective flattening".

Aristotle's poetic elements	Affective flattening components
Plot	Unchanging facial expression
Character	Paucity of expressive gestures
Ideas	Decreased spontaneous movements
Diction	Lack of vocal inflections
Music	Poor eye contact
Design	Affective non-responsivity
	Inappropriate affect
	Global affective flattening

Table 2. Connecting the schizophrenic negative symptoms to the performance's elements

"Dramatherapy Performance Evaluation" can be used for an evaluation of a therapeutic project based on objective circumstances (since it can be observed through video documentation), as well as for a subjective assessment by the dramatherapist at different points throughout the therapeutic work. For example, it can be used to measure the presence of a client's symptom, such as "unchanging facial expression", in the six poetic elements of a performance at a certain point in the therapeutic process, i.e beginning and closure. In other words, it can measure the level of the client's "unchanging facial expression" present during the plot of a performance, while playing characters, while expressing the characters' ideas, while uttering speech, and while responding to or creating the music and design of the performance. Also, it can be used to measure the change in this symptom throughout a dramatherapy performance project. For example, how did the client contribute to the performance's poetic elements? How did the client's presence of "unchanging facial expression " appear in the plot, the character, the ideas, the diction, the music and the design of the sessions, and what changes were noted from the first session to the last? Some clients could have made an improvement in their expression through gestures during the enactment of certain characters, rather than while using props or making music. Table 3 shows a part of the questionnaire.

After observing the video sample for individual X, please rate the following.
(1. not at all, 2. mildly, 3. moderately, 4. markedly, 5. severely)
e.g. Client X presents an unchanging facial expression

a) During the plot of the scene   1-5
b) During the display of a character   1-5
c) During the flow of the character's ideas   1-5
d) During the flow of the play's diction   1-5
e) In relation to music or sound effects.   1-5
f) In relation to his/her use of props and scenery   1-5

Table 3 – Questionnaire for the item "unchanging facial expression"

Hence, a chart can be designed to relate the clients' symptom appearance to each of the performance's elements. The lower the total score is, the less apparent are the client's symptoms and the healthier and more creative the client's performance is. An example of measurements follows with qualitative comments on the client's performance (Table 4).

Name: Leto Date: 4/6/2003	Unchanging facial expression	Paucity of expressive gestures	Decreased spontaneous movements	Lack of vocal inflections	Poor eye contact	Affective non-responsivity	Inappro-priate affect	Global affective flattening	Total score
Plot	5	4	4	4	3	2	2	3	27
Character	5	4	4	5	4	3	4	4	33
Ideas	5	3	3	3	3	2	2	3	24
Diction	5	4	4	4	4	2	3	4	30
Music	5	4	4	3	3	2	2	3	26
Design	5	4	4	4	4	3	3	4	31
Total score	30	23	23	23	21	14	16	21	171

Table 4. Quantitative measurements
Example of rating

Example of interpretation of this chart in relation to the clients' presence in the group:
Qualitative comments: Leto's blunt affect influenced all the poetic elements of this performance noticeably. Her contribution was mainly through her participation in the Ideology (Dianoia) of the play. Her comments were thoughtful, sincere and important for the group. Her attempts to create Character (Ethos) were unsuccessful (Character score is the highest) and she held an almost mute part (high score in Diction) on stage, playing a girl in the company as she sang with the rest of the chorus. Her contribution to the Music (Melos) of the play was better than the rest of her performance, since she made a genuine effort to be tuned in harmonically with the rest of the members, even if not in a particularly animated manner. Her contribution to Design (Opsis) was restricted, with a limited use of space and props, as she was often hiding behind others on stage. Among Leto's expressive components the most severely affected was her "facial expression" which was almost unchanging throughout the whole play. Much less influenced (moderately) were her "appropriate affect" and "affective responses", which indicated her positive intentions towards the group work and established her as a sympathetic presence within the group.

Application and Results
As a pilot study, this tool was first applied to four Dramatherapy performances devised in a similar way within psychiatric settings, in order to modify its final applicability. Then, the developed "Dramatherapy Performance Evaluation" was used to investigate aspects of psychopathology in relation to the "Dramatherapy Performance" in the Athens University Day Hospital for clients with psychotic disorders, resulting in a body of quantitative and qualitative data which was analysed. This became part of the fieldwork of a PhD project in Dramatherapy which was completed at the University of Hertfordshire (Yotis, 2002).

The client group of this project was formed by 15 members: young adults, male and female, with schizophrenic psychopathology and without any organic disorder, mental retardation or drug misuse or dependency. All clients were under anti-psychotic medication, which was kept more or less unchanged during the project. The project lasted for four months and there was a follow up period of three months thereafter. There was a control group in the same Day Hospital matched for the clients' characteristics, the average dose of medication and the duration of illness and hospitalization. Apart from the clients' "Dramatherapy Performance Evaluation", clients of both the dramatherapy and the control group were assessed through the BPRS scale (general psychopathology), the Zung depression scale, the SANS scale (negative symptoms), the Robson self-esteem scale and the SOS – significant others scale.

"Dramatherapy Performance Evaluation" focused on the cluster of negative symptoms: "affective flattening". This framework permitted a qualitative evaluation of the following research areas:

1. The dramatherapy process and performance event in relation to the creative process of its core elements: Plot, Character, Ideology, Diction, Music and Design;
2. The individual contribution of each client to the aforementioned poetic elements of the "Dramatherapy Performance" and the effect of their affective flattening on each one of them;
3. The total contribution of this client group to each of the Performance's elements. This analysis resulted in information that indicated which performance areas can be useful therapeutically and which are more problematic for individuals with schizophrenia.

A quantification of the qualitative data indicated which changes in the performance elements had a statistically significant positive correlation (r0.5, p.01) and which were influenced independently of each other within the therapeutic process (their distributions differed significantly, $p<.01$):

i) The clients managed to create a united and coherent performance, all the particular poetic elements of which – Plot, Character, Ideology, Diction, Music and Design – showed a statistically significant positive correlation ($0.759 < r < .981$, $p<.001$).
ii) The Plot, the Ideology and the Diction of the Performance were created more through verbal processes. These elements showed a significant interconnection, influencing in the same way the clients' affective flattening, which was

demonstrated in a similar way in these performance elements.

iii) Music and Design had an interconnection, as they were created mainly through nonverbal processes. The clients' affective flattening was less apparent in these two performance elements than in the other elements that were mostly based on verbal processes.

iv) Character, which included verbal as well as nonverbal processes, was positively correlated with all of the above elements, indicating that the common unifying element was character creation, manifested as individual role-playing.

v) The Ideology was conveyed in a similar way through both character and chorus representations. However, this study showed that the more functional clients (whose general psychopathology and overall dysfunctioning, as measured by the BPRS and the SANS scales, scored lower) were more apt to present individual characters and, thus, to contribute to the play's dialogic parts, the "episodes" than the more dysfunctional clients. Clients who were assessed as more dysfunctional presented a greater ability to participate in the plays' chorus than to create characters. Therefore, their contribution to the dialogic parts (episodes) was restricted, though they had a strong presence during the "stasima", the chorus parts of the play. Thus, the Poetics' quantitative elements, episodes and chorus, within the cathartic structure of the play, enables clients with various levels of psychopathology and functioning to co-exist within a therapeutic process and to contribute to a whole dramatic event.

In general, clients whose negative symptoms were manifested through affective flattening were helped more when the "Dramatherapy Performance" project focused on the nonverbal processes as being important for enhancing the verbal ones. Moreover, a quantitative evaluation was also undertaken, analysing the impact of this dramatherapy project on the clients' schizophrenic symptoms and their relationships with self and others, as measured by common psychiatric research tools.

This instrument's initial formulation referred to the schizophrenic symptoms. However, it can be used for any psychopathology, once as the therapist defines what the tragic conflict for the client is. For example, if the client has an affective disorder (i.e. mania and depression) the "tragic conflict" could be emotional stability versus instability and the symptoms for observation throughout the performance elements would be related to emotional control. Future research could inform us of how this instrument could assess and evaluate therapeutic processes with other client groups.

Summary

A specific tool for the evaluation of "Dramatherapy Performance", as a specific model of dramatherapy practice, was developed. The evaluation tool was based on theatre semiotics, more specifically on Aristotle's Poetics. Aristotle's Poetics was used as a metaphor within the contemporary context of Dramatherapy for individuals with schizophrenia. The use of this metaphor was based theoretically on the notion of "tragic conflict", which can be seen as the drama that individuals with schizophrenia experience within the context of their societal norms, and their struggle towards rehabilitation and reintegration into society, from which they have been cast out because of their stigmatizing disorder. The concept of catharsis was specifically re-examined within the framework of Dramatherapy practice. The notion of catharsis was viewed as a provider of structure and containment and not merely as a means towards the emotional relief of the participants in the performance. A model of Dramatherapy was proposed, which culminated in a performance that had therapeutic goals. The total process had a "cathartic" structure, which was evaluated using the six Aristotelian poetic elements of Tragedy: Plot, Characters, Ideology, Diction, Music and Design. A system of evaluation was devised specifically for clients with schizophrenia in order to correlate changes in the clients' negative symptoms and, in particular, their "affective flattening" in relation to the poetic elements of a "Dramatherapy Performance" construction. This evaluation system, named "Dramatherapy Performance Evaluation" is designed to be applied:

a) to the whole Dramatherapy process,
b) to the performance event,
c) to the individual contribution of each client within the performance creation.

This evaluation instrument was used in a clinical trial which took place at the Athens University Day Hospital for clients with psychotic disorders. This research investigated the impact of the "Dramatherapy Performance" on the clients' schizophrenic psychopathology and, in particular, their "affective flattening" – a specific cluster of their "negative" symptoms during a four-month therapeutic period and a three-month follow up. This project showed that:

- There was an interconnection of verbal processes (Plot, Ideology and Diction), as well as an interconnection of nonverbal processes (Music and Design) during the performance project.
- Therapeutic work on Character creation was correlated with all the rest of the performance's poetic elements.
- The performance's Ideology was conveyed through Character – mostly apparent in the performance's dialogic parts (episodes) – for more functional clients and through chorus participation for less functional clients with schizophrenia.

Thus, the ancient Greek sign-system of Aristotle's Poetics can stand as a basis of inspiration for dramatherapy evaluation in our post-modern world. The use of quantitative (sequential parts) and qualitative elements (intrinsic processes) can form a "cathartic structure" within a therapeutic process. This therapeutic structure can be assessed, evaluated and interpreted by the new instrument "Dramatherapy Performance Evaluation". This instrument can be especially helpful when working with clients with schizophrenia, where the main objective is to create structure and find meaning in chaotic expression and communication.

References
Andreasen C.N. (1982). *Negative versus positive schizophrenia*, Arch. Gen. Psychiatry, 39: 789-794
Bielanska A., Cechnicki A., Budzyna-Dawidowski P. (1991). *Drama Therapy as a means of*

Rehabilitation for Schizophrenic Patients: Our Impressions, Am. J Psychotherapy, 45 (4), 566-575

Butcher S.H. (1920). *Aristotle's Theory of Poetry and Fine Art with a critical text and translation of the Poetics*, London: Macmillan

Carson R.C. (1996). *Aristotle, Galileo, and the DSM taxonomy: the case of schizophrenia*, Journal of Consulting & Clinical Psychology, Dec; 64 (6): 1133-9

Cattanach A. (ed.), (1999). *Process in the Arts Therapies*, London: Jessica Kingsley Publishers

Chronopoulos C. (2000). *The Aristotelian Tragic Catharsis*, Athens: Kardamitsas

Drakakis J. and Liebler N.C. (eds.) (1998). *Tragedy*, London & N.Y: Longman

Elam K. (1980). *The Semiotics of Theatre and Drama*, London: Routledge

Else G. (1967). *Aristotle's Poetics: The Argument*, Leiden, published in cooperation with the State Univesity of Iowa: E.J.Brill

Emunah R. (1994). *Acting for Real*, NY: Brunner & Mazel Publishers

Grainger R. (1999). *Researching the Arts Therapies*, London: Jessica Kingsley Publishers

Jenkyns M. (1996). *The play's the thing*, London: Routledge

Jennings S. (1994). *The Handbook of Dramatherapy*, London: Routledge

Johnson D.R. (1980). *Effects of a Theatre Experience on Hospitalized Psychiatric Patients*, The Arts in Psychotherapy, 7: 265-272

Johnson D.R. and Quinlan D. (1993). *Can the mental representations of paranoid schizophrenics be differentiated from those of normals?* Journal of Personal Assessment, 60 (3), 588-601

Jones P. (1996). *Drama as Therapy–Theatre as Living*, London: Routledge

Landy R. (1995). *Drama Therapy Theory: Concepts and Practices*, Springfield, IL: C. C. Thomas

Langley D. and G. (1983). *Dramatherapy and Psychiatry*, London: Croom Helm.

Lyketsos G.(1980). *The Ancient Greek Tragedy as a means of Psychotherapy for Mental Patients*, Psychotherapy Psychosomatics, 34: 241-247.

Mitchell S. (1992). Therapeutic theatre: A para-theatrical model of Dramatherapy, in *Dramatherapy Theory and Practice 2*, (ed. Jennings S.), London: Routledge.

Yotis L. (2002). *Dramatherapy Performance and Schizophrenia*, PhD Thesis, University of Hertfordshire, UK.

ERNA GRÖNLUND, BARBRO RENCK AND NITA GYLLANDER VABÖ

DANCE MOVEMENT THERAPY FOR DEPRESSED TEENAGE GIRLS

Introduction

Depression is a frequently occurring psychiatric disorder with a prevalence of approximately 5% in the general population. It is estimated that at least one third of all individuals are likely to experience an episode of depression during their lifetime. Evidence now available suggests a link between stressful life events and adolescent psychiatric disorder. In an epidemiological Swedish study from the 1990s, 2300 schoolchildren, 16-17 years old, were screened for depression and previous suicide attempts. The results showed that 6% of the boys and 17.9% of the girls had high depression scores in self-evaluation (Olsson & von Knorring, 1999).

The Swedish National Board of Health and Welfare (2001) has noticed how mental illness of teenage girls has seriously changed for the worse. An increasing number of teenage girls are using self-destructive behaviour, frequently cutting or burning themselves to get rid of inner pain and anxiety. Among young people suicidal attempts and fulfilled suicides have increased and death by suicide is today the most common cause of death among young people in Sweden. Major Depressive Disorder (MDD), which is uncommon before puberty, increases in adolescence and its co-morbidity with other psychiatric disorders is high. The frequency of MDD for adolescents is four times higher for girls than for boys. Depression can start with a traumatic life-event and then has an acute debut, but it can also come creeping step by step. The heredity for depression is strong and it is not unusual that family-members also suffer from depression. Therefore it can, for example, sometimes be difficult for a depressed mother to be aware of the depressive symptoms of her daughter.

It is noticed that depressive adolescents is a group that has a great need for help but the treatment that is offered is neither adequate nor enough. In Sweden medication with antidepressants, such as Zoloft and Cipramil, has increased for young people. However, there is a discussion among many medical doctors whether to prescribe antidepressants or not to youngsters, because both of the risk for side effects and for addiction. Thus proper medication should not be treated as the only or sufficient treatment of depression. Recent research (Olsson & von Knorring, 1999) points out that the level of serotonin, that is very low in depression, can be increased by natural means like doing physical exercises. That is a good reason for using dance movement therapy (DMT). Cognitive therapy, which is trying to break the negative pattern, has had some good effects but there are very few cognitive therapists at the child and adolescent psychiatric clinics in Sweden. Mostly the depressed adolescents are offered antidepressants together with verbal therapy. For some girls that is an effective treatment. Others don't want to talk about their problems and they soon drop out of therapy. Perhaps dance therapy could then be an effective alternative treatment? We decided that it was worth trying. In the study a goal oriented DMT with a strength's perspective was used to help the depressed girls to develop positive coping strategies and to increase self-esteem. As we see it, DMT has a good chance to be of help for the depressed girls because DMT is working with the body through rhythm and energy lightening movements. It is also working with the depressed girls' poor concentration, trying to increase memory and attention.

The girls were above all helped to get in touch with and express difficult feelings – such as sadness, aggression and shame. The main goal for the treatment was to try to change the depressive girls´ negative attitude to life.

Specific criteria of depression for adolescents are:
Depressed mood
A depressed adolescent can either be very sad or irritated and angry with sudden outbursts. When she is angry it is sometimes hard for the parents to understand that there can be a depression underneath.

Lack of joy and initiative
The depressed adolescent has lost initiative, nothing is interesting and joyful
The thoughts are negative and she finds no meaning in life.

Low self-esteem
The self-esteem is very low and the depressed girl often looks at herself as ugly and worthless. She is not loveable. That gives her feelings of both guilt and shame

Inability to concentrate
The depressed teenage girl has lost her ability to concentrate. She can´t follow the teaching at school and she can't do her home-work as well as she used to do before depression. That starts a negative spiral and often leads to truancy. She soon drops out of school.

Tiredness – sleeping problems
The depressed girl is extremely tired. Sleeping problems can be of various kinds: either she sleeps too little and can't fall asleep in the night or she is sleeping too much and can be lying down on the sofa all the day. The parents may look at her as lazy and nag at her. That will not make the situation any better.

Psychomotoric inhibition
The depressed girl moves very slowly. The movements are without energy and direction. The face is stiff without expression. She speaks low and slowly if she speaks at all.

Eating disorders
When being depressed the teenage girl often loses her appetite and there is a risk that she will get anorexic. On the other hand it might be the other way around – the depressed girl may start eating uncontrollably and become bulimic.

Self-destructiveness and suicidal thoughts
Many depressed teenage girls are self-destructive and can cut or burn themselves. It is not a suicidal behaviour but on the contrary a way of surviving by getting rid of inner pain and anxiety. However, this behaviour is contagious and must be stopped by the grown-ups. It is not unusual that depressed teenage girls often have suicidal thoughts and frequently make attempted suicide. Therefore it is important to listen seriously to the signals and give professional help as soon as possible.

Aims of the study
The comprehensive aim of this study was to evaluate the effect and value of dance therapy for young girls diagnosed as having a depression related to DSM IV.
When studying the dance therapy process we wondered if DMT could help the depressed girls to increase their self esteem and get back their energy and lust for life.
Another aim of the study was to try to identify those interventions in the dance therapy that had a positive effect. We were also interested in looking at turning-points in the dance therapy process.

Design of the project
We started with a one-year pilot-study. After that came the main study that lasted for two years. Two dance therapists together led the DMT, which took place in a clinical department of child and adolescent psychiatry in Karlstad, a middle-sized Swedish town.
Eleven girls were offered dance therapy once a week, either in group or individually. The girls who were between 13-17 years old all had the diagnosis Depression. Some of them also had other diagnosis such as Asperger´s syndrome, Morbus Chron or eating disorders. Two of the girls had been sexually abused.
The median length of a depressive episode in young patients is 8 – 9 months, so we wanted the dance therapy treatment to go on for that long – that is over two terms. Unfortunately it was not always possible to fulfil that plan since the girls could not leave school for that long. Thus the treatment went on for between six weeks and two terms.

Qualitative research methods
The research in this study is interdisciplinary with researchers from three areas co-operating – dance therapy, public health and psychiatric medicine. The study is both an effect and a process study and consequently both quantitative and qualitative methods are used. Multiple data sources were used to triangulate data and increase validity. The results from the dance therapy process are presented in cases which are based upon interviews and video-observations.
Since the parents are seldom aware of symptoms of depression and anxiety in their children – they might be blocked by their own depression – as a researcher you may not get a trustworthy result when just interviewing the parents. Therefore to get the adolescents' own feelings we interviewed the adolescents themselves, sometimes complemented with parents' interviews.
The girls were interviewed before and after DMT and for the first group the girls

were also interviewed three years after, in order to see what they remembered and if some healing effects were still left in the body and mind.

All the sessions were video filmed, more than a hundred hours, which gave us a unique picture of the whole process. The films were used both in the supervision and in the research. In the interviews after DMT most of the girls assured us that they were not disturbed by the camera. They told us that they forgot the camera when occupied by the group and their own inner process. However, the dance therapists said that sometimes it was troublesome for them to be scrutinized by the camera.

Questionnaire and instruments

We used a very short socio-demographic questionnaire with questions about the family situation – the age of the parents, the education for the parents and work situation. Another question was whether or not the girls had medical problems. Other self-reported scales we used in this study were Strengths and Difficulties Questionnaire – SDQ, Sense of Coherence – SOC-scale, Depression Self-Rating Scale – DSRS and I Think I Am Questionnaire – ITIA. The scales were used both as pre- and post test and we can compare the differences.

SDQ is a behavioural screening questionnaire divided between 5 scales of 5 items each: Hyperactivity scale, Emotional symptoms scale, Conduct problems scale, Peer problems scale and Prosocial scale. The scores for hyperactivity, emotional symptoms, conduct problems and peer problems can be summed to generate a total difficulties score ranging from 0 to 40, with a normal score between 0 and 13. The prosocial score is accounted separately. Five items examine for psychiatric help and one item calculates the burden for the family and friends (Goodman, 1997).

SOC – scale was developed by Antonovsky (1987). He is very well-known in the area of public health and he has introduced the concept of Sense of Coherence as an integrated perception of one's life as being comprehensible, manageable and meaningful. SOC describes a personality disposition in terms of stress resistance resource. In this study we used the short version of SOC with 13 items. The SOC scale total score range is 13 to 91. A high SOC-scale value indicates a high level of well-being.

DSRS was developed by Birleson et. al.(1987) in clinical practice and measures depression in children and adolescents. The scale contains 18 items, some worded positively and others negatively. A value between 0–36 can occur. Birleson recommends a cut-off point of 15 for depression. A higher value indicates depression.

ITIA is a self-reported questionnaire containing 72 items which cover five domains of self-esteem: Physical characteristics, skills and talents, psychological well-being, relations to parents and family, and relations to peers and teachers (Ouvinen-Birgerstam, 1999). A high value indicates a high self-esteem.

Results

The p-value measures the significance of the difference between pre- and post-test. In statistics, significant means that, given the hypothesis, the obtained results are unlikely to have been due to chance, at some specified level of probability.

SDQ. There are positive changes in most of the subscales but only emotional symptoms are significant (p<0.01). SDQ total decreased from 18.5 to 14.9 (p<0.05). Both impact rating and burden rating has decreased but the differences between pre- and post-test are not significant.

SOC. In our results we see a higher mean value after dance therapy, 46.6 to 49.2, but the difference is not significant.

DSRS. There was a significant difference between mean value pre- and post-test (18.2 to 13.9; p<0.05). Five girls showed after dance therapy normal scores. For seven girls the DSRS-value has decreased after dance therapy.

ITIA. There are positive changes on three of the five sub-scales but only the difference between pre- and post-test for psychological well-being is significant (1.45 to 2.80; p<0.05). The total score has increased from 2.64 to 3.30; not significant.

Summary
The results from the quantitative data indicate a trend in a positive development. All the scales show positive changes. However, there are a few limitations in the quantitative part of the study:

1. The study group is very small.
2. There are differences in the length of the dance therapy for the groups.

One question is also if there are differences between individual dance therapy and group dance therapy. Perhaps the qualitative analysis of the DMT- process can give us an answer? When this paper was presented at the ECArTE-conference, in 2005, the analysis of the comprehensive video films was not completed. However, we noticed that quantitative and qualitative data give unanimous results. There was a clear positive trend: A relief of the depressive symptoms and an increased state of mind. During the dance therapy process most of the girls´ energy and activity obviously increased, so too did their emotional openness. From the joy of movement followed a lust for life. For most of the girls the depression has diminished. Anxiety and aggressiveness have decreased and the psychic stability has been much better. In the interviews after dance therapy the girls confirmed that they were helped by dance therapy and that the goals with the treatment were reached.

A case-study
In a case study a fifteen-year old depressed girl's dance movement therapy (DMT) is presented. The girl's progress in the DMT is illustrated by a short video sequence. Both the girl and the girl's parents have given us the permission to show the video and talk about the girl in the DMT.
The girl is called Eve, but that is of course not her real name. Eve had two diagnoses, besides Depression she was diagnosed as having Asperger´s syndrome. She also had a serious social phobia and she dared not to go out among people.

She had stopped to go to school and was taught at home. She longed for friends but was unable to go out.

Before she got her depression her great joy was to take dance classes. Dance then was an important part of her life. When I first met Eve she looked upon herself as ugly and worthless. She thought of herself as an outsider. No one could love her. Eve's self-esteem was very low. She also had difficulties to talk about her problems. As a dance therapist I was aware of Eve's need of finding a new way to express her feelings. Could dance therapy, that is a non-verbal creative treatment, perhaps be a way to loosen her tensions and release her hidden feelings?

When Eve started dance therapy she was very shy and afraid of physical contact, so I had to be careful not to touch her suddenly and to come too close. Eve used the room in a very cautious way. She moved slowly with no energy and preferred to stand in the corners of the room. However, step by step Eve felt safer and more trustful. Increasingly, she used the whole room in improvisations and different dance forms.

Eve had dance therapy for two terms and when after some time in the second term Eve seemed to feel safe with me I made up my mind to try flamenco in order to let her get in touch with her feelings. I chose flamenco because that dance is about being proud of yourself, of who you are and having the courage to express strong feelings. To dance flamenco would hopefully be a way of increasing her self-esteem. It showed that introducing flamenco led to a turning-point and then on to an important change.

When the film starts Eve is sitting on the floor with her hands in her knees and her eyes closed. She is waiting for me to come with a surprise for her. I placed a flamenco-dress in her knees and she examines it with her eyes still closed. When she looks up and sees the red dress she is delighted and says: – *Oh what a beautiful dress!* She wants to put it on and I help her with that. When I myself had also put on a flamenco-dress we danced together. After a while I asked her if she wanted to look at herself in the mirror. She nodded yes and I took away the curtains. In the mirror she could see herself dancing and she seemed glad to see that she looked beautiful in the red dress. When Eve realized that, it was obvious that she felt proud. That was a turning point, and a step in increasing her self-esteem.

When the DMT was finished, Eve wanted to show her parents what she had done and learnt in the DMT. We decided to show them some video sequences from her dance therapy. On the video one could see how Eve at the end of DMT integrated her poems, written by herself, with her dance. With strong movements and with power in her voice she sang and danced her poems. The last line in one of her poems goes like this: – *I am who I am and here I am!* When Eve's father saw and heard this he started to cry.

In Sweden we celebrate the International Day of Dance one day in the spring with dance performances, seminars, workshops and lectures at different places all over the country. This year Eve was able to join a dance group again and she took part in a performance in front of a big audience. She was indeed proud of herself.

Today Eve is 18 years old. She has finished high school and has got a job. She is working with small children. She says that she has been helped greatly by DMT and she is looking on her future with confidence.

References:
Antonovsky, A. (1987). *Unraveling the Mystery of Health*. San Francisco: Jossey-Bass
Birleson, P., Hudson, I., Gray Buchanan, D., Wolff, S. (1987). Clinical evaluation of a self-rating scale for depressive disorder in childhood. *J. Child. Psychol. Psychiat. 28(1),* 43-60
Goodman, R. (1997). The Strengths and Difficulties Questionnaire: A Research Note. *Journal of Child Psychol. Psychiat.* 38(5), 581-586
Olsson, G. & von Knorring, A-L.(1999). Adolescent depression: prevalence in Swedish high-school students. *Acta Psychiatric Scand.* 99, 324-331
Ouvinen-Birgerstam, P. (1999). *Jag tycker jag är. Manual.* [I think I am. Manual]. Stockholm: Psykologiförlaget AB
Swedish National Board of Health and Welfare – Socialstyrelsen (2001). Folkhälsorapport. [Public Health Report]. Stockholm: Socialstyrelsen.

MATHILDE A.M. TUBBEN

GROUNDED VISION: A MATTER OF 'MAKING EXPLICIT', OR BRIDGING THE GAP BETWEEN PRACTICE AND THEORY

In this article the process of constructing an observation instrument out of an observation task used in drama therapy is described. In describing this process of constructing, the author will emphasize all the steps of 'making explicit' necessary to bridging the gap between practice and theory. The psychometric outcomes of the pilot research with the constructed instrument are satisfying. A national norm and validation study has started after the pilot project and is ongoing. With this observation instrument, 'the building of a hut', conclusions can be drawn about the social emotional development of children from seven up until and including twelve years of age.

Have you ever built a hut? – In the garden, in the attic, on a building site nearby, or just under the table? – In the clinical practice of drama therapists many huts are built by young clients. What do drama therapists consider to be important information concerning this drama task, and what is the aim of observing clients building a hut?

This article deals with building huts, those constructed in the practice of drama

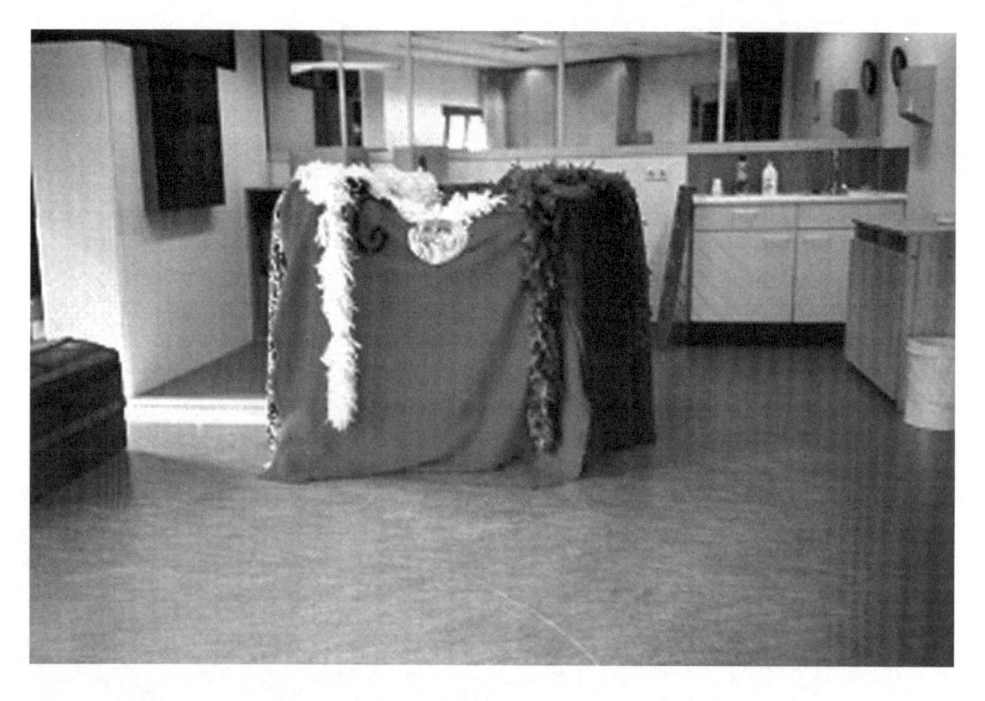

Hut: girl of 11 years of age

therapy by clients varying from 7 up until and including 12 years of age. It is about building huts and about constructing a scientifically-based observation instrument.

Introduction
As a drama therapist I have seen many huts built by children undergoing therapy. I saw large and very small huts, open, friendly looking houses and fully armed fortresses. The huts belonged to kings, beggars, vagabonds, as well as to animals or just ordinary children. The huts were situated on mountaintops, in woods, in slums, in a backyard. Mothers pass by these huts, or police officers, football stars, or animals. The stories children told about their huts varied from cheerful, superficial, and fierce to very sad.

All these different huts and the stories about them provide much useful information about the constructor: the client. Therefore, the observation of children building a hut may be used for diagnostic purposes. But what diagnostic conclusions can be drawn? If a hut is stable, may we conclude the child him/herself must be stable? In the case of a hut showing strong emphasis on the outside and no attention paid to the inside, may we consider the child is embellishing the outside in order to hide his or her inner self? Some children show extreme fear of failure and don't manage to construct any hut at all, so the diagnosis seems obvious: fear of failure. The conviction that the observation of a child constructing a hut is revealing seems understandable, but when the findings refer to different aspects of psychological functioning every time, it becomes hard to draw clear and transparent diagnostic conclusions.

Although my colleagues loved the stories which I told them about the huts, and although they thought my findings always very interesting, we could not really communicate any clear conclusions. The hut-observations did not have the diagnostic impact which I was convinced they could (and should) have. I could not clearly and explicitly formulate proof. I couldn't ground my vision!

This refers to the title of this article, *grounded vision – a matter of 'making explicit', or bridging the gap between practice and theory*. In this article the grounding of a vision is described.

First the social relevance for adequate and reliably diagnostic procedures will be mentioned. Then the process of construction of the observation instrument 'the building of a hut' will be described in five steps, with each next step 'making more explicit what exactly is measured and how'. The article ends with a short description of the ongoing national norm and validation study with the observation instrument, 'the building of a hut'.

1. Social relevance
1.1 Psychosocial measurement for young children
Diagnostic research is an important part of the socio-psychological healthcare. Good diagnostic research is necessary for efficient and effective treatment of clients. Good diagnostic research depends on sound diagnostic instruments, which must be reliable and valid. If it comes to measuring the intelligence of young Dutch children, a reasonable number of tests are available, qualified as reliable and valid by the Commissie voor Test Aangelegenheden (COTAN). COTAN is a national board that documents all tests and test research (Evers at al. 2000, Kievit

et al 1992, Walsh 1990). However, for measuring the social-emotional development of primary school children, very few reliable and valid instruments are at hand. There is, though, an offer of sound instruments, the inquiry forms or questionnaires, which indirectly measure the social-emotional development of young children. But they have two disadvantages: Because of the verbal capabilities needed, the tests can only be administered by children older than nine years of age. And because of this verbal basis of the tests, linguistically deprived children and children with some sort of deficiency in language skills, like dyslexia for example, will have more problems with inquiry forms. And the question arises: do these tests give a good measurement of the psychosocial development by young children?

To make statements about personality traits or the psychosocial development of young children, diagnostic researchers often use instruments based on projective techniques. The disadvantage of most of these projective tests is the subjective judgement and the non quantified scores. Reliability and validation are therefore unsatisfying. For this reason the Children's Apperception Test (CAT), the Rosenzweig and Columbus are eliminated by the COTAN out of their last published documentation (Evers et al. 2000). Another diagnostic tool used for measuring psychosocial development is the clinical view. But here also the disadvantages of subjective assessment and non quantified scores apply. As a diagnostic instrument, the clinical view lacks transparency, just as many of the projective tests.

1.2 Measurement in drama therapy

The significance of systematic observation and standardized procedures is revealing, because it enhances the transparency of diagnostic research and treatment. In the clinical practice of drama therapists no such systematically described and standardized observation instrument with quantified scores is at hand for children from seven up until and including twelve years of age.

The observation instrument 'the building of a hut' as a diagnostic instrument follows the hypotheses testing model (van Strien, 1986). Such a model provides a systematic and standardized procedure. Beforehand hypotheses are formulated which are tested with the instrument. The observation-instrument 'the building of a hut' provides outcomes on two levels of diagnostic research.

- A global screening with an overview of the broad psychosocial functioning of a client as outcome
- An assessment of the functioning on itemized areas of the psychosocial development with an outcome specified on these developmental areas

And so the scores on the subscales of the observation instrument 'the building of a hut' offer the opportunity to formulate explicit treatment targets and to re-adjust already formulated treatment targets. The instrument also gives the possibility for use as an evaluation instrument, but this demands further research first.

The construction of the test is a previous project, we now do a national norm and validation study, after which the observation instrument 'the building of a hut' can form a multi applicable, effective and efficient diagnostic instrument for young children. Organisations benefiting from this research are all the youth health care institutions, like Bureau Jeugdzorg (an national ambulant health care organisation) or child psychiatry centres. Special schools can also benefit and insert the instrument into the indication basement procedure. A side effect of this research will be a positive impetus on the professionalizing of drama therapy, not only for the workers in the field, but for the educators as well.

2. The process of construction of the observation-instrument 'the building of a hut'

The process of constructing the observation instrument 'the building of a hut' contains five steps. The steps are based on professional knowledge, practitioner theory and psychological theories. The whole of subjective knowledge and personal findings about drama therapy is meant by practitioner theory (de Vries, 2004). Practitioner theory is always the result of (reflection on) one's own experiences. Professional knowledge refers to the generally shared knowledge concerning drama therapy among educated dramatherapists. This knowledge is more or less explicitly described. Psychological theories are well described theories often based on research.

2.1 First step in grounding the vision: standardizing the procedure

The task of building a hut is introduced differently by every therapist and even by the same therapist on different occasions. What exactly is asked of a client with this procedure? What precisely is the client expected to do? The building task needs to get a standardized introduction. And the introduction is explicitly formulated and prescribed. In the guideline the standardized method of administering the procedure is described as follows:

'After a tour through the working space and introduction to the materials, the child is asked to build a hut. "You may use all the materials available here to build your very own hut. I will not interfere, but if you need help or have any question at all please let me now. Only then I will go into action". After the child has completed the outside of the building, he/she is invited to equip the hut: "you may now equip your hut by gathering things you would like to have inside your hut". When this is finished, or the time allowed for it has run out, the child is asked three questions: "just imagine, if you were to fantasize to whom this hut belongs, who could live there? And where is this hut situated, where does it stand? And who is passing by this hut, at that very place?" After giving his/her answers, the child is invited to make up a short story about the owner of the hut, about the hut itself, and where it is situated, and about the person passing by. This told story is played out, whereby the child always plays the role of the owner of the hut and the therapist the role of passer by'.

I had to decide for which diagnostic purposes I wanted to use the instrument.

In the diagnostic practice there are 4 central questions, each of which indicates a specific form of diagnosing:

- What is the matter with this child?   (descriptive diagnosis)
- Why does this particular child has a problem? (explaining diagnosis)
- Which treatment or therapy will fit best?   (indicating diagnosis)

- Does the therapy have the wanted effect?　　　(evaluative diagnosis)

Considering the aim of my research, the first two questions were important to me. To answer the first question I had to provide reliable and relevant information, which would adequately reflect the problems of the child. But what is reliable, what is relevant? To answer the second question I needed to gain insight into the conditions causing the problems. For this, I needed psychological knowledge, knowledge of pathology of the psyche, some medical knowledge, and knowledge of family therapy. So in the observations I had to focus on reliable and relevant information. Before being able to do so, I had to state explicitly what I considered reliable and relevant.

2.2 The diagnostic use of the observation-instrument 'the building of a hut'.
From the moment a client enters the therapy room, a process of interpretation starts. We all know that neutral, objective observation does not exist. The diagnostic observer processes information, using all sorts of theories, based on scientific insight, professional knowledge, experience and intuition. Very often this process of interpretation remains implicit.
Grounding a Vision is to make explicit: It means gathering information in a systematic and functional way, in which the methodology needs to be explained explicitly. Grounding a Vision means bridging the gap between practice and theory: research that increases the (body of) knowledge by a methodical cyclus (Kievit et al, 1992).

2.3 The second step in grounding the vision:
This second step of 'making explicit' is based on <u>practitioner theory</u> as well as <u>professional knowledge</u>. In 'building a hut' we can distinguish four levels of expression. In arts therapy a distinction between the art product and the art process as a diagnostic tool is a common one (Smeijsters, 2000; Malchiody, 1998). To these well known art product and art process criteria, I added two more levels of expression as observation criteria.

1. expression on the level of *the product* (the 'thing' hut):
   —What does the hut look like? Is it a big or small hut, is it open or closed, is it comfortable or not?
2. expression on the level of *the process* (the way the hut is built)
   —Is the whole working space used or not? Does the client ask for help or not?
3. expression on the level of *giving meaning* (the answers to the three posed questions in the standardized procedure, and the story based on these answers)
   —Does the client dare to invent role-figures for the hut-owner and passer-by? Are the invented role-figures logically connected in a story?
4. expression on the level of *thematic play* (the playing out of the told story by child and therapist)
   —The told stories can change while playing them out. For instance: one client invented a story about a little girl (hut-owner) who taught a witch

(passer-by) a lesson, but did not dare to do so in playing out this story. Instead she invited the witch in for a cup of tea.

This ordering in levels of expression form the observation criteria of the observation instrument 'building of a hut'. (See Figure 1)

Product
Process
Giving meaning
Thematic play

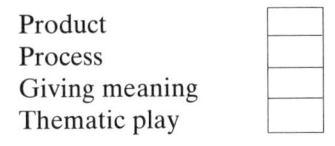

Figure 1: Egostrength measured on levels of expression

However, what can be measured by observing these criteria?
Can diagnostic conclusions be drawn concerning this observation task? Can something be asserted about personality trait, developmental dimension or skill?

2.4 The third step in grounding the vision:
The third step is based on practitioner theory:
The question of exactly what conclusions can be drawn from this observation has been answered by an analysis of observation reports concerning the task of building a hut. More than twenty observation reports of clients building a hut revealed that often expressions to describe the client were used like "is sure of himself" or "doesn't stand very firm" or "seems to have an unstable basis" or "cut herself off from her environment". The psychological concept all these descriptions apply to is called *ego strength*. Egostrength is a psychological concept that is often referred to in the psychological literature.(Nixon, 1982; Carver, 1988, Eurelings-Bontekoe, 2003). However, an instrument that directly measures the amount of ego strength of children does not exist. Such an instrument exists only for adolescents and adults (for sixteen years and older), the Barron ES-scale (Barron 1963).
The observation task of building a hut provides information on the degree of ego strength measured on the four levels of expression.
The psychological construct is insufficiently described by 'standing firm' or 'having a stable basis'. Again, in wanting to ground the vision, one has to make things very explicit. The question of what this 'standing firm' looks like refers to the descriptive diagnosis. And the question of why one child feels sure of him/herself, while another does not, refers to the explaining diagnosis . Both questions need to be answered by a sound diagnostic instrument and therefore the vision needs to be made more explicit before being soundly grounded.

2.5 The fourth step in grounding the vision:
This fourth step is based on psychological theories:
In literature about egostrength, we meet two opposing theories: the psychodynamic versus the dispositional theory. Most convincing and most workable, with

regard to the observation instrument, was the psycho-social developmental theory of Erikson (Erikson, 1964, 1987).

The psychodynamic theory offers perspective for growth of the egostrength, whereby the dispositional view of egostrength is a static one. Egostrength in this conception is seen as a stable and constant trait. Apart from that the observation instrument 'the building of a hut' is based on a projective technique. Projective techniques stem from psychodynamic theories and not from the dispositional ones. Questionnaires stem from trait theoretical or dispositional views (de Zeeuw, 1978; Evers et al., 2000).

2.5.1 Egostrength according to Erikson
Egostrength according to Erikson (Erikson, 1987) is the weighted sum of a number of so called qualities of feeling. These qualities of feeling refer to the effects of the completion of the developmental stages. Erikson distinguished a number of developmental stages, from which the first four are relevant in the frame of the observation instrument because of the age of the target group. In every stage, a conflict between opposite poles has to be worked out, which result in an adaptive psychological quality which, in turn, result in qualities of feeling. (See Figure 2)

Conflict	**Adaptive Psychological Quality**	**Quality of feeling**
1. Basic trust vs mistrust	Basic Trust	Hope
2. Autonomy vs shame, doubt	Autonomy	Having a will of one's own
3. Initiative vs Quilt	Initiative	Purposive
4. Industry vs Inferioty	Industry	Competence

Figure 2: Developmental stages of Erikson

Successfully solving the conflict doesn't mean the scale has to tip completely to the positive side: having some feelings of mistrust can be very adequate. One should not trust everybody in this world! The balance is not fixed for the rest of one's life. People meet these conflicts again and again, and every new solution influences the acquired qualities of feeling. However, the way the conflicts are solved first affects the quality of subsequent solutions.

Summarizing thus far: the observation instrument 'the building of a hut' is an instrument for measuring the degree of egostrength. Four levels of expression are observed: *product, process, giving meaning and thematic play*. The diagnostic conclusions about egostrength are based on four developmental dimensions: *basic trust, autonomy, initiative* and *industry*.

2.6 The fifth step in grounding the vision:
The next step was inspired by an expert panel. A list of indicators was formulated with the help of a number of experienced drama therapists and lecturers in the methodology of drama therapy. For every cell (*basic trust – product; basic trust – process, etc.*) an observable item was carefully devised. Often during this process, it became clear that more than one meaningful item could be placed in each cell. So next to the divisions we already had in place, regarding the levels of expression and in developmental dimensions, it was decided to make a third division: the so-called umbrella indicators were born.

The following umbrella indicators were defined as: *taking space, making contact* and *integrating*. The introduction of these umbrella indicators gave the score form, for the observation instrument, its final structure. (See figure 3).

Each of the indicators mentioned in the cells can be scored on a 7-point scale. A manual has been drawn up explaining each individual indicator.

		Taking space	Making contact	Integrating
EGOSTRENGTH				
Basic Trust	product / process / giving meaning / thematic play			
Autonomy	product / process / giving meaning / thematic play			
Initiative	product / process / giving meaning / thematic play			
Industry	product / process / giving meaning / thematic play			

Figure 3: score form observation instrument 'the building of a hut'

The observation instrument 'the building of a hut', an instrument for measuring ego-strength of children in age of seven up and until twelve, had come alive!

4. National norm and validation study
In the pilot study it turned out that the observation-instrument 'the building of a hut' discriminates between clients and a norm population. The estimates of

reliability and validity, however, were very satisfying. As a result, this pilot research was extended into a national research project, which is currently taking place. The aim of this research is to set up a standard for scoring. A team of eleven dramatherapists are administering the observation-instrument with at least 750 children, aged 7 to 12 years, all over the country. A parallel validation study is taking place: the instrument will also be used by the clients of the eleven therapists together with other instruments which measure the psycho-emotional development, in order to validate the observation instrument.

The observation instrument 'the building of a hut' is planned to become a standardized observation instrument to measure the amount of egostrength and the amount of basic trust, autonomy, taking initiative and industry. At the same time the instrument offers outcomes concerning taking space, contact making and integrating. All these are important aspects in the psycho-emotional development of children. The best thing about the instrument is its nonverbal character. In this way, verbal abilities do not interfere with the test scores and I consider that this makes the observation instrument a more appropriate assessment method for children than existing verbal questionnaires.

5. Conclusion

I do not plead that every professional in the field of psychological health care should become a scientific researcher. But I do think that these professionals should be able to formulate their methodology more explicitly than is often the case now, by describing their frames of reference on the levels of professional knowledge, practitioner theories, psychological theories, experience and know-how and intuition. I am convinced that this will enhance greatly the grounding of very valuable visions of dramatherapists, or arts therapists in general.

References

Barron F. (1963). *Creativity and psychological health.* New Jersey: D. van Nostrand Company, Inc.
Carver C. S. & Scheier M.F. (1988). *Perspectives on personality* .Boston: Allyn and Bacon, Inc.
Erikson, E. H. (1964). *Het kind en de samenleving* Utrecht: Het Spectrum
Erikson, Erik H. (1987). A way of looking at things. Selected papers from 1930 to 1980. in Stephen Schlein (ed). New York: W.W. Norton and Company
Evers, A., Vliet-Mulder J.C.van, Groot C.J. (2000). *Documentatie van tests en testresearch in Nederland, deel I en II.* Assen: van Gorcum & Comp. World Wide Web page
Eurelings-Bontekoe, E.H.M. & Snellen, W.M. (2003). *Dynamische Persoonlijkheids Diagnostiek.* Lisse: Swets&Zeitlinger B.V.
Gabel, D., (1995). National Association for Research in Science Teaching (NARST) *An introduction to action research* from http:www. physicsed.buffalostate.edu/danowner/actionrsch.html
Kievit, Th., Wit, J. de, Groenendaal, J.H.A. & Tak, J.A. (red.), (1992). *Handboek psychodiagnostiek voor de hulpverlening aan kinderen.* Amersfoort: College uitgevers
Malchiody, Cathy A. (1998). *The Art Therapy Sourcebook, art making for personal growth, insight and transformation.* Illinois USA: NTC/ Contempory Publishing group, Inc.

Nixon, S.J. & Kanak, N.J. (1982). Ego-Strength and methods of learning associations. *Bulletin of the Psychonomic Society,* 19, No 4, 205-208

Reason, P., & Torbert, W. R. (2001). Toward a Transformational Science: a further look at the scientific merits of action research. *Concepts and Transformations,* 6(1), 1-37 *World Wide Web page*

Smeijsters, H. (2000). *Handboek Creatieve Therapie.* Bussum: uitgeverij Coutinho

Smith, M.K. (1996; 2001). *'Action research', the encyclopedia of informal education,* from http://www.infed.org/research/b-actres.htm

Strien van P.J. (1986). in Kievit &Tak *Handboek psychodiagnostiek voor de hulpverlening aan kinderen.* Amersfoort: college uitgevers. *World Wide Web page*

Vandermeulen, J.A.M. *Practische facetten in het kruisveldvan neuropsychologische behandeling bij niet-aangeboren hersenletsel.* from: http users.pandora.be/vvo/artikelvandermeulen.pdf *World Wide Web*

Vries, Y. (2004). *Onderwijsconcepten en professionele ontwikkeling van leraren vanuit praktijktheoretisch perspectief.* Dissertation from.http://www. library.wur.nl/wda/dissertations/dis3541.pdf

Walsh W.B. & Betz N.E. (1990). *Tests and Assessment* (second edition). New Jersey: Prentice Hall, Inc.

Zeeuw de, J. (1978). *Algemene Psychodiagnostiek I en II. Testmethoden en Testtheorie.* Amsterdam: Swets & Zeitlinger

EDITH LECOURT AND VIOLETA HEMSY DE GAINZA

RESEARCH IN ANALYTIC GROUP MUSIC THERAPY: ANALYSIS OF A WORKSHOP IN ARGENTINA. THE FOREIGN LEADER AND THE QUESTION OF TUNING THE EMOTIONAL INSTRUMENT IN THE GROUP

The experience of analytic group music therapy presented in this article is an illustration of research carried out over the last 25 years on how music production is an expression of the psychic structure itself. The theoretical backgrounds are the Freudian psychoanalysis enriched with analytical concepts developed in group analysis (Foulkes, 1964, 1975; Bion, 1961; Anzieu, 1975; Kaës, 1999), and musicology. The original method presented here (with recording and feedback) is used to give the necessary material for a precise analysis of the relationship between acoustic/music elements and structures, and psychic elements and structures emerging in group dynamics. The comparison of the evolution of two groups is a method that helps to distinguish the influences of individual and group differences, from those of the setting itself. The especial interest of this article is the exploration of the influence of intercultural difficulties in the processes of group communication, which is a very present day clinical preoccupation.

Through hundreds of such experiences our research has promoted concepts to describe the general states and movements in groups, their acoustic/music supports, expressions, and their psychic significances.

In August 1995, as a French group analyst and music-therapist, I was invited, along with an Argentinean music teacher, who happens to be the president of the Argentine Association of Music Education, to lead two workshops on group analysis in Buenos Aires. This experience gave us the opportunity to realize and analyze the role of language and cultural differences in group dynamics, particularly when there is a difference of language and culture between a group and its leader. It also led us to analyze the problem of the "handling" and the tuning of emotion within a group.

I. Presentation

To make the understanding of these experiences easier for the reader, we will, in the first part, give a summary of the development of each of these two groups – a diachronic approach – and then, in the second part, use a transversal approach to develop the principal issues raised by the comparison of the two groups. We will call these two groups "C" and "D" in the text. Thus the readers, who choose to go directly to the second part of this paper, will have the possibility to go back to the first part, should they need details for a better understanding.

The framework
Both workshops were organized by "Pedagogicas Musicales Abiertas", with the collaboration of the Argentine Association of Music Therapy and the Collegium Musicum of Buenos Aires. They were held in a room of this institution.

They were presented as experiences of sonorous communication in a group, based on Edith Lecourt's procedure. This procedure had already been tested in France and in different countries (1987, 1993, 1994), and the participants wanted to be trained in this approach which was new to them.

The general purpose of these workshops was first, to explore what is communicated in a group through sonorous sensoriality and, second, to observe the way the group-structure is constructed through sonorous communication.

Violeta Hemsy de Gainza, the Argentinean music teacher responsible for the promotion of the workshops, participated in the group's work, but only as an observer.

The setting: general principles
Sonorous improvisations in a group used as a tool to analyze group communications follow the same pattern: Each sonorous improvisation is limited to ten minutes and is recorded. It is followed by a free verbalization time. Then comes the listening phase, during which the subjects are invited to listen to their sonorous production. Finally, there is another verbalization time. Therefore the non-verbal and the verbal periods are alternated.

The rule for improvisation is expressly stated as follows: "Try to relate through sounds using non verbal expression". In the case of these two groups this rule was completed, after the first improvisation, by the command: "close your eyes". This facilitates the concentration on relationship through sounds and deepens the exploration of the sonorous world.

Although some simple music instruments (mainly of the percussion type) were at the participants' disposal, it was clearly understood that the purpose of the workshops was not to play music and that the instruments should be used "if necessary".

The leader did not participate in the sonorous productions, since she was here as the group-analyst.

The composition of the groups
The two groups were composed of professionals from both the musical field (professional musicians, music teachers, composers), and the clinical field (music therapists, psychotherapists, psychiatrists and psychoanalysts). It was possible to enter the workshops either as an active participant or as an observer. This is an unusual situation since normally there are no observers, as such group-experiences demand privacy. As a consequence we set up the following procedure: after each improvisation, first the observers, then the participants were requested to express themselves about their perceptions.

The program
The program was the same for the two groups: four sessions of group improvisations alternated with "sonorous dialogues" between two persons only.

The protagonists had to keep their eyes closed. This helps refine the sonorous exchanges between people and helps make their relational values manifest.

Each workshop lasted for ten hours (spread over two days for the first group and over three days for the second group). The musical instruments and the rooms were the same.

The encounter of two different cultures gave rise to certain peculiarities

Right from the beginning, the difference of languages between the leader (French) and the group (Spanish) appeared as a major difficulty. Only the presentation of the workshops, the rules and the syntheses were translated. No translation was given during verbalization times, although the translator, Segio H. Garcia, was present throughout the workshops. He took notes which were later transmitted to the leader.

This choice had a double function: to let the dynamics of the process take place (translation can take a very long time, especially during the moments of free verbalization), and to let the participants work through the language difficulties (verbal versus non verbal).

The fact that the translator was a professional musician, a composer, influenced the quality and the precision of the exchanges. Moreover, the couple leader/translator reflected the two professional components of these groups.

It was peculiar to observe that in both groups, because of the language difference, the experience focused on the issue of emotional expression within the group and of its *containment,* when the sharing of the same verbal code is missing. This difficulty was overcome in a way that is akin to the emotion that pervades the whole of Argentinean daily life and that was close to Argentina's musical roots (as was demonstrated by a vocal document from the aborigines of the north-west of Argentina, which displays intense emotion).

II. Summary of the two groups
Group 1 "C"

This group was composed of eleven participants, five men and six women (comprising music teachers, composers, music therapists and psychoanalysts) and of five observers, all of whom were music therapists.

After some questions and answers on small percussion instruments, the improvisation time (C1) began. The drum started, the tambourine answered followed by the whole group. Their production was very sonorous but its intensity was broken by two decrescendos and silences, then by three moments of "jamming". This term refers to a peculiar sonorous production which appears when everybody is shaking or rubbing their instruments (a very special sound indeed). A lot of energy emerged from the group, sustained by a binary rhythm in the background, running from one instrument to the other. The same rhythm served as a basis for the next sonorous productions.

The leader then suggested a sonorous dialogue: two women volunteered and played on two different tambourines; it sounded like a musical question and answer time; the sounds alternated from one instrument to the other, sometimes similar, sometimes complementary. This musical exchange was characterized by a relative shyness.

The second improvisation (C2) began in a very different way. Another element was introduced: the body, in the form of breathing sounds. Then came the sound of the "quiros", then the cymbals, then the voice. Two participants, a man and a woman, started singing. Their duet led the group to produce a sonorous ensemble. In the end, the group accompanied themselves by beating the floor with their hands. It is worth noting that once again it was a three-part structure, with two crescendos and a moment of silence.

In the verbalization time that followed two opposite reactions were successively voiced by the group: first, a feeling of satisfaction expressed in these terms: "it is fabulous, perfect!", which is typically the psychological effect of "group illusion" described by D. Anzieu (1975). "Group illusion" is a special moment in group dynamics which can be observed through the auto-satisfaction of the group: all the members are very pleased and speak of them as making a very "good group". D.Anzieu analyses this state as the expression of a fantasy of fusion (illusion of being "one"), a defence mechanism against the fear of lost of identity, of aggression ("break fantasy"), fears generally present at the beginning of a new group.

The second reaction was situated at the very end of the improvisation. It was the perception of a danger, of something threatening. This can be referred to as "break-fantasy", which is the opposite of group-illusion (for this author: these two fantasies are two faces of the same phenomenon: anxiety ("break-fantasy", which is a fantasy of chaos, destruction) and defence against anxiety ("group illusion")).

The emotional impact of the introduction of the voice was commented upon and a discussion started about the participants' opposite perceptions at the end of the production. Some of them spoke of "chaos, destruction", whereas others mentioned a "creative process". One of the participants even resorted to her professional identity, reminding the group that she was a "composer", to evaluate the artistic quality of the production. Thus, the problem of the differentiation of two levels of experience, one corporal, the other aesthetic was introduced.

The group started the third improvisation (C3) before the leader could recall the rules, thus creating a "sonorous carpet" that began with a participant we will call Xavier's continuous random-like playing of the xylophone. The breathing sounds were introduced again and the same couple as before introduced a litany which created a second temporality. While the sonorous carpet was sustained by a rapid ceaseless tempo, the litany was slow. The emphasis was laid on the sonorous continuum which was reinforced by the maintaining of a sharp vocal sound throughout the improvisation. These characteristics can be understood as a search for linkage after the risk of disorganization created by overwhelming emotions.

All that influenced the two following sonorous dialogues. The first was an exchange between a man and a woman. The woman played the tambourine and the man the "quiros". He was to be as surprised as the group by the possibilities of expressions offered by this instrument. For the observers, this dialogue conjured up the images of a "wedding ceremony" or of "a civilized conversation", which can be interpreted both as a satisfaction and as the assessment of a need for formality, made necessary to cover up the aggressiveness of the group.

For the second dialogue the leader asked the group to explore the role played by the instruments in a dialogue by trying to improvise without instruments. Two men volunteered. A fairly sonorous corporal expression was introduced which engendered two sorts of comments: on the one hand the dialogue was qualified and categorized as "civilized, human", on the other as "savage, animal". Once again, this reveals the need of the group to categorize as in C2.

Finally the fourth and last group improvisation (C4) began. It was endowed with the same energy as the first (C1). The timbre of the cymbal, then the drum which set up a precise recognizable rhythm facilitated the introduction of voices. It was followed by three vocal movements ending with a succession of chromatic glissendi, with some disorganization of voice timbres. This production evoked very clearly the Argentinean native culture: it was a reference to the "malambo" rhythm and to the "chacarera," a song of the north-west of Argentina. On hearing them a general feeling of satisfaction ran through the group.

Overall we can say that this group showed a lot of energy. This energy was channelled by their technical knowledge of music. Thus, music was used in a rather conventional way, which reduced possible explorations. In such a short experience, the need for mastering was the predominant element, categorization of the productions served as a defense against emotions perceived as disorganizing.

Group 2 "D"

This group was composed of eight participants only one of whom was a man (four music therapists, two music teachers, a body-therapist and a psychologist.) and of four observers (both music therapists and music teachers).

The first group improvisation (D1) began, before the leader could state the rules, by Lydia clapping her fingers. From the very first minutes a very smooth, delicate and intimate ambiance prevailed, with glissendi on the xylophone in triple piano! With this basic background sound the voice appeared as subdued as the ambiance itself. By listening closely we were able to identify right from the very first sounds the cues of the rhythm of Carmen's song (Bizet): "L'amour est enfant de Bohême", a rhythm that was to be asserted later on. Yet, it is only afterwards, during the detailed analysis of the recordings of the sessions, that this permanency became obvious, enhancing two opposed movements: that of rushing into the experience, and that of restraint.(Lydia said that she had to take the leadership and could not wait for any rule to be stated.)

The sonorous dialogue that followed played a central part in the workshop. A man and a woman volunteered. The woman, that we will call Sirene (mermaid) took the tambourine. The man, that we will call Ulysses, took a tambourine with cymbals and sat in front of the woman. Sirene started producing a vocal lament endlessly developed and repeated. Ulysses tried to relate musically, to contain the lament (with rhythm, for instance), but in vain. He relied basically on the instrument, offered rhythmical propositions and in the end, he tried a vocal accompaniment which led to some moments of duet. But very quickly he felt distraught and anxious. The insistent and monotonous lament went on and on and pervaded the group. Contrary to group improvisations, in the case of a sonorous dialogue, there is no rule setting a time-limit for the improvisation. The rule says: "You begin when you feel ready, and you end whenever you like". In the present case, however, the leader had to stop the exchange: the fairly emotional content of the dialogue and the hysterical dimension of the production created a feeling of anxiety within the group. This feeling was reinforced by the "mise en scène" of the dialogue: a couple, within a group.

The analysis of the recording shows that the voice gradually introduces itself. It begins with descending melodic movements, as a charming voice, a true mermaid's voice; then it repeatedly changes into breathing and rattling sounds until it becomes an expression of rage. All that creates a closed, repetitive discourse. An observer described the lament as "a permanent wailing" and the group perceived this experience as a failure and a threat. Sirene pretended that she had not heard the rule and that she had felt abandoned, left to herself, compelled to sing this never-ending lament, which she had gradually transformed into an attack against the setting.

The second group improvisation (D2) began. Ulysses pulled a diapason from his bag. He seized an "anklung", a bamboo instrument from Indonesia, examined it closely, and, with his diapason, tried to verify if it was tuned. Then, he decided to use only the diapason throughout the improvisation. It started with sighs, as if echoing the preceding dialogue, then the voice was introduced with a "speak-sing" ("parlando") vocalization that developed into a siren-sound (up and down movements as in a fire-alarm). Meanwhile the instrument kept setting a rhythmical movement in which the rhythm of Carmen's song was clearly heard. The voices tuned by singing a chord and from that a choir developed, improvising a sort of litany, accompanied by this sustained rhythm. This ten-minute improvisation was spontaneously brought to an end by the group through a decrescendo. It was the source of a genuine aesthetic emotion. This group can be said to have created an authentic composition starting from this painful, crude and authentic lament, progressively integrated in a musical form.

About the first part of the improvisation, the members of the group spoke of "a collective catharsis" in which an attempt had been made to speak an unknown language. They pointed out the musical richness of the improvisation and they recognized in it a simple African rhythm, the "habanera".

One of the participants, a woman, then asked the leader if she could explain the chapter that she had written in D. Anzieu's collective book on "psychic envelopes" (1987) "The musical envelope". In this chapter I argue that music is a form of protection against not only chaos, but also the intrusiveness of noises and sounds, it offers an organised foresighting world (offering a containment like an "envelope"). It is a psychic construction like the other "psychic envelopes" described by D.Anzieu. I underline also the other sonorous risk, which is to feel overflowed by corporal or emotional sounds (cries, weeps etc.), with which Sirene felt particularly concerned. As the participant used the title of this chapter "the musical envelope", it can sustain the interpretation that the problem of a "container" for emotions was central to this experience.

The third improvisation (D3) began in the same way as the first, with the same discretion, the same pattern of questions and answers. It was well-mastered and led by Lydia, the participant who had at the beginning of the workshop (D1) anticipated the enunciation of the rule. This time, the group stopped before the allotted ten minutes, anticipating the end which normally is marked by a signal from the leader. The first part was a polyphonic production (third rhythm and pantatonic chant in major C, with a peculiarly timbred voice) in which the "anklung" played a fairly sonorous part. It was followed by two sonorous dialogues. The first was between Lydia and Ariane, two assertive personalities. It sounded like an extremely expressive children's play and was spontaneously applauded by the groups. It offered a relief to the tension engendered by the dialogue between Sirene and Ulysses. The second was between Cecilia and Paula. It was very sensitive, even intimate. It took the form of an emotion-filled duet and was perceived by the group as the expression of the development of a love relationship). Some participants commented on it with great sensitivity and emotion.

The fourth improvisation (D4) started. The "anklung" was passed around the group before being taken by one participant. The sonorous production began with the successive entrance of several instruments until a group performance was achieved. There was a murmur, then a silence, then another murmur followed by a choir developing from two musical themes, one rhythmic, the other melodic. This is when the cultural reference clearly appeared in the form of music from the Andes (binary rhythm, minor pentatonic)."We are going to the north" was the message the group members heard and commented upon. It meant a return to their origins.
The physical journey of the group can actually be heard in the music. It is a nostalgic "Good bye!". The song starts with the vocalization of the lament sustained by a dynamic, rapid and vital rhythm, with the rhythmics of Carmen's song in the background. This composition is obvious when one listens to the recording of this improvisation. The group dedicated the choir to the leader. They presented their performance as a compliment to the foreign leader, as an echo of her personality and they offered her their music as a gift.

Thus, in this group, we could observe the search for a containment of emotion, an elaboration of the lament and its symbolization which led to a musical creation. Contrary to what happened with the first group, whose work remained under control, in this second group emotion prevailed and they took relational risks, elaborating on emotions to compose music.
The difference of functioning of these two groups can be explained by their composition. They were different as regards sex-ratio (we will come back to this point later) as well as regarding professional activities. The first group, in which there was a greater number of professional musicians, stuck to activities and a way of listening that was more technical than relational. In the second group emotion prevailed.
The question of difference, symbolized by the presence of a foreign leader, and the question of emotional expression in a group thus became the link between these two workshops.

III. Thematic analysis
As we don't have enough space to develop all the different items of this analysis in this article, we have chosen to present some reflexions on emotion and the role of the musical instrument in these situations.

The emotional pattern:

It is obvious that some sort of emotional language had sustained these two groups. Couldn't then, the emotional expression be seen as a "common denominator" to the different cultures? This assumption may explain the importance given to the emotional language by these two groups.

Because of the particular situation created by the absence of translation, analogical communication, even if it is generally considered as secondary to verbal exchanges, was put to the forefront. Some participants were particularly attentive to gestures, mimics, eye-contacts etc. They concentrated to be sure they were understood by the leader, while others talked at great length without bothering to establish any contact with her. On the part of the participants, as on the part of the leader, the listening task was highly influenced by this unusual situation. In fact, the first group had already "chosen" to create a composition, using different levels of expression and categorizing them. They were concerned by the distinction between corporal and aesthetic expressions. Let us recall that, with the entrance of the voice, the end of the second improvisation (C2) was perceived by some participants as a risk of destruction. This occurred when the composer's identity was verbally expressed in the group. Thus, the production of the group was really "composed" and the "Afro-style" voice (myxolidian mode, in G second) engendered a musical play on chromatism and scales which led to the mixing in the third improvisation (C3) of the two levels: the sonorous carpet and the chant. But this little vocal incursion did not go very far. The fourth improvisation (C4) asserted once again the musical and cultural identity of the group. It is actually a desire for mastery that governs the group. The emotional dimension recognized by the group through the introduction of the voice remains on a group level.

The second group was very different. As we have already seen, emotion was expressed through Sirene's massive demand, which was perceived by the group as depressing, bottomless, and highly distressing. At first it was just the emotional expression of one member of the group, but gradually the question of giving shape to and containing the emotion took a central place in the group's experience and their play with vocal sirens expresses directly the urgency of the situation. They gave their emotion a shape by using the "Afro" rhythm known as "habanera". But they also contained it and this containment is expressed by the fairly elaborated endings (codas) of each improvisation. Their progressively attained mastery is obvious in the next two dialogues: they are very sensitive on the relational level and at the same time contained in duration as well as in musicality. The musicalization of the initial lament has thus totally engulfed the group's composition task up to the final choir in which a song, elaborated from the lament but with a vital rhythm efficiently sustaining the depressing effect, can be recognized.

The bamboo instrument, a metaphor:

The "anklung" is a bamboo instrument from Indonesia. It is composed of three bamboo pipes which slip on stems fixed to a closed frame. When it is shaken the pipes produce deep sounds by knocking against the stems. It creates a sort of "sonnailles" or chiming. The importance for the groups was that it was a foreign instrument. It was used with relative indifference by the first group as trivialized by professional knowledge and skills. The second group clearly manifested its curiosity for the instrument as an object. In their first improvisation (D1) they used it to a limited extent.. In their second improvisation (D2), they introduced it by asking questions about how to handle it, how to play it and how to tune it. They passed it around until it became central to the experience. In the second group the "anklung" took the role of the foreigner, became the actual double of the foreign leader. It also symbolized what remains unknown and strange within emotional expression.

Once more it can be observed that the second group showed a very different sensitivity and a greater availability to metaphor than the first group which seems to have stayed within the limits of what it could master.

Let us now reconsider the place and status given to this Indonesian instrument, "the anklung" which appears at the end of this analysis as a metaphor for the body as emotional instrument.

Its fragility (bamboo), the way it is shaken to produce sounds, the approximation of its sounds and of its tuning, which make it difficult to control, are all characteristics that bring it closer to the emotional experience. This instrument produces an approximate language that must constantly be decoded or interpreted. In opposition, the deep-rooted percussion instrument, the "caja" drum, gives an image of a solid body with a clear expression. These two instruments illustrate two different aspects of corporal experiences: solidity, energy and control on the one hand and fragility on the other. Finally this very part of the experience referred us all to our difficulties of language.

These two groups dealt with the difficulties in very different manners. The sexual ratio of each group certainly accounts for that. In the first group there was a balance between the number of men and women, whereas in the second group there was only one man. We can assume that the first group set itself mainly on the genital level, around the couple. The couple appeared in the vocal duet, in the couple of leaders, with a progressive passage inside the group from a feminine leader to a masculine one. In this group the question of the instrument was raised in the heterosexual sonorous dialogue, about the big drum taken by the woman and the small instrument – but with new capacities – chosen by the man ("quiros"). This dimension of couple was also, in this case, an echo of the leader/translator couple organizing the group.

The second group can be situated on the pregenital level: the fusional experience of the first sonorous dialogue, the search for an envelope as well as the question of instrumental tuning are all features linked to this level. The diapason as a musical instrument was not, in this perspective, opposed to a bigger instrument, but addressed fundamentally the emotional tuning with the group, with the leader.

This tuning refers to the original tuning to the mother which is the first form of understanding.

After the failure of the first heterosexual dialogue (Sirene/Ulysses), the image of a couple appeared in this group: It was a homosexual couple (Paula/Cecilia). However one will remark that Ulysses started with small instruments (woodblock, diapason), and finished the experience by asserting himself on the "caja" drum. What a progression in this women's group!

In the same way, as regards the introduction of emotion, we have seen how it appeared as group-based in the first group whereas it was initially individual in the second (with Sirene).

Let us recall here O. Avron's works (1986, 1990, 1991) on "group emotionality". After Bion, Ophélia Avron is a psychoanalyst especially interested in the emotional level in group dynamics. She considers that there is a basic "interactional rhythmic emotionality" between individuals (stimulation/reception) which can be even viewed as an impulse, different from the sexual impulse – an impulse to search human contact. The Sirene/Ulysse 's dialogue is a good illustration of this rhythmic, emotional interaction.

The notion of "group emotionality" would apply here more to the first group than to the second, except if we consider the minimalist improvisation (D1), which preceded the Sirene-Ulysses dialogue, as a putting into resonance this restrained emotion, before the emergence of an individual dimension through Sirene. As we have already seen, what followed was a work of containment, of composition, a working through, a transformation, up to the level of aesthetic emotion.

These experiences with Franco-Argentinean groups and their analyses situate cultural differences on the pregenital level. In any case it is the second group that showed the necessary mobility to investigate language, culture, otherness, and foreignism of emotion. It is also the one which was more sensitive to the transfer dimension. Couldn't the quotation-which remained implicit-of Carmen's song "L'amour est enfant de Bohême... Si tu ne m'aimes pas, je t'aime...Prends garde à toi!", a song whose rhythm pervaded the group, be considered as a sort of group "air dans la tête" (a tune that remained stuck in their minds)? The final song, which expressed the return to the origins, could be considered as the only manifest part of the discourse. And this double hearing reflects the synthesis of emotional and cultural aspects (traditional music and classical music combined). Bearing this interpretation in mind, the "gift" is to be received with caution. The lament was integrated and musically transformed into a demand for love, for reciprocal love, in transfer reaction to the restraint manifested by the leader toward the productions of the group.

References

Anzieu, D. (1975). *Le groupe et l'inconscient*. Paris: Dunod

Anzieu, D. et al. (1987). *Les enveloppes psychiques*. Paris: Dunod. (*Psychic envelopes*, London: Karnac Books, 1990; *Gli involucri psichici*, Milano: Dunod/Masson, 1997)

Avron, O. (1986). "Mentalité de groupe et émotionnalité groupale". *Revue de psychothérapie psychanalytique de groupe*. 5-6, pp. 67-75

—1990 « Le groupe : émotionnalité rythmique ». *Psychanalyse à l'université*. 15, 60, 55-66

—1991 « Le processus participatif scénique ». *Revue de psychothérapie psychanalytique de groupe*. 17, pp. 63-74

—1996 *La pensée scénique, groupe et psychodrame*, Toulouse: Erès

Bion, W.R. (1961). *Experiences in groups and other papers*, London: Tavistock

Foulkes, H.S. (1964). *Therapeutic Group Analysis*, London: Allen and Unwin.

Foulkes, H.S. (1975). *Group Analytic Psychotherapy: Methods and Principles*, London: Gordon and Breach

Kaes, R. (1993). *Le groupe et le sujet du groupe. Eléments pour une théorie psychanalytique du groupe*, Paris: Dunod

Kaes, R. (1999). *Les théories psychanalytiques du groupe*, Paris: P.U.F.

Lecourt, E. (1986) « L'émotion musicale, entre art et thérapie ». *Actes du festival Art et thérapie: Sur les chemins de l'émotion. Bruxelles, 21-23 février*, pp.42-49

—1987. « Identité culturelle et création groupale polyphonique, une expérience franco-marocaine ». *Revue de psychothérapie psychanalytique de groupe*. 9/10, pp. 57-78

—1990. « Una musica antica come l'Umanita, Experienza di communicazione sonora psiccoanalitica a Napoli. *Musicoterapie/Fone*. Editnews. 4, 17-31

—1993. *Analyse de groupe et musicothérapie. Le groupe et le sonore*. Paris, Editions Sociales Françaises (ESF). *Analisis de grupo y musicoterapia, el grupo y lo sonoro*. 2005. Victoria-Gasteiz (Spain) PRODUCCIONES AGRUPARTE. Assise (Italia) : La Citadella 1996 *Analisi di gruppo e musicoterapia, il gruppo e il « sonoro »*.

—1994. « Modèles de groupes et cultures : la musique comme révélateur ». *Connexions*, 63, 1, pp. 159-168.

—2005. *Découvrir la musicothérapie*. Paris : Eyrolles pratique

—2006. *Découvrir la psychanalyse*. Paris : Eyrolles pratique

—2006. *Le sonore et la figurabilité*. Paris : L'Harmattan

—2006. *El grito esta siempre afinado. Vinetas de la clinica musicoterapeutica*. Buenos Aires: Grupo Editorial Lumen

—2007. *La musicothérapie analytique de groupe*. Courlay (France): J.M. Fuzeau

VICKY ZERVA-SPANOU

PASSAGES TO TRANSFORMATION

This paper aims to outline the process of a child-centered Play Therapy intervention with a young woman named Pollyanna[1] who had difficulty in sharing emotions, in recollecting experiences of her early childhood, avoided body contact and resisted sexual arousal. The therapeutic use of creative tools allowed her to reveal symbolically her early life traumatic experiences and emotions that had, until then, been repressed. Through the metaphors of play she made sense of her experiences and expressed difficult feelings connected with them. At around the twentieth session she described her therapeutic process as "Passages to Transformation" by drawing a caterpillar just about to transform into a colourful butterfly.

Play therapy in contrast to psychoanalytic child psychotherapy, structured ('problem focused') play therapy or narrative therapy does not attempt to guide or alter the client's experiences but allows, with the use of different ways of metaphorical communication such as drawing, embodiment, clay, stories, narratives, puppetry and role play, the creation a safe and trusting space where experiences and emotions can be expressed and contained.

The intentional use of creative activities as a healing process is what makes the Play Therapy intervention therapeutic, and differentiates therapy from the simple participations in play or art, for their own sake (Cattanach, 1999). The therapist respects the client's ability to create through means of expression more suitable to their personality, uses interpretation only as clues for further exploration, respects the client's space and time, stays with the feeling of the client and co-constructs a relationship with them that is mediated through the medium of play.

Case study

Pollyanna was an attractive young woman, in her early twenties, the first child of a middle class family with a brother three years younger than herself. Both her parents were highly educated. She was at that time studying to become a dance-music teacher; she had rather few friends and lived for the last couple of years with a partner five years older than her.

Pollyanna was referred for Play Therapy by her Physician. Although her symptoms were physical, they were believed to be psychogenic in origin, caused by anxiety and tension, and so psychological intervention was recommended. She had had both eyes operated upon after the retina was detached – something unusual for such a young age; had just recovered from pestilent mononucleosis, had suffered from persistent headaches and several times had experienced numbness when trying to stand up for her rights.

It is worth mentioning that when taking her case history, Pollyanna could hardly recollect any of her early life experiences. She had then described her infancy as

---

[1] the name and demographic information has been changed and it was given written consent for the presentation as well as the art work.

being good enough, her parents as "a piece of gold", naïve and caring. She had no special events to share apart from staying for long periods of time with her grandparents, the feeling of being afraid of her father for reasons she could not remember and jealous of her brother, whom she said their mother treated as a favoured child. She also shared her 'illogical', as she characterized it, fear, since early childhood of a feeling of being swallowed or eaten up by snakes or sharks that could come out of the bath tub or the sea. Therefore she would avoid taking a bath or swim in an open sea.

In her early twenties Pollyanna gave the impression of a joyful, rather extraverted, fashionably dressed young woman. While moving her body stayed stiff and withdrawn; her face hardly changed expressions when sharing emotions and she generally avoided physical closeness. There was the impression that her body communicated what could not be spoken or articulated through words at that time (White, 2004).

Metaphorical forms of communication (stories, narratives, sand play, drawing, role-play and puppetry) rather than conventional talk seemed more appropriate in the exploration of her experiences and processing of her feelings. The respect for the client's ability to create means of expression most suitable to their personality, competencies and emotional life is at the heart of non-directive Play Therapy intervention.

Play Therapy sessions took place once a week for an hour, initially for twenty sessions. The intervention was then extended for over a year. The first sessions were focused on taking her case history and building trust and confidence in the therapeutic relationship. Little information about her infancy was shared at that point. The questions, however, raised many different issues concerning her early childhood that she was later going to explore at her own pace and in her own time. At the fifth session Pollyanna came in a state of panic. She was breathing heavily and was mostly uncomfortable on the seat. She could not make any connection between experiences she might have had lately and the stress she was experiencing. The therapist suggested she draw a symbol to describe her feeling, to give it a shape, colour it, and think of its speed and weight. Drawing is a preferred expressive medium Play Therapists choose in order to make visible and manageable very troubling current experiences and memories.

> 'To find a symbol means detaching from the object it represents and this aesthetic distancing is critical for the safety of the abused child.' (Cattanach, 1992: 43)

Though the projection may at first glance appear to have nothing to do with the client or her life, it is "out there", safe. It is often called a "defense mechanism", a defense against hurt to the inner self, a disclosure of the self; a projection that may express fantasies, anxieties, fears, avoidances, frustrations, patterns, resistances, guilt, wishes, needs, feelings (Oaklander, 1988).

She chose brown and black crayons and created what she called a bowl full of rain. Her drawing, as she then explained, represented the fear of an impending menace. Containing it in a bowl enabled her to deal with it. By giving concrete representation to her inner reality and having thus taken appropriate distance from it, she was then encouraged to explore further characteristics of the menace. It was a hard menace, heavy as an iron, hanging over people's head. The menace kept coming and going without any notice. Sometimes it hurt people for no reason and its whereabouts and next target were unknown. People had to be very cautious and aware of its warning signs in order to avoid it; they had to be observant, cool blooded, fast moving and needed to create a shield made of strong, hard, undissolvable metal, in order to defend themselves. The "menace" did not mean any harm though. It was in its nature to oppress. It was once created by opponent sadistic forces, and it had itself experienced violence. It had no age. It was there eternally, it was and it would stay there. In order to get close to people it changed forms, it could take a liquid form, and thus intrude without being noticed.

She then structured her description into a narrative:

"Once upon a time there was a menace. People were frightened and shivered upon its coming. They were scared in case they would meet it accidentally in the street as they walked without concern. They neither knew where nor when it would come. As the menace was unpredictable and awesome, the people were very scared of it. They created strong shields in order to defend themselves and that was how they carried on living".

In the following session she connected her art creation with memories of her infancy.

> 'Working with "line/colour/shape" drawings clearly bypass the mind and its intellectualization and go directly to the source of the feelings, [they] also allow the clients a unique opportunity vividly to capture "feelings" on paper and to visualize their emotions.' (Jennings, 1995:126)

Pollyanna shared experiences of domestic violence in her family. Her father used to force both children to obey his commands by smacking them both hard in the presence of their mother, who remained a mere observer. He often chased his son with a kitchen knife threatening to cut off his ear. It was during one of those terrifying incidences that Pollyanna hid herself under the kitchen table and tried to scream for help but no sound came out. Her body had gone stiff, her limbs were unable to move and cold air was surrounding her skin. Several times she was threatened to have her skin burnt by her father's cigarette ash. In order for her torture to end she would plead with him to get it over and done with. She neither knew when her father would get upset nor the reason that would trigger his anger. Pollyanna remembered being hit on the hand, by an olive branch or a "fly killer". She remembered being hit up to her teens.

Another important aspect of the father's behaviour that made things even more complex for Pollyanna was that her father often stared at her with lust, made sexual remarks about her appearance and insisted on being hugged and kissed by her, against her own will. Pollyanna shared feelings of guilt for accepting, not resisting and giving in to his demands. She had not considered, until then, that a child cannot be in control or exercise free choice with an adult.

'Adults have more power than children. This is an immutable biological fact. Children are essentially a captive population; totally dependent upon their parents or other adults for their basic needs...thus they will do whatever they perceive to be necessary to preserve a relationship with their caretakers'. (Herman, 1981: 27)

It was very important at that time for me the therapist not to identify with the victim or with the offender and allow the client free expression so that she might understand her own feelings in her own time. Thus she was able later to identify with a father who had also been a source of caring and affection in her life.
On the tenth session she shared a dream:
The heroine of the dream was a young girl, round about her age that had to save her boyfriend who had been kidnapped, imprisoned and tortured by brute people who captured anyone that did not share their personal views.
In order for the therapist to clarify the themes, conflicts, difficulties, coping resources and emotional states, several questions were cautiously asked.
It was discovered that the heroine travelled by a big ship at night, in deep darkness, among strangers in order to reach the place the rascals lived. Just before reaching the shore a black and white striped devilfish attacked the ship and nearly capsized it. The heroine got in a cage made of glass. That cage saved her and enabled her to reach the shore. There she confronted the 'rascals' who were racist, oppressive, tough, violent and imprisoned all who differed from them. The heroine had at first experienced fear, panic and distress, but she then used her brain, intuition, speed, swiftness and ability to communicate in their language and thus managed to save her friend.
It was proposed to draw the dream in six parts according Mooli Lahad's BASICPh. The parts followed the questions: who was the main character of the story, what was the task of that character, who or what helped in that task, what were the obstacles in the way, how did the main character go about it, what was the outcome of the story.

'The assumption is that by telling a projected story based on the elements of fairy tale and myth, we may be able to see the way that the self projects itself in organized reality in order to meet the world'. (Lahad, 2000: 99)

The connection of that story with Pollyanna's experiences and her ways of coping with both hers and her parents' opponent sides (good and bad), her coping methods (glass cage-numbness, powers) were more than obvious in that story.
During the next couple of sessions the first described "piece of gold" naïve and caring parents kept taking different names: "monsters, bloodthirsty beasts, disgusting figures that devoured their victims", as well as "special and precious characters".
On the fifteenth session the therapist suggested that Pollyanna choose some miniatures in order to represent her family members and then to create a short imaginary story using those chosen figures. She chose four miniatures for that task:

- a dwarf with a stupid, twisted, slimy looking face(father),
- a sensitive but powerful fairy (herself),
- a vicious witch who wanted to get rid of the fairy (mother),
- a weasel that bit and occasionally helped the witch (brother).

The narrative she structured follows:
All four characters lived in a forest where warriors were imposing the laws. The dwarf wanted to extinguish the warriors and be the only one to exercise power in the forest. In order to accomplish his aim he tried to persuade the fairy, using his familiar seductive vision, to hand over her powerful magic filter. The fairy was deluded and handed the magic filter over to him. Thus the dwarf fought against the warriors and won. Soon after the witch and the weasel, who was the witch's lawful and loyal servant, helped the dwarf to capture the fairy. They imprisoned her in a cave. The fairy called out to her friends, the forest's good spirits, for help. They lent their powers to her and so she managed to escape. Having regained her strength she was empowered and went to face the dwarf. She ordered him never to enter the forest again.
The story reflected different aspects of the client's inner realities. At that point it was important to notice that though the fairy had had very troublesome experiences, she had managed to escape and to face her offender.
Inspired by that story in the next session Pollyanna brought a song she had written during that week, as well as the music she had composed to accompany it. The title was: "The Opposite of Zombiefication"; she left the manuscript with me. It follows exactly the way she had written it:

The Joy is over!
No more happy days
The deads are back
From their heavy graves.

Don't worry, they won't hunt you
They haven't come for you
It's other things they're after
Though they remember you!

The dead are little children
That you buried alive
You forced them to become
Something they didn't like.

Don't worry, they won't hunt you
They haven't come for you
It's other things they're after
Though they remember you

The deads are back!
The deads are little children
That you buried alive
You forced us to become
Something we didn't like

Don't worry, we won't hurt you
We haven't come for you
It's other things we're after
Though we remember you.

She explained that the emotions that emerged from the story she had created in the previous session had inspired her imagination and thus the words and the music to accompany the song came quite naturally.

She wanted me to listen to the song. She shared how difficult and painful the process of composing, singing and listening to her own voice had been. She was still feeling the pain there and then. It was hard to bear feelings that hurt like a burning iron.

She connected her feelings with a documentary film she had once watched on the television. It was about a tribe that lived on a Caribbean island. As far as she remembered the witch doctors of that tribe were giving poisonous herbs to youngsters to render them unconscious. They then buried them alive. The youngsters could feel the process of being buried alive but were unable to react. A few seconds before dying the witch doctors would take them out of their graves and give them the antidote that brought them back to life. These youngsters were called 'zombies'. The experience of being alive yet unable to react as they were buried, stayed vivid for as long as they lived.

Pollyanna went even deeper that day. She recollected a nightmare she often had when she was a child. In that nightmare her parents were hitting her so hard that she would fall into a deep sleep. The pain experienced in those dreams was still vivid after waking up. She herself commented that, like the zombies, her own life experiences of abuse were so strong that she had to freeze many of her feelings in order to bear them.

Inspired by her song in the next session she decided to draw instead of talking.

She created a blur picture using crayons with no borders; black, red and blue curly lines running all over the page; she gave it the title "Hell". Symbols are highly likely to be fragmented and confused when emotional events and situations are complex (Slade, 1994).

She talked about her drawing and said that though it had many different colours, it represented a dark space that contained tension and movement. She discerned four figures, three on the left, one on the right, that could probably represent her parents and her. There was a jelly sort of substance in between them. Amidst that jelly substance laid all the episodes she had witnessed during her childhood. In the session, she experienced a feeling of suffocation, quite similar to the feeling she experienced as a child. She did not want to share more at that point.

During the next few sessions there was no further mentioning of her past. She was bringing everyday situations mainly difficulties that had occurred in relation to her mother, brother, partner and friends.

On the twentieth session she shared feeling tense. It was a tension, similar to the one that kept coming and going every now and then since she was a child. The therapist asked her whether that tension was connected to a situation. She described it as a reaction to an intimate body contact that would last more than she could endure. In these situations she had the feeling that her body itself reacted towards a coming danger.

I decided to use embodiment play to get her closer to that feeling, to facilitate her gaining further sensory experience. She initially used words to create a picture – a picture of her hands tightly embracing her body and creating a shield of protection.

In order to get even closer to that feeling I suggested she let her body take that position and experience there and then the feeling she had just described. She was then encouraged to slowly breathe the feeling in through the nose for a count of three and out through the mouth. To facilitate a transformational change I then proposed to her to adopt an opposite posture – a posture in which her body would feel loose. She then experimented with the breathing in and out exercise. Questions about the colour, the weight, the sound, the speed of both feelings were then posed that were followed by two drawings. The first drawing representing the tension was named *"The Grip"* the other was named *"Colours"*.

While choosing pencils, memories of her mother's attitude during her adolescence arose. She recollected her mother denying the changes of her body during her adulthood. It was becoming clear to her that her mother denied her physical potential to grow. The use of a razor to eliminate the growth of hair was forbidden. She was chastised for asking to buy a bra, her mother commenting that she had nothing to put in it. The word boyfriend was a taboo never to be mentioned. Pollyanna herself connected the tension of her body with the impression just shared: her needs as a child completely diminished as well as ignored by her mother. Her journey through puberty was lonely; she had to find her way through it all by herself, searching for answers, craving for fragments of love from a mother who refused to accept her daughter's passage from childhood to adulthood, as she said.

On the next session she shared a very vivid sensation of her body being a caterpillar just about to shed its skin and become a butterfly. The necessary innate seeds of change were beginning to develop.

She talked about the caterpillar and its process of change. It was a colourful, small but happy caterpillar as it knew that one day it would transform into a beautiful butterfly. Though most people did not like caterpillars, it learnt to ignore that notion as it knew for sure that transformation was to come. It needed though to work hard for it.

It had to look after itself, to search for food, keep warm, create a shelter to hide from danger and be cautious when coming out into the sun. On several occasions birds tried to eat it up as it looked so delicious. On other occasions, people nearly stepped on it as they did not like it. It got in their way. Both birds and people kept trying to extinguish it. It always managed to escape though… and one day it discovered the way to hide from them. It built its own safe place, where no one could enter and thus slowly – slowly it started to transform. Time did not matter, it could take as much time as it needed. The result was what counted and it would be rewarding. Time went by and one day it looked at the mirror and saw itself! It was transformed! It had become a pretty, big, colourful butterfly. Joy overfilled its heart!

That narrative represented more or less Pollyanna's process of the transformation she had gone through in Play Therapy. She realized that more issues of her past were to be revealed and that the journey had to carry on going in order to resolve past experiences and let go negative influences. Therefore we both decided to carry on after the twentieth session for as long as needed. We both respected the gentle pace we had to follow for new resources to be integrated into her life.

Conclusions

More detailed approaches used in this process were not discussed in depth in this presentation. The intention was to focus on the means of creative work used by the client to externalize internal experiences and memories of her past that was hard to bear and difficult to verbalize. The Play Therapist and the client established a relation together and mediated that relationship through different medium of play.

In the early stages of therapy familiarity, boundaries and trust were established. Having gained a sense of emotional security in a therapeutic relationship that contains, sustains, accepts, respects the client's pace, time and abilities, the client was enabled not only to explore experiences of the past but also to discover her own mechanisms of coping, dealing, facing, and gaining mastery over those experiences.

As she was becoming more confident, she started giving concrete representation to her inner reality. By the use of mostly projective and embodiment play she was enabled to bring up memories of her childhood, recognized their reality and prepared defenses so as to be more assertive. The scenes of domestic violence, as well as behaviours that were both inappropriate to relationships and to her age, were externalized, understood and assimilated. She symbolically externalized issues and feelings she identified with and clarified them without reducing or simplifying them.

The passages to transformation were revealed as the therapy progressed.

The horrifying memories had to be contained in a bowl and while they were projected 'out there', it was possible to explore them safely. By structuring narratives conflicts and difficulties, coping resources were expressed, understood, explored and clarified. It was thus that the "deads came back from their graves and faced their offenders". The pronoun 'they' became 'we' (not yet 'I'). The client then dared to come closer to her own experience of 'dying alive' and 'freezing' in order to survive the abuse.

Complex emotional tensions that were first symbolized as fragmented and confused were then experienced through embodiment play. The body started getting sensory experiences. Those experiences were witnessed in all their fullness by both herself and the therapist. We were both constructing a relationship gaining access into her internal world and memories of her past. She described the passages to transformation of that Play Therapy process sharing the sensation of being a caterpillar shedding its body in order to become a colourful butterfly. She had found her inner seeds of change and was at the threshold of experiencing a less distorted sense of self and others, gradually leading her way to find forms of resolution. She had recognized the inner ability to heal by using forms of art. The inner resources lying dormant within her had become alive.

References
Cattanach, A. (1992). *Play Therapy with Abused Children*. London: Jessica Kingsley Publishers Ltd.
Cattanach, A. (1994). *Play Therapy Where the Sky Meets the Underworld*. London: Jessica Kingsley Publishers Ltd.
Cattanach, A. (1997). *Children's Stories in Play Therapy*. London: Jessica Kingsley Publishers Ltd.
Cattanach, A. (1999). *Process in the Arts Therapies*. London: Jessica Kingsley Publishers Ltd.
Herman, J.L (1981). *Father-Daughter Incest* .Library of Congress Cataloging in Publication Data, Harvard College
Jennings, S. (1993). *Playtherapy with Children*. Oxford: Blackwell Scientific Publications.
Jennings, S. (1995). *Dramatherapy with Children and Adolescents*. London: Routledge
Lahad, M. (2000). *Creative Supervision*. London: Jessica Kingsley Publishers Ltd.
Oaklander, V. (1978/1988). *Windows to Our Children*. New York: The Gestalt Journal Press
Slade, A. (1994). 'Making meaning and making believe: their role in the clinical process' In A. Slade and D.P. Wolf (Eds) *Children at Play*. Oxford: Oxford University Press, 81-107
White, K. (2004). *Touch, Attachment and the Body.* London: Karnac (Books) Ltd.
Wilson, K., Kendrick, P. and Ryan, V. (1992). *Play Therapy: A Non-Directive Approach for Children and Adolescents*. London: Bailliere Tindall

KATERINA COUROUCLI-ROBERTSON

IN SEARCH OF AN IDENTITY: INDIVIDUAL DRAMATHERAPY WITH A CLIENT SUFFERING FROM PANIC ATTACKS

In the following paper I will present the case of a client who wished to overcome her fears and become more self-sufficient. The vignette that follows is based on a two-year Dramatherapy intervention.

People suffering from panic disorder experience sudden extreme terror. This is called a "panic attack." A person may feel as if they are in great danger or even think they are dying or losing their mind. This can become an obsessive fear, with the result that they are constantly worrying about having an attack in an enclosed space. A consequence of this is that they develop agoraphobia and are afraid to leave home.

Panic disorder clients have a tendency to interpret benign bodily sensations as signs of impending physical or mental catastrophe, such as a heart attack or a psychotic decompensation. (Beck & Emery, 1985; Clark, 1986). Once such a misinterpretation is made, the individual succumbs to a vicious cycle in which the panic reaction triggered by the misperception is taken as further confirmation that some type of physical or psychological catastrophe is imminent.

According to Bergin and Garfield (1994) there are currently two prominent models of panic pathogenesis. The neurological model which postulates a defect in brain function, possibly related to the part of the brain that orchestrates infant separation responses. This defect is thought to be best described by characterizing physiologic processes, such as neurotransmitter abnormalities and hormonal or metabolic imbalance. Then there is the cognitive-behavioural model, which postulates that panic occurs because of a psychological mechanism in which conditioned reactivity to bodily sensations occurs, mediated by a conditioned fear response or cognitive misinterpretation of interceptive cues. They go on to say that a third integrated model can be constructed using principles of each of the others.

My client, whom I will refer to as Ali, suffered from high blood pressure and tachycardia and sometimes paralysing panic attacks. The panic attacks usually took place when she was travelling. The most common occurrence was when she drove to work along the motorway.

During Dramatherapy Ali was also keen to investigate her sexual identity. Before her marriage she had had a passionate affair with a woman. This relationship came to an end after the interventions of both her mother and fiancé.

While working with Ali I found that it was best to concentrate on the themes she brought to each session rather than focus on her panic attacks. My dramatherapy techniques needed to be adapted for Ali as she felt self-consciousness in role-play and movement. Ali was best facilitated with projective techniques, sand-play, drawing, stories and clay. Her dreams were also very good material to work with and focusing on them helped her avoid her tendency to intellectualise.

The reason I chose this client was because Ali has puzzled me. It would appear that there was an issue in Ali's life regarding control, which was mirrored in our relationship. One minute she needed total control and the next she handed over the reins. It is likely that this behaviour stems from her losing her father at the age of seven before she had been able to develop into a whole personality. At that time, she also lost her home because of financial reasons. She was separated from her mother most of the day, as she had to start working to support her family. This issue of control was apparent throughout Ali's treatment. At the end of her therapy she gained control over our relationship by discontinuing at a time when I believed she was still very vulnerable.

Ali was in her early forties, a professional, mother and wife. She had had experience of psychotherapy in the past, with the result that she would always stand up to leave after the 50 minutes were up. She said that in her previous therapy she had suffered because she did not like being told her time was up. During our meetings, especially at the beginning, she always needed to terminate the session herself.

Ali said that her aim during her therapy, with me was to overcome her constant panic attacks, which made it difficult for her to function alone. She said she wished to be in control of her life and not depend on others. Ali lived in a small two-bedroom flat with her husband, her two teenage children, a girl and a boy, as well as a Rumanian girl, who I will refer to as Mirela. Before five years, the family had lived in a slightly larger flat, where they had looked after Ali's grandmother, who needed care. Mirela had been hired to nurse her. When the grandmother died two years previously they moved to a smaller flat. Ali felt sorry for Mirela, on whom she had become dependent, and invited her to stay on.

At the beginning of her therapy Ali was concerned about her dependence on Mirela. She needed her to accompany her on almost all her journeys outside the house. Going to work was a problem, as she was forced to travel on her own and she dreaded the possibility of getting a panic attack while driving.

During one of our earlier sessions, Ali made a picture of her family with small objects. She chose a peacock to represent herself and placed Mirela, in the form of a doll-like figure, closest to her. In her book *Women Who Run With the Wolves,* Pinkola Estés (1992: 85) refers to the doll as a symbolic *homunculi,* little life. It is the symbol of what lies buried in humans that is numinous. It is a small and glowing facsimile of the original Self. Superficially, it is just a doll, but inversely it represents a little piece of the soul that carries all the knowledge of the larger soul-Self. Perhaps for Ali, Mirela in the form of a doll represented an ideal part of herself. On her other side she placed her children, represented by two hippos embracing. Further away, on the same side, she placed her husband as a fat man and at the back she placed her mother as a soldier. When she looked at her composition she said that she would have preferred her husband to be further away from her. Also Ali said that her relationship with Mirela tired her. It was like having a third child in the house, one that was more demanding than her own. Ali went on to say that when Mirela first came to live with them they had a brief sexual relationship. This was no longer the case but she knew that Mirela saw her as her partner.

The idea that Ali might be a lesbian was totally alien to her, even though she had never enjoyed sex with her husband. She occasionally endured his sexual advances and complained that he was inadequate. She said that she could not possibly be a lesbian because she fantasized about having sex with a prominent politician. We talked about the image of herself as a peacock, which was obviously male. Ali said that she had chosen that image because she wanted to feel proud of herself. Her husband did not think highly of her nor did her mother, whereas Mirela admired her. Then Ali talked about the image of her husband. In reality, he was not fat. He was tall and thin, but she felt that he took up too much space. Her children she saw as happy hippos. Her son, the youngest was very close to her, while her daughter was more independent. She had chosen the doll image for Mirela because she was like a child but she was larger than the other two and required more attention. Ali did not mention the figure of her mother as a soldier!

Ali's panic attacks continued during the first year of her therapy, but they were not as paralysing as they had been. She was able to inhibit their intensity when she felt them coming on. She also had very high blood pressure on a few occasions, and twice when she had been alone at home she telephoned her husband to come and be with her even though it meant him leaving work in the middle of the day. When I asked her how she felt about her husband responding to her plea for help, she said that even though it inconvenienced him he liked coming to her rescue. Ali felt that he treated her as his child and admitted that she behaved like a child with him. She believed that perhaps this was connected to the fact that she had lost her own father at a very young age.

Ali remembered many of her dreams. One she had had, around the 15th session, was about 'A journey without boundaries', as she called it. It was complex and ended with her desire to see her old girlfriend, Nata, just for a day.

In the next sessions Ali talked about Nata again and referred to dreams about her that involved sexual fantasies. What may have caused these thoughts was the fact that Ali was going to meet Nata again at some social business gathering. Nata had worked in the same line as Ali but had been transferred to another town and only in the last few months had she returned to Athens. Ali was in a quandary whether she should go to the meeting or not. She wrote a long letter that she wanted to send to Nata but instead she brought it to her therapy. In the letter she complained to Nata for having disappeared from her life. Storr (1989) maintains that when exaggerated, the drive towards attaining order and control is destructive of spontaneity, and may eventually paralyse action. Obsessives actively defend themselves against such feelings and strive to master both themselves and the external world. Ali decided to keep the letter as her attempt to keep the order. Eventually the day of the meeting came and mustering her courage Ali went; she faced Nata and even had a brief conversation with her. After that meeting Nata ceased to occupy her mind.

Following the encounter with Nata and what Ali referred to as her 'dethroning', a new chapter started in Ali's life. Internet surfing became a passion and Ali started entering various chat groups. She began entering a Greek lesbian group and had controversial conversations with them. One day she was told that she was homophobic so she left that group and joined another.

Next, Ali moved to a broader chat group with a variety of topics. She found some interesting people to chat with, and after about a month she 'came out' and told them that she was a lesbian. There were several reactions from the various members. Some supported her and others didn't. There was a particular woman, whom I will refer to as Dimi, with whom Ali started to correspond on a frequent basis. Soon, Interneting became an obsession with Ali. She spent hours at it, both at work and at home. She began to neglect her family and her household duties. She rarely cooked, mostly having food delivered. This chat forum had different rooms and one could follow the movements of other members and their conversations with other people. There was also a private line that Ali and Dimi used in order to talk privately to each other. Ali fell passionately in love with Dimi. Her emotions were so strong that nothing else in her life mattered. Landy (1993) characterised this state of overwhelming emotion by the term underdistance. When underdistanced, the client is unable to work dramatically and think through her dilemma. Underdistance is characterised by an over-abundance of emotion which, when expressed, brings neither relief nor insight. This was reflected in Ali at the time, who needed the whole session to tell me what was happening to her. Finally, one day I received a distressed signal from Ali. She wanted to see me sooner than our scheduled day. At this meeting Ali told me of her great shock. Dimi announced that she was not a woman. She was a man and he would make Ali fall in love with him. Ali was devastated but continued to communicate with Dimi. Storr (1989) mentions that since identity implies difference, it follows that the affirmation of identity requires a modicum of self-esteem. Ali was at a loss and at the time possessed very little self-esteem.

Slowly Ali became accustomed to the fact that Dimi was a man and put up with his previous deceit because his writing fascinated her. Ali became totally infatuated by Dimi the man, to the extent that she gave him her mobile phone number. Dimi said that he lived in another town of Greece and he would like to meet Ali on some beach. Then he said that he lived in another country and he would like Ali to visit him. This was a big test as Ali was frightened of flying. The situation was becoming out of hand and I was worried about Ali. Dimi was playing with her feelings and her trust and Ali began to feel insecure, with her panic attacks becoming more intense and more frequent. Dimi insisted that they met and threatened to tell Ali's husband about her. Ali was scared, not so much about her husband finding out that she was a lesbian, but because she had begun to think that Dimi was a rather disturbed person. Then, suddenly, one day Ali gave up the internet, changed her mobile and started to lose weight. It was a bit like some people give up smoking from one day to the next and never look back. Laing comments:

> 'A strong sense of one's own autonomous identity is required in order that one may be related as one human being to another. Otherwise, any and every relationship threatens the individual with the loss of identity.' (Lanig, 1960: 106)

Ali had felt this threat so strongly that she was able to give Dimi up completely. When Ali ended her relationship with Dimi she suggested that she paid me more money for her sessions, as she had heard that other people charge more and my price had not changed in a year. I told her that she was not to worry about my fee and that it was my job to let her know when the price went up. It was as if, having lost control in her relationship with Dimi, Ali needed to have the upper hand in our relationship.

Gradually Ali's life started to return to normal. She began to take notice of her family again and also started cooking. Slowly, however, she began to realize that she was not happy with her domestic life. She no longer believed that she was a lesbian, but this did not alter the fact that she wanted a divorce. She announced her decision to her husband and children who humoured her because they did not take her very seriously. Her son was more concerned and became very affectionate demanding more physical contact with her. As the weeks started to pass and she continued to say that she wanted a divorce, her husband began to get angry. Ali arranged for them to go and see a divorce lawyer and ended up going on her own. The children started to discuss which parent they would like to live with, but Mirela was not mentioned.

At the next session, Ali announced that she had told Mirela to start looking for alternative accommodation. Storr (1989) maintains that the obsessional person's failure to integrate or control his aggressive impulses may lead in either of two directions; towards submission, on the one hand, or towards tyranny on the other. Ali fitted both parts at different times. Ali was determined about her divorce, but she decided that she would wait until her son had finished his university entrance exams. She wanted to be near him while he was doing his exams and she did not want to upset him. During this time Ali worked with some cards I use for story-making to gain some insight into her deeper thoughts. This technique I learned from Dr. Mooli Lahad in 1999 during a workshop in Athens. It involves the following:

A pack of story-making cards are given to the client to shuffle and the therapist cuts. Then the client takes the first card and places it face down on the table. This is followed by a second card, which is placed face down above the first card. Next, a third card is placed beneath the first one. Next, a fourth is placed to its right and finally a fifth card is placed to its left, thus making the form of a cross. The position of each card has a specific interpretation. The first one represents the client's problem generally, the second one the client's history, the third a wish or a fear, the fourth the problem concerning the client at that time and the fifth the problem the client is working with during his/her therapy. The differences between each theme are not very distinct but they give the client the chance to be creative and free associate. These cards are used to help clients make connections with their feelings. In their book 'The Aeolian Mode' Murray Cox and Alice Theilgaard (1987:99) suggest that metaphor exerts its mutative effect by energising alternative perspectival aspects of experience. This means that material, which the patient has endeavoured to relinquish, avoid, or deny so that it is 'safely' categorised, and 'filed away', appears again in the 'pending action' file. Through these cards such material emerges and becomes more comprehensible.

Ali's cards were:

1. Her problem generally – The picture showed two people who fall in love.
Ali said that she could only connect this card to Nata but that was over now and

the female body disgusted her. When she felt she was a lesbian it was different, but now she knew she was a heterosexual she could not be attracted to another woman.
It was interesting how she connected the act of falling in love with Nata and at the same time condemned the female body. It was as though even though Ali was an educated and broad-minded person she could not accept being a lesbian herself. She had started reading religious books, which condemned homosexuality with the result that maybe deep down Ali felt that homosexuality was a sin. Storr (1989) found it interesting that Freud's supposition that paranoid delusions arise from the denial and projection of homosexual desires is better supported by research than are many of his theories.

2. Ali's history – This picture showed a village.
Ali talked about the neighbourhood she had been brought up in with nostalgia. The family home had been torn down and now the place had filled up with apartment blocks. It was all totally different.
Ali's family had been much better off before her father was taken ill. They had lived in a house with a garden and her memories were happy ones. During her father's illness they had to sell their house so he could be taken to England for treatment. After his death they had lost their home and her mother had to start working as a seamstress.

3. Ali's fears or hopes – This card showed death.
Ali was not frightened by death. She said that this card represented the death of her fear to leave her husband.
Ali interpreted this card, which could have been frightening, in a positive way. Maybe she felt it represented the death of an era. She did not want to connect it to the death of her father. She said that that was a wound that had healed.

4. Ali's problem at this time – This card had a picture of a ring.
Ali interpreted the ring as the engagement of fear to her new life. She said her new life was going to be difficult but she was not going to let her fear hold her back.
Maybe this card represented commitment to her decisions and respect for her personal feelings.

5. What Ali was working on in therapy – This card depicted a road.
This for Ali was the road to her new life. She was pleased with this card and felt strong enough to face it.
After this session Ali telephoned saying that she wanted the next session to be our last. I said we could discuss it when we met. On the day she said that she no longer needed our meetings and that she had finished with her therapy as she had overcome her panic attacks. I believed that this was not the best time for her to end her therapy, but I respected her choice. During this session we made a journey of retrospection through all her Dramatherapy. She said that when she started she had been a wreck with her fears and her panic attacks. Now these had gone completely she was no longer frightened when dealing with bank clerks, the

police or anybody official. She could drive on the motorway and she could even drive into Athens during the rush hour without any fear.

Ali said that during her Dramatherapy she had resolved her issues with her mother and was now able to become the child and yet, at the same time, help her mother out as she was getting older. She said that she had overcome her father's death as much as this was possible. Ali said that she had made a dive into lesbian circles not because she had been attracted to other women, but because she felt that women were superior to men. As far as her feelings for her husband were concerned, these had not changed. She still wanted the divorce. Her separation with Mirela was difficult. Mirela had moved out, but came to visit at regular intervals and often stayed the night. The difference was that Ali invited Mirela to come, not because she needed her, but as a friend. Before the end of the session, I suggested that we meet in two months' time to check out her feelings and Ali agreed. When the session was over, Ali forgot to pay me, the first time ever.

Conclusion

Bergin & Garfield (1994) maintain that studies assessing the efficacy of psychodynamic techniques for panic have not yet been conducted. However, they suggest that psychodynamic treatment is well suited to address the interpersonal problems and pervasive anxiety states that disturb many panic disorder patients.

The two years with Ali had been fascinating. I cannot say that she resolved all her problems or that she had found her true identity. She had convinced me that she was a suppressed lesbian and when she rejected this idea it was almost too sudden for me to take in. I then realized that it made no difference how I thought of her identity because it was hers and hers to enjoy as she wished. Jones (1996: 152) maintains that within Western culture, the relationship between an individual's identity and their body can be characterised by a tradition of duality. He goes on to say that there is a tension indicated between identity, body and society. This was certainly the case with Ali. I believe, however, that just by allowing herself to contemplate the possibility that she was lesbian was enough to give her more self-confidence, with the result that the panic attacks had stopped. Miller (1987) in her book *The Drama of Being a Child*, maintains that not knowing who we are, what we feel, and what we need, even as grown-ups we remain subject to the expectations placed upon us from the very beginning of our lives, expectations we fulfilled not for love but for the illusion of love. Without that illusion, we could not have survived childhood. In the case of Ali, her symptoms had ceased, so something had changed inside her. She was planning on living without crutches in the form of a husband or a girlfriend. A number of therapists have suggested that interpersonal, particularly marital, differences play an important part in the development and maintenance of a patients' phobic symptoms (Goldstein & Chabless, 1978; Hafner, 1982). Furthermore, it has been suggested that a change in phobic symptoms through treatment may have a negative impact upon the patient's marriage (e.g. Hafner, 1982).

I did not feel that Ali had made the best decision to end her therapy when she did, but I was in no position to force her to continue. Ali had lost her father prematurely and she was leaving her therapy prematurely. It was my hope that if she found herself in trouble she would contact me again and that is how we left it. She needed to be in control of our meetings. Laing (1960:28) maintains that:

> 'the main goal of human research is to identify those concepts which both indicate the interaction and interexperience of two persons, and [which] help us to understand the relation between each person's own experience and his own behaviour, within the context of the relationship between them.'

In my relationship with Ali, my belief was that giving her control of our meetings would help in her struggle for independence.

Using dramatherapeutic techniques helped Ali on her journey because she was able to move away from verbal analysis, with the result that she was able to feel more and think less. These techniques enabled her therapy to become more tangible. Ali was an intensive and intelligent person, so just using talking therapy could have been a hindrance. Jung (1963) believed that creativity was essentially therapeutic and that it allowed for a synthesis between the artist's inner world and external reality. The artwork is an integrative combination of inner and external realities, which inspires a feeling of completion and determination.

Jennings (1990; 1993; 1998) and Landy (1986; 1992) talk about the creative process not only in dramatic improvisation but in other dramatherapeutic techniques, for example, working with stories, sand-play, painting, mask-making, movement and so on. They maintain that facilitating artistic work with regressive material such as sand, clay, pebbles and water has a liberating effect on the clients. With Ali this was certainly the case, especially when working with small objects and story cards. I do not know how close this paper has come to the conference title of 'Grounding the Vision'. In fact, 'grounding' in this case was very difficult to arrive at. Ali was an impulsive person, who needed to be in control. However, through the projective work in her Dramatherapy sessions she was able to gain insight into the conflict between her need to be conventional and her natural proclivities. Ali may not have finished her therapy, but she had overcome her panic syndrome and this had made her a stronger person.

References

Beck, A.T. & Emery, G. (1985). *Anxiety disorders and phobias: A cognitive perspective.* New York: Basic Books

Bergin, A.E. and Garfield, S.L. (1994). *Handbook of Psychotherapy and Behaviour Change* New York: John Wiley & Sons, Inc.

Clark, D. M. (1986). A cognitive approach to panic. *Behaviour Research and Therapy, 24,* 461-470

Cox, M. & Theilgaard A. (1987). *Mutative Metaphors in psychotherapy The Aeolian Mode.* London: Tavistock Publications

Goldstein, A. & Chambless, D. (1978). A reanalysis of agoraphobia. *Behaviour Therapy, 9,* 47-59

Hafner, R.J. (1982). The marital context of the agorophobic syndrome, in Chambless D.L. & Goldstein A. J. (Eds.), *Agoraphobia: Multiple perspectives on theory and treatment* New York: Wiley

Jennings, S. (1990). *Dramatherapy with Families, Groups and Individuals.* London: Routledge.

Jennings, S. (1993). *Playtherapy with Children: A Practitioner's Guide* Oxford: Blackwell Scientific.
Jennings, S. (1998). *Introduction to Dramatherapy Theatre and Healing,* London & Philadelphia: Jessica Kingsley Publishers
Jones, P. (1996). *Drama as Therapy: Theatre as Living,* London: Routledge
Jung, C.G. (1963). *Memories, Dreams, Reflections,* London: Routledge
Laing, R.D. (1960). *The Divided Self* London: Tavistock Publications
Landy, R. (1986). *Dramatherapy- Concepts and Practices,* Springfield, Illinois: Charles C. Thomas
Landy, R. (1992). 'One –on-One: The Role of the Dramatheapist Working with Individuals', in Jennings, S., (Ed.) *Dramatherapy – Theory and Practice II,* London: Routledge
Landy, R. (1993). *Persona and Performance* London: Jessica Kingsley
Miller, A. (1987). *The Drama of Being a Child*, London: Virago Press. Trans. Ruth Ward.
Pinkola Estés, C. (1992). *Women Who Run With the Wolves,* London: Rider. Publishers
Storr, A. (1989). *Churchill's Black Dog,* London: Harper Collins Publishers

LIA ZOGRAFOU

THE DRAMA OF ADDICTION AND RECOVERY: APPLYING THE RITUAL MODEL OF DRAMATHERAPY IN QUALITATIVE RESEARCH WITH MEMBERS OF NARCOTICS ANONYMOUS

This paper is based on a qualitative research project, a small-scale group case study, I conducted as part of my MA thesis in Dramatherapy for the University of Surrey, Roehampton. Apart from a brief outline of my methodology and design I present a more detailed discussion of the findings in the hope of enhancing dramatherapy practice within 12-step programmes.

A. Rationale and purpose of the study:

The Narcotics Anonymous model is one of the most widespread and most effective drug addiction treatments (Flores, 1997). It is highly unlikely that any arts therapist working in the field of addictions will not come into contact with the principles of the Anonymous Fellowships at some point in his/her professional life (Fisher, 1990).

The Narcotics Anonymous programme of recovery from drug addiction is a self-help model which relies exclusively on self-diagnosis. Recovery occurs under the guidance of the 12-step treatment programme which relies on the acceptance of addiction as a pervasive and progressive illness that attacks the person mainly on a spiritual level, rendering him/her unable to exercise mindful choice and control on all levels, emotional, perceptual and behavioral alike. The person is never fully recovered, but always in the process of recovering (Flores, 1997; Rasmussen, 2000), renewing their contract to remain sober every day, as illustrated in the NA slogan "just for today".

The purpose of my study was to investigate the phenomenological dimension of dramatherapy by extracting participants' perceptions of addiction and recovery before and after the dramatherapy intervention in order to identify whether and how any change took place.

Despite criticisms of NA's inflexibility (Larkin and Griffiths, 2002), we cannot ignore its phenomenological dimension. Thune, a staunch supporter of the phenomenological perspective on addiction, (in Flores, 1997) highlights the need for a phenomenological research perspective which complements other perspectives in order to understand better the way the addict defines self and world and the mechanisms of therapy. The purpose and rationale of my research fit precisely this need.

As Larkin and Griffiths (2002) state, subjective accounts of individuals' experiences of addiction are vitally important to our understanding of addiction but largely neglected by psychological research. The 12-step programmes, despite being criticized as being too prescriptive or cognitively based, do, however, recognize the affective, experiential dimension of addiction (Larkin and Griffiths, 2002).

My study investigates the application of the ritual model of dramatherapy (Mitchell, 1996; Mitchell in Cattanach, 1999; Rebillot and Kay, 1993) which employs character and myth making, dramatization and role play in the context of creating and preparing a personal monomyth or hero's journey. (Campbell, 1993). The reasons behind my choice were manifold. The body of arts therapies research in addiction contains numerous examples of successful treatment and methodological innovation (Cox and Price 1990, Fisher 1990, Gallant and Holosko 1997, Hanninen et al 1999, Johnson 1990; Julliard 1995; MacKay 1987, Matto 2002, Moffet and Bruto 1990, Moore 1983, Treder-Wolff 1990, Wilson 2002). There is, however, a gap in research that specifically takes into consideration participants' self-reports on their addiction, applies phenomenological research methods in extracting the essence of meanings inherent in them and then matching them to the dramatherapeutic intervention.

Marion Woodman (1982:29) most aptly offers the connection between ritual and addiction:

> 'Many people in our society are being driven to addictions because there is no collective container for their natural spiritual needs. Their natural propensity for transcendent experience, for ritual, for connection to some energy greater than their own, is being distorted into addictive behavior.'

Ritual is at the heart of dramatic expression while recovery from addiction implies a substantial inner struggle to control one's impulses, thoughts and behaviour for the sake of a healthier, freer identity. As Campbell explains (1993), the adventure of the hero in the monomyth involves leaving the world of habit in order to enter a world of supernatural wonder where forces beyond one's control are encountered in challenging battle so that a final victory may be achieved that will allow the hero to return home renewed and full of knowledge and power. The compatibility between the dramatic structure of the monomyth and the efforts involved in recovery from addiction is obvious.

Moreover, the ritual model of dramatherapy employs dramatic structures for the exploration of different forces within the person. Participants in the model, as Mitchell explains in Cattanach (1999), create heroic characters that possess the resilience to take on the subversive, oppositional forces exemplified in the Demon of Resistance whose aim is to undermine the whole project of self-renewal and discovery. I considered this dramatic premise appropriate for this project since the process of recovery from addiction implies the negotiation between the participants' dual experiences of being both addicts and in recovery, both contaminated and clean, both in need and in control.

B. Methodology and Design

The aims of my research were:

- To identify participants' perceptions of recovery and addiction prior to the dramatherapy group experience
- To identify participants' perceptions after the dramatherapy experience and specify whether any change has occurred

- To recognize key moments that participants identified in the dramatherapy process as facilitative of change in perceptions

I employed Clark Moustakas's (1994) method of using semi-structured interviews before and after the experience of dramatherapy. Verbatim interview accounts were clustered according to themes and composite textural structural descriptions were extrapolated to reveal the meanings and essences of the participants' experiences. The post-group interviews contained an additional section where participants reexamined and evaluated their artwork made during the dramatherapy group and took place 4 months after the dramatherapy group closed. Force majeur prevented the group and the therapist from conducting the interviews earlier and the time lapse certainly poses questions as to what is an appropriate time margin for retrospective analysis. However, process research in psychotherapy was conducted by Somer and Somer (1997) with client interviews taking place 8 months after termination of therapy.

The participants were interviewed individually by the therapist prior to and after taking part in the dramatherapy group. The interviews lasted approximately one hour, were taped and transcribed. The questions focused on participants' experience (sensations, memories, perceptions) of life and self prior to addiction, during their years of active drug use and after their decision to recover. During the second interview participants were invited to look at all their art products from the dramatherapy group (drawings, writings) and identify moments of insight, struggle or change in perception. Both sets of interviews were held in the therapist's studio, where the group also was conducted. The dramatherapy group lasted for 10 weeks, at one and half hourly sessions held weekly.

The therapist kept detailed clinical notes throughout the dramatherapy group. These were referred to later in order to triangulate the data generated by the participants.

Selection and description of the participants

The research group was comprised of four participants. Participants were randomly selected from a group of Narcotics Anonymous members who demonstrated a willingness to take part in a dramatherapy group. I intentionally selected two males and two females so as to avoid gender bias. I decided to limit the number to four due to time and procedural constraints imposed by my Master's programme. All participants joined the research project voluntarily. Ethical considerations, such as obtaining written consent and establishing rules of confidentiality and protection of the identity of participants were observed and maintained.

All four participants started using drugs in early adolescence, eventually progressing to serious heroin addiction. I noted the step level of each person at the time of the first interview. Names have been altered to preserve their anonymity. The participants were:

Anna, 32 – Step 1, had been clean for 9 months, 13 days.
George, 40 – Step 6 , clean for 4 years

Philip, 41 – Step 10, clean for 7 years
Iris, 37 – Step 7, clean for 3 years

C. Analysis of data

For the analysis of interview transcripts I followed Moustakas' method of phenomenological analysis (1994) which relies on horizonalizing, i.e. identifying and reproducing statements from verbatim accounts that were relevant to the topic, which in turn were clustered into larger themes to avoid repetition. The ultimate essential meanings of the phenomenon studied were revealed by employing the processes of phenomenological reduction (bracketing), imaginative variation (approaching the phenomenon from a variety of perspectives in order to illuminate the 'how' of the experience) and finally reaching a synthesis of meanings (Moustakas 1994, 90-101).

I then compared the results of the first set of interviews with those of the second to reveal what, if any, change has occurred and with regard to which particular structural theme. Participants' comments on their images and/or writings were compared to my clinical notes to identify significant moments in the process and determine any agreements or discrepancies with regard to the identification of key moments of change.

D. Discussion of findings

The interviews pre and post dramatherapy revealed the following essential common themes underpinning the perceptions of addiction and recovery (for the sake of brevity and clarity, headings of themes are followed by the main feelings, sensations or subjective processes in bulleted form):

1. *Addiction as a lifelong process/traumatic childhood experiences*
   - Isolation/alienation
   - Loss/trauma
   - Depression
   - Need to belong
   - Lack of knowledge
   - Escape into fantasy
   -

2. *The split self – intolerance of ambiguity and discomfort/easy access to escape*
   - Confusion
   - Self-doubt
   - Unease
   - Anxiety
   - Temporary pleasure

3. *Non-participation – progressive double bind/the need to belong leads to further isolation*
   - Social isolation
   - Lack of self-awareness
   - Meaningless relationships

4. Loss of meaning – filling the void with repeated use
- Inauthenticity
- Secrecy/duplicity
- Self-loathing
- Guilt/shame
- Loneliness/depression
- Inner chaos – battle for control

5. Willful self-restructuring/The new 'addict' identity
- Self-recognition and self-acceptance
- Tolerance of ambiguity/owning disparate identities and aspects of self
- Firmness of beliefs
- Relationship restructuring
- Spiritual restructuring
- A new foundation/addicted to NA ideas of recovery?

The following theme emerged after the second interviews and relates to processes with which participants engaged in the group:

6. Participation – the subject in communication with self and others
- Spontaneity
- Expression
- Intrapsychic and interpsychic communication
- Self-exposure
- Intimacy

Differences in perceptions of addiction and recovery that the participants identify
There was no change in perceptions of addiction and recovery as outlined in the first 5 sections above. All participants adhered strongly to NA definitions of illness and recovery and all reported that the main supportive structure in maintaining their renewed identity were the 12 steps. However, the 2nd interview revealed change in the ways participants perceive certain aspects of their polarized self-definitions along with an increase in insight.
For instance, Iris reported greater acceptance and self-regulation, which she attributed to her experience of dramatherapy:

> What I remember most vividly is the balancing of the two sides of myself, the good and the bad, the recognition first and the acceptance afterwards that it's okay to have a bad self, I don't need to be afraid of it, …It is I who have them and I can choose … it's up to me. And this has directly to do with addiction.

Iris expanded on her attitudes toward her conflicting sides by recognizing that she had, in the past, tried to cover up her bad self whereas in the dramatherapy group she "sat and listened" to it.
Anna reported the most obvious change in the theme of tolerance of ambiguity, as a result of her experience of dramatherapy. In summary, she reported feeling

more together, more able to withstand inner conflict or discomfort and more "carefully carefree". She experienced considerable tension while getting in touch with her Demon character in dramatherapy and was overcome by feelings of inadequacy and inability to contain the dark influence of her Demon, Satanious. This culminated in a serious threat of relapse in session 6 which is further discussed below.

Anna's progress is a testament to the potential compatibility of NA treatment with the ritual model of dramatherapy, especially with clients working through the 1st step's challenge to recognize their helplessness over their addiction. Anna's threat of relapse was a serious reminder that the Demon is not easily vanquished. She admitted her helplessness but also managed to remain clean. During the post-group interview Anna investigated her written work and drawings. She marked her discovery of a new point of balance in her life:

> Here is the dialogue between them. Look, here, at some point where my two extremes, my good and bad selves function, let's say, either one or the other operates, and here, let's say, they meet...And I think a balance will be struck, and so it happens. And, you know, Satanious, rules the mind a bit and then the emotion a bit, because I've been very emotional and this didn't help me. And here is the harmonious coexistence of the two, which I can say now represents me. I mean, sometimes I need to be both, both selves, but, you know, not at the same time, yes, but also at the same time perhaps. Not to be careless and fancy free and leave myself exposed, nor to be isolated. And I am like this now. I somehow function with both of them.

Participants reported that dramatherapy enhanced their awareness of change in their perceptions of intimacy, self-exposure and spontaneous expression. Specifically, George responded emphatically that he overcame his "terrible problem taking part in any kind of drama". His experience of dramatherapy dispelled his fear.

> As if I got rid of some taboos, some complexes, let's say, a weight I carried, as far as having fun goes, amusing myself, interacting with others, expression. I've always had an issue with theatre, something I never quite, which I never understood, what was that craziness about? Something grabbed me, a strange thing, a kind of paralysis, regarding anything theatrical, and I think I certainly overcame it.

Philip stated in his second interview that he had not connected the experience of the group as directly related to his addiction. However, when pondering the question "which issues regarding your addiction and recovery did you address" he made the connection between how isolating addiction is and how the group experience functioned as a "catalyst" that brought him "one jot closer to my fellow human beings, this is how it helped". Moreover, Philip evaluated his performance in the group as a "measure... of my development, my progress in relation to the past".

Iris commented on how the group experience elucidated her concerns with participation and intimate relationships and facilitated her deeper awareness of the process of addiction.

> It was a kind of test, to be able to let go, to open up and dive in while the other three people, whom I don't know this way, also do the same. And I learned a lot from that. ... I saw results of addiction in others, I recognized some things which perhaps are also in me but I couldn't see them, and I saw how addiction can work in different people and the faults that there can be. ...I felt afterwards that I have something in common with those people, to bind us together, we have been together in very intimate moments.

What is the change due to that participants identify?
The answers to the question "what do you attribute your recovery to" revealed one common factor. All participants are very much indebted to NA for giving them the foundation to continue their progress. Additionally, they mentioned their own personal will and determination, their relationships, their spiritual practice. To the final question "is there anything else you would like to mention with regard to your experience of dramatherapy" the participants identified cultivation of spontaneity and experiential awareness through play as the attributes of dramatherapy that were most helpful to them.

Anna:
> It was very good, regardless of how I hurt or how exposed I felt, it doesn't matter. It is, for me, it is knowledge, which I lack. Where would I get knowledge from? From nowhere? Since I didn't exist in my life. I was a stoner. And from drama, ... I hold on to the playing, and it was very nice sometimes, and I got out things which stayed with me. But what stuck with me most, is that I don't need to be very open to everybody, even in a group. When I thought I was obliged to be.

George:
> Yes, and I don't know how there was somehow the motivation to open up emotionally, on a more intimate level, let's say. I somehow had the stimulation to open up. This isn't so much on a conscious level but I believed played a role.

Iris, however, mentioned that she did not feel that the dramatherapy experience contributed substantially to her recovery. Her statement, apart from touching upon her own difficulty with group process and participation, raises a provocative challenge as to how dramatherapy can address the needs of clients who are long-term NA members and advanced in their step work.

> I don't think I got substantial help in this process, as far as recovery goes at least. Why? ... I think it was because... I've exorcised the greatest part of the past through the steps. So the work we did here was too light for me... There were some pleasant moments that also worked therapeutically on some little themes, but no essential changes. ...I have sorted out the heavy stuff... if

there is still in me something regarding addiction and hasn't been explored yet, I think would need more sessions to begin with but also deeper work. I think I could do some work on my own, but not with other people.

What are the key moments participants identified in therapy?
The key moments, extracted from subjective accounts, fall into two categories:
1. moments related to personal process, facilitated through dramatic structures that pertained to the creation of personal characters. More specifically, participants reported that the symbolic representation (through drawing, mask-making and dramatization) of issues participants were grappling with, such as their home life, employment and relationships, facilitated personal insight and spontaneity.
2. moments related to group process, whereby participants felt playful and relaxed, challenged or comforted by the other members of the group or the therapist.

Key moments in the individual and group process identified by the therapist
My observations of individual and group process highlight a very significant issue regarding therapeutic practice and the systematic study of therapeutic process that further research could explore. The study contains limitations, some inherent in the phenomenological paradigm, such as the emergent nature of the design and the non-universality of conclusions. (Giorgi et al 1971, Moustakas 1994).
My dual role as practitioner and researcher was an integral part of the process, which inevitably affected the life of the group. The information I gathered as researcher from the interviews was often inconsistent with or different from the data I gathered as practitioner. Methodological limitations, such as the absence of an independent observer who could have contributed to the triangulation of data, (Aldridge, 1994, Smeijsters 1997), could have elucidated potential pitfalls of bias or unmitigated countertrasferential reactions to the participants.
I therefore present my own observations as practitioner advisedly, hoping to stimulate further debate on how best to address in research the dual presence of the practioner-researcher and identify more precisely the therapeutic tools which render dramatherapy effective with such populations.

a. Individual processes
Anna
In addition to her relapse crisis which she also identified, I note three additional incidents.
The first is her disclosure in session 5 that she did not remember playing as a child. In her 1st interview she had described herself as a very lonely, sensitive child who was more concerned about others rather than herself. Managing to incorporate both desire for play and inner vulnerability, Anna created her Hero, Ag, who was spontaneous, expressive, sensitive and innocent: "In my soul live the souls of many young children, and purity, play, movement and energy are my foundations and I live through them".
The second moment was in session 9 when she disclosed sexual abuse in adolescence by a male friend of her father's. She spoke very angrily about the

"rage inside" her and her indignation about "what this jerk did" to her. This ownership and direct expression of feeling came in marked contrast to the self-destructive ways Anna had employed to cope with the pain of abuse in the past:

> And (pause), basically the first time I used was when I wanted to take revenge on my dad, because...he was a very violent man, who, you know, insisted to always get his way, and I ... wanted to punish him ..., and my mother who put up with this and my sister who never said anything. I said, now I'll make you all dance, alright, I'll sort you out, I'll make you all jump.

The third key moment was again in session 9 when Anna, instead of getting into her familiar habit of assuming the worst and fantasizing about how others might actually be feigning interest in order to manipulate her, asked Philip for clarification about a statement which she had assumed was maliciously directed at her. This was the first time Anna engaged in some reality testing in the group, confronting her interlocutor in the here-and-now.

George
An important moment was during the 6th session, as I tried to manage the relapse crisis with Anna. Although the group had agreed to my proposal to extend the hour, George became very angry with me and accused me of being too directive. In his general irritation he accidentally knocked down a lampshade in the studio. After the group had closed, he insisted on staying behind to fix the lampshade. Was George trying to assuage his guilt for having confronted me in the group? Not wanting to jump to premature interpretations of his resistance and transference to me, I didn't address this with him there and then. In the following session, however, when we discussed the aftermath of Anna's crisis, George apologized for his behaviour and explained that he realized his aggressive reaction to me was due to his habit of mistaking assertiveness in women for aggression.
The second key moment relates to George's confrontation with his Demon in session 9. He treated the incident as a cartoon fight and diminished its importance. During the dramatization of his dialogue, George beheaded his slimy, amorphous Demon with a swift stroke of his sword but the demonic energy was not exterminated. I asked him if a sword was the appropriate weapon to attack slime. He reacted by letting out a roaring war cry, which surprised him and convinced him he had no trouble at all being expressive. He then said that perhaps "chemicals to burn the slime off" would be a more appropriate method. I noted there that George was tottering on the dividing line between two opposing tendencies in him. His need to scream expressed an impulse to express rage and/or desperation at not being able to beat his Demon. In a flash he resorted to disembodied and magical solutions to his problem. His warrior Hero had no access to chemicals in his script. Where would the chemicals come from? Isn't this how George had coped with his conflicts when he was an active drug user? I did not carry the discussion further because I had already seen how resistant he was to the confrontation and any possibility of communication or integration between his Hero and Demon had evaporated. I elected to let him stay with the two inner

characters still in unresolved opposition. I noted that George experienced difficulty staying with discomfort and decided that, should the opportunity arise in future, I would encourage him to explore uncomfortable feelings further.

This opportunity arose in what I identified as another key moment in session 10. He was recapitulating on his entire experience in the group when Anna laughed about something unrelated. George took offence and felt diminished. I encouraged him to stay with the feeling and his introspection led him to memories of being humiliated by other children in the playground. He disclosed that as a child he felt insecure, helpless and paranoid about how others saw him and this was something he was still grappling with.

Philip

He was generally very cooperative and enthusiastic in the group, a very "good" client, always punctual and very supportive of me during the aforementioned incident with George. Although at the 2nd interview he spoke of dramatherapy as a "pleasant event", I do note two key moments that were not so pleasant and which he did not mention. One had to do with his disclosure in session 3 of feeling betrayed by a member of his family and the other with his disclosure in session 7 that he often felt he undermined himself by his self-destructive anger. He used the metaphor of an 'upside down drill' that he turns onto himself instead of directing outwardly. This makes him waste energy by raging against others rather than focusing his energy to soothe himself.

Iris

Iris's Hero was a perfect creature, without any weaknesses or passions but when she tried to embody her heroine she painfully realized: "I have passions and I cannot be perfect". Iris was resistant to personal disclosure throughout the process, did not participate in the dramatization of the confrontation between Hero and Demon because she wanted to "protect" herself and complained in the 2nd interview that she did not receive enough stimulation to open up about her deeper personal issues. I refrained from pressing her or offering her comforting solutions. I do, however, note that in dramatherapy Iris experienced a direct conflict between the spiritual principles of NA and the discovery that she was inwardly unable to meet her Christian standards of conduct. She understood how this fuelled her perfectionism and intensified feelings of inadequacy.

Group process

Anna's relapse crisis in session 6 greatly challenged the group emotionally and was a pivotal moment in revealing group resistance. This was expressed in terms of the threat of relapse in the face of intrapsychic threat from an inner demon (Anna) as well as in terms of conflict both among group members and with the therapist. George and Anna were visibly upset, the former expressing anger at my interventions, the latter extreme anxiety at having met her Demon. Iris and Philip were less visibly upset and took a supportive stance toward the therapist. The group was split in two. The splitting of the group mirrored the participants' inner polarity as expressed by the creation of two conflicting characters, the Hero and the Demon of Resistance.

I accepted that the group was not in a position to move on to complete the monomyth as planned. I followed Flores's advice to stay with the resistance when it appears (Flores 1997) and elected to address it by calling for a process check-up (Yalom 1995: 352). The group remained at the point of confrontation between the two opposing characters and the following 3 sessions were devoted to exploring just that with the final session reserved for closure. This raises another important matter to consider when working with members of NA. According to their perceptions of recovery there is no final victory in the confrontation between heroic and demonic qualities. The struggle is renewed every day. Practitioners, therefore, who apply the ritual model may consider alternative ways of framing and presenting the struggle so as to contain it "just for today". Moreover, the multiple manifestations of the struggle, both in terms of dramatic action and in terms of group process suggest that additional care be exercised to remain aware of the metaphors that inform the life of the group and illuminate the understanding of resistance and transference-countertransference issues.

E. Conclusion

In conclusion, the study revealed that for the most part, these NA members adhered strongly to the ideas and perceptions of addiction and recovery embraced by the Fellowship. The ritual model facilitated the recognition and concretization of disparate and conflicting aspects of identity (Anna, Iris, Philip) and further assisted their integration, though not always conclusively (George). Although we cannot draw decisive conclusions about the applicability of this model to particular NA steps, all participants, irrespective of step level experienced change in the qualification and subtle management of self-perception and self-regulation.

References

Aldridge, D. (1994). *Single-case research designs for the creative art therapist.* The Arts in Psychotherapy, 21(5), 333-342

Campbell, J. (1993). *The hero with a thousand faces.* London: Fontana

Cattanach, A. (ed.) (1999). *Process in the arts therapies.* London: Jessica Kingsley

Cox, K. & Price, K. (1990). *Breaking through: incident drawings with adolescent substance abusers.* The Arts in Psychotherapy, 17, 333-337

Fisher, B. (1990). *Dance/movement therapy: its use in a 28-day substance abuse program.* The Arts in Psychotherapy, 17, 325-331

Flores, P.J. (1997). *Group psychotherapy with addicted populations: an integrated 12 step approach.* New York: Haworth Press.

Gallant, W. & Holosco, M. (1997). *The use of music in counselling addictive clients.* International Journal of Alcohol and Drug Education, 42(2) retrieved from EBSCO databases at URL:www.ebscohost.com

Giorgi, A., Fischer, W.F. and von Eckartsberg, R. (eds.) (1971. *Duquesne studies in phenomenological psychology*: vol 1. Pittsburgh, PA, Duquesne U. P.

Hanninen, V. & Koski-Jannes, A. (1999). *Narratives of recovery from addictive behaviours.* Addiction, 94(12) retrieved from EBSCO databases at URL: www.ebscohost.com

Johnson, L. (1990). *Creative Therapies in the Treatment of Addictions: the Art of Transforming Shame.* The Arts in Psychotherapy, 17, 299-308

Julliard, K. (1995). *Increasing chemically dependent patient's belief in step one through expressive therapy.* American Journal of Art Therapy, 33(4) retrieved from EBSCO databases at URL: www.ebscohost.com

Larkin, M. & Griffiths, M.D. (2002). *Experiences of addiction and recovery: the case for subjective accounts.* Addiction Research & Theory, 10(3), 281-311

Matto, H. (2002). *Integrating art therapy methodology in brief inpatient substance abuse treatment for adults.* Journal of Social Work Practice in the Addictions, 2(2) 69-83

MacKay, B. (1987). *Uncovering Buried Roles Through Face Painting and Storytelling.* The Arts in Psychotherapy, 14, 201-208

Mitchell, S. (ed.) (1996). *Dramatherapy: clinical studies.* London: Jessica Kingsley.

Moffet, L.A. & Bruto, L. (1990). *Therapeutic theatre with personality disordered substance abusers: characters in search of different characters.* The Arts in Psychotherapy, 17, 339-348

Moore, R.W. (1983). *Art therapy with substance abusers: a review of the literature.* The Arts in Psychotherapy, 10, 251-260

Moustakas, C. (1994). *Phenomenological research methods.* Thousand Oaks, CA: Sage.

Rasmussen, S. (2000). *Addiction treatment: theory and practice.* Thousand Oaks, CA: Sage.

Rebillot, P. & Kay, M. (1993). *The call to adventure: bringing the hero's journey to daily life.* USA: Harper San Francisco.

Smeijsters, H. (1997). *Multiple perspectives: a guide to qualitative research in music therapy.* Gilsum, NH, Barcelona Publishers.

Somer, L. & Somer, E. (1997). *Phenomenological and psychoanalytic perspectives on a spontaneous artistic process during psychotherapy for dissociative identity disorder.* The Arts in Psychotherapy, 24(5), 419-430

Treder-Wolff, J. (1990). *Music therapy as a facilitator of creative process in addictions treatment.* The Arts in Psychotherapy, 17(4), 319-324

Wilson, M. (2002). Art therapy in addictions treatment: creativity and shame reduction. In Malchiodi, C.E. (ed.). *Handbook of Art Therapy.* New York: Guildford Press.

Woodman, M. (1982). *Addiction to perfection: the still unravished bride.* Toronto: Inner City Books.

Yalom, I.D. (1995). *The theory and practice of group psychotherapy.* 4th edition. New York: Basic Books.

IV
ESSAYS IN THEORY AND PRACTICE

PAULINE MCGEE

DOES ENGAGING WITH THEIR OWN ARTWORK PROTECT ART THERAPISTS, WORKING WITH CHILDHOOD SEXUAL ABUSE FROM VICARIOUS TRAUMATISATION?

Introduction

My interest in this topic arose through years of experience of working in the field of childhood sexual abuse as an art therapist, manager, trainer, consultant and political campaigner. Within each of these roles I came to know the anger, cynicism, despair and sense of hopelessness that can affect workers, communities and organisations when complex issues of engagement are not addressed.

McCann and Pearlman (1990), noting the pervasive effects of long term engagement in trauma therapy on identity, worldview, beliefs, memory system and psychological needs of the therapist coined the term 'vicarious traumatisation'. They recognised vicarious traumatisation as a process over time pertinent to many professionals engaged in trauma work.

In *Trauma and The Therapist* (1995) Pearlman and Saakvitne further explore the risks to therapists, clients and organisations when the effects of working with trauma are not properly recognised and addressed. *Trauma and The Therapist* focuses specifically on the area of childhood sexual abuse for the following reasons:

- More survivors of abuse are now seeking help in addressing disrupted childhood experience therefore more therapists will be working with this client group.
- The complex coping strategies survivors have adopted can prove challenging and confusing to both client and therapist.
- Development of a therapeutic relationship can prove difficult and threatening for survivors whose boundaries and trust were violated at an early age.
- The secrecy, fear and cultural taboo surrounding childhood sexual abuse, carries powerful related affects and defences. Transference and counter transference issues will therefore be continually challenging.
- Many survivors themselves choose to become therapists and face unique challenges in relation to transference and vicarious traumatisation.

Pearlman and Saakvitne identified early literature on therapist's responses to working with war veterans. However whilst recognising the valuable contribution this makes to our understanding of trauma, the focus of work tended to be on individual clients and not long-term cumulative effects on the therapist.

Childhood sexual abuse

An overview of the literature on work with survivors of childhood sexual abuse acknowledges the complexity of counter transference issues, Bass & Davis (1988), Courtois (1998), Davies & Frawley (1991), Herman (1992) and Woodward (2000) with strong, often negative, reactions within the relationship expressed by the therapist.

Art therapists working in this area have illustrated counter transference through the therapeutic relationship and production of powerful, painful imagery, Case & Dalley (1992), Greenwood (2000), Hagood (2000), Moon (2002) and O'Brien (2003). Other art therapists have recognised the potency of working with and through imagery, referring to the powerful nature of 'witnessing', Bannister (2003), Burt (1997) and Learmonth (1994) which can continue to affect art therapists beyond the session. Vicarious traumatisation is referred to in literature by two art therapists, Hagood (2000) and Greenwood (2000). Others recognise the effects of 'burnout', McNiff (2004) or Post Traumatic Stress Disorder, Bannister (2003).

Despite recognition of the affect on the therapist of long-term engagement in therapeutic work with survivors there is little information serving to address possible vicarious traumatisation.

Working as an art therapist with child victims and adult survivors of childhood sexual abuse I have experienced the 'Witness' role on a variety of levels, each impacting upon the other. I have witnessed excellent workers in this field reach a point where they could no longer engage meaningfully in the work. Some have left taking with them years of skills and knowledge, which are difficult to replace. I have seen organisations come and go when abuse dynamics impacted upon teams culminating in blame culture. In this respect no one could do the job well enough, competently enough or for long enough. I have witnessed media blaming and shaming of workers when yet another child suffered or died at the hands of a perpetrator. I have witnessed communities rise in response to media reporting and taken justice into their own hands, often with dreadful consequences. I have known only too well personal feelings of exhaustion, anger, sadness and inadequacy in engaging with this work. Sometimes I recognised my limits but often I didn't.

In retrospect I recognise how unequipped and ill prepared I was for engaging in work with survivors on completion of what was in 1987 a one-year postgraduate training in art therapy. It has since been recognised that many professionals feel ill equipped to work with the complexity of issues surrounding childhood sexual abuse (Nelson 2001).

Art therapy training courses with their historical grounding in psychoanalytic theory have been slow to incorporate other theoretical viewpoints. Whilst acknowledging the crucial theories which formed the backbone of our profession, students should also be encouraged to review and critique thinking which has had lasting impact in negative or detrimental ways. Freud for example in retraction of belief in his clients' abusive experiences had set a precedence of denial, which has had immense implications for survivors (Hall & Lloyd 1989, Warner 2000), for organisations and for society.

The feminist movement, in the 1970's, by opening its eyes and ears to the reality of women's experience of violence also opened the floodgates to the shocking extent of childhood sexual abuse. The feminist movement has been crucial not only in defining sexual abuse and domestic violence but also in fighting for legislative change which names such violence as crime.

Art therapists therefore are not only likely to be exposed to painful and graphic images of childhood abuse and torture, but to bear witness to the unfolding detail of crime perpetrated against a child. This affects how we work within teams and organisations (O'Brien 2003). It has huge implications for the confidentiality and boundaries of therapy. The ongoing social, political and ethical dilemmas involved in this work will inevitably affect us over long term.

There is still a lot of ground to cover in understanding the wider social and political implications of working with survivors. Susan Hogan's book Feminist *Approaches to Art Therapy* (1997) provides a welcome and much needed contribution to the literature with other art therapists providing insightful feminist perspectives through case study material (Waldman 1999).

Professional isolation

Art therapists often find themselves the lone therapist within multidisciplinary teams where they have to define and exemplify their role to others. Support and supervision, if not provided by another art therapist, may prove inadequate or frustrating through lack of understanding of the task. Edwards (1994) highlights that art therapy supervision has numerous definitions and is open to differing interpretations. Inevitably, feelings of professional isolation can arise for the art therapist, which can be exacerbated when working with the complex needs of survivors of childhood sexual abuse. They may unknowingly work beyond their limits losing a sense of balance in tending personal needs. Pearlman and Saakvitne (1995) recognise the dangers inherent to therapist and client by a return to silence and denial of the impact of abuse. They remind us of the subversive and detrimental effect of this work in which we "name and address society's shame" (1995:2).

Media reporting can strongly influence how survivors, and those who work with them, are viewed within society. Informed and sympathetic reporting can encourage those who have never sought help to do so, while ill informed reporting or 'victim blaming' perpetuates dangerous myths around lies and fantasy which leave children and adult survivors vulnerable and without access to services. Professionals and organisations working with survivors have often suffered societies backlash of fear and disbelief, through high profile media reporting of child abuse 'scandals'. Child protection workers in Britain in the 1980's were publicly humiliated by the media, ostracised and in some cases ensured their career in child protection was ended (Itzin 2000; Bacon and Richardson 2001). Heather Bacon and Sue Richardson (Bacon & Richardson 2000:273, in Itzin 2000) report on the subsequent controversy and fear of becoming the next media target which "inhibited workers from uniting in defence of their own and children's interests."

Childhood sexual abuse has always been around, but inevitably the social taboo and disbelief, which surround it force it out of public conscience until the next 'scandal' unfolds. However for every high profile case, which may have reached court, there are thousands of disclosures, which are never made public. Professionals working in this field face a difficult balancing act between belief and hope in the work they do and fear of the consequences of 'witnessing'. Herman (1992) highlights that even within the confines of therapy any disclosure of abuse may result in public disclosure and is what perpetrators work hard to prevent.

Herman also refers to 'traumatic counter transference' or vicarious traumatisation wherein the therapist experiences helplessness or is in conflict with professional colleagues. Working with secrets, anger, rage and shame is bound to impact upon any team, regardless of levels of awareness and professional competency.

Pearlman and Saakvitne (1995) define the various aspects of counter transference, which impact upon work with survivors and upon the life of the therapist recognising organisational counter transference as one aspect, which may ultimately lead to vicarious traumatisation. These authors stress that although the issues are powerful they are rarely addressed. They indicate that institutional re-enactments between therapist, client and organisation are a parallel process, which are complicated yet important to track. However I believe that if art therapists are finely tuned to their own responses within organisations and aware of all the counter transference issues that affect therapeutic work, then the cumulative effects of vicarious traumatisation may be transmuted through their personal engagement with artwork.

Art therapists have at their disposal the unique and personal language of image making. Although supervision does not stress the need for engagement in art making The Health Professions Council (HPC) state that for continued registration art therapists must "recognise that the obligation to maintain fitness to practise includes engagement in their own arts-based process" (2003:7,1a.7).

How this will be monitored and assessed remains to be seen but it is interesting that art therapists are being asked to speak their own language, keeping the art in art therapy. In the words of Gilroy (2004:78) continuing to engage in personal artwork "maintains the uniqueness of the discipline and of the individual". Her research paper, *On Occasionally Being Able To Paint* (2004:77), illustrated that a number of art therapists continued with their artwork not solely because of their own need but "because of the risks to their work as art therapists of not doing so". The potency of the image invested with symbolic meaning made me increasingly aware of the risks art therapists were exposed to in working long term with survivors of abuse. Pearlman and Saakvitne (1995) remind us that the need sometimes for survivors to recount horrific images of their experience can contribute to the therapist's vicarious traumatisation. We can internalise vivid descriptions which reappear to us as clearly as if they were our own. Although they do not refer specifically to art therapists, I wonder whether working with actual images of abuse or our visual capacity to recreate detail would make us more susceptible to vicarious traumatisation.

Counter transference
Although art therapists have increasingly acknowledged the importance of counter transference within the therapeutic relationship, I believe it plays a significant part in working with survivors of childhood sexual abuse.

Disempowerment, shaming, secrecy and isolation from others, which form the core of abusive experiences, make future reconnection through relationship particularly difficult for survivors. Committing to a therapeutic relationship poses real threat of feeling disempowered again. Tackling this imbalance requires transparency and honesty from the therapist, in order that transference and counter transference issues are identified and worked with. When the therapist addresses her own fallibility and limitations within the relationship she introduces the idea of respect and negotiation. A survivor's belief system of being bad, unlovable or even toxic leaves little room for belief that anyone would want to be with her, never mind help her work toward a greater understanding of herself. Reenactment of early relationships can impact endlessly upon the therapy requiring ongoing vigilance.

Pearlman & Saakvitne (1995) recognised five needs, which appear most sensitive to effects of psychological trauma:

- **Safety.** Sexual abuse in childhood, often by someone in a caring role, creates an inability to feel safe anywhere. A survivor may also believe that the therapist will be unsafe by association or by their feelings of badness and toxicity.
- **Trust/ dependency.** Betrayal and fear of abandonment for the child can become internalised. Inability to trust their own feelings and responses in any situation creates huge barriers to therapy.
- **Intimacy.** Sexual abuse violates a child's body and mind. Intimate connections with others are difficult to tolerate. Self-care can be neglected and self-harm may become a coping strategy. The boundaries of therapy are often pushed.
- **Self esteem.** Survivors often believe they could or should have protected themselves. They cannot value themselves or the therapist.
- **Control.** A sense of helplessness in interpersonal relationships may create a strong need to control others. The therapist may be accused of being too authoritarian or not directive enough. Dissociation may continually be used to control feelings and memories.

These same issues will affect the therapist at various times and degrees through ongoing work with survivors. The therapist may experience vulnerability and fear for their own safety and safety of loved ones. Trust in self-capacities and trust of others can become disrupted. Self esteem, intimacy and self control may all be affected in confusing and distressing ways. However, disruption in the therapist's sensory system although mentioned in literature pertaining to sexual abuse (Hall and Lloyd 1989, Herman 1992) requires a greater level of understanding and may be where art therapists are particularly vulnerable.

Dissociation has often been regarded as an essential coping strategy in dealing with unbearable physical and psychological pain (Hall and Lloyd 1989, Herman 1992, Warner 2000). However, Herman (1992) highlights research, (Cardena and Spiegel, 1994; Marmar et al. 1994) indicating that use of this defence in the face of overwhelming terror may be a significant contributory factor in long lasting post traumatic stress disorder.

Within therapy a client can experience dissociation as threatening or comforting.

It may arise in response to fear of memory or intimacy with the therapist. A parallel process may arise within the therapist when fear, shame, horror or rage threatens to overwhelm. Identifying our own dissociation is crucial to connection with the client's experience, our humanity and our coping strategies. Not recognising counter transference can lead to emotional distance and numbing, which feeds the clients identity of being bad, worthless and contaminating, all of which may lead to sudden endings in therapy.

For the art therapist, overwhelming counter transference responses can feel shaming and destructive to professional, competent identity. Case (1994) highlights the work of Racker (1968) in identifying lack of research into counter transference and our difficulty in looking at it because it makes us personally and professionally vulnerable. For this reason many art therapists may be reluctant to identify counter transference issues within their supervision.

The therapist who is new to work with survivors may experience great anxiety in not recognising feelings of blame, shame, anger and helplessness, which may be transferred to the client. Sudden ends to therapeutic relationships can therefore feel like personal attacks. Pearlman and Mac Ian (1994) also found that those new to work with survivors were more likely to experience intrusion of client's imagery upon their own thought processes.

Sensory impact

As Schaverien (1990) points out we all enter this work with needs of our own. Past experience shapes our identity as therapists and shapes our understanding of the potency and power of creativity. Past experience also shapes our sensory perception and sensitivity to the experience of others. Working with survivors of childhood sexual abuse exposes us to the helplessness of childhood and the wickedness and evil intent of perpetrators.

Herman (1992) notes that it can shock the sensitive, caring and encompassing nature of the therapist who comes face to face with their own capacity for evil through expressions of anger, scorn, shame and hatred directed toward perpetrators. These feelings not only impact upon a therapist's identity but also bring a whole range of undercurrents or re-enactments into the relationship wherein the client senses the therapist as being in the role of perpetrator, victim or rescuer.

The creative, active and alert imagination, which forms our core of being an art therapist, can also leave us open to destructive sensory stimulation, which requires attention and processing. Therapists working with survivors often refer to sensory intrusion (smells, touch, images and taste) to which they can ascribe no immediate connection. Some have become ill through symptoms that appeared to have no medical grounding. I have personally experienced uncomfortable and disturbing sensory intrusion, which was difficult at the time to define or comprehend. However I believe that continual processing of images, my own and those of clients, through art making enabled me to continue in therapeutic work whilst offering balance in my life.

The images I produced were made in response to a particular feeling of anger, sadness, frustration, uncertainty or joy. I instinctively knew that the act of creating, making a mess or playing made me feel better and able to function the next day. If I neglected my art over a period of time I became lethargic, feeling low and depleted. Just being with the materials in my own space could make such a difference to fluctuating feelings. Time would fly past and I really felt I had grounded my senses. In retrospect it enabled me to engage in working with survivors for such a long time.

An example of personal sensory intrusion was when I had a continual feeling of presence of a third person in the room while working with a client. My paintings at the time were of three heads in close proximity. Often only one of the faces had their eyes open. I called these paintings 'See No Evil' although I was not consciously aware of how they related to my work experience. Months later on reading Herman's book *Trauma and Recovery* (1992:7) I came across the following definition of the perpetrator who "Appeals to the universal desire to see, hear and speak no evil."

The presence of a third person would of course be the client's abuser who commanded that the secret of abuse never be revealed. Making sense of this image had a powerful impact on how I related to clients whenever this fearful presence intruded upon us. They intuitively knew what I was talking about, allowing us both to move forward from a less fearful position.

In her article *Captivity and Terror in The Therapeutic Relationship,* Greenwood (2000:53) highlights counter transference in response to her work with two women who had experienced abuse and torture. The honest and powerful defining of her countertransference responses was affirming and greatly reassuring to my own experience of "a disquieting sense of evil, more extreme than I could ever have imagined".

She cites motivation for writing the article as an attempt to understand moments of terror in therapy when she felt in danger of jumping out of her skin. It is a feeling I personally identify with and my hope is that further honest recognition and detailed exploration of the impact of working with survivors of abuse will allow more art therapists to find ways of maintaining their core identity.

Reconnection

If art therapists are recognising the sensory impact of this work upon their being, it makes sense that reconnection to personal artistic exploration will offer a sustaining and energising outlet for processing graphic imagery. However, there appears to be continual debate as to why or why not art therapists lose touch with their own creativity. Dudley, Gilroy and Skaife (2000) comment on the paralysis around therapists' priorities and attending to personal art making as a way of maintaining that which makes art therapy unique. By highlighting this dilemma in the context of student training, a pertinent point is being made with regard to future practitioners. If trained therapists struggle to maintain connection to art making, then what message is being relayed to students? How can educators advocate that art making sustains health and fitness to practise when so many skilled practitioners do not make it a priority?

Rogers (2002) suggests that the art made by art therapists is a massively under-valued resource, not only in bringing our own unconscious dynamics to the fore, but in making the art of our discipline the crucial element of empathic engagement. She emphasises that processing counter transference issues through her artwork was not intentional but essential to working with losses in her own and her clients' lives. By so doing she was able to prevent over identification with their feelings of helplessness.

McNiff (2004) in highlighting the serious problem of burnout endemic in caring professions asks us to look to the chemistry of the creative process, which he stresses does some of its best work with the extremes of emotion. We know this instinctively in our work with clients so what leads us to neglect our own creative chemistry? Moon (2002) requests that we challenge one another to keep engaging with our art as an intentional, disciplined practice. In this way, she suggests, we will come to know intimately the stories of our own lives, enabling us to empathise with the stories of others.

In her article *On Occasionally Being Able To Paint,* Gilroy's research highlighted a number of reasons why art therapists maintained, or not, their connection to personal image making. Although the article was first published in 1989 the reasons given are universal enough to justify republishing the same article in 2004. With emotional demands of the profession cited as reason for not continuing to engage with art, it is still heartening to read that many found their own art work to be a source of refreshment, self discovery and insight. Crucially Gilroy's research highlighted that a number of people continued with their own art because they believed there were risks inherent to their work as therapists of not doing so.

Individuals enter therapy with a sense of hope, no matter how distant, that they can change their way of being in the world. Pearlman and Saakvitne (1995) highlight that depletion of our identity, as 'good enough therapist' is part of the continuing process of vicarious traumatisation wherein losing life balance depletes our sense of hope. Warner (2000) reminds us that hope is born out of reflection. Recovery, she adds, can only become a reality for survivors if we therapists can look to our own future with a sense of hope. Reconnection with our core artistic identity is crucial in realigning us with a sense of balance. Reflection through artwork is what we instinctively know and, by processing horrific, disturbing imagery, we will not allow it to impose upon our private lives. Reflection will allow us to prioritise, to reground and rebalance our own relationships, instilling hope that we are 'good enough'.

Conclusion

Recognising the process of vicarious traumatisation is the first step in addressing it. It seems crucial therefore that the teaching of art therapy students addresses aspects of self-care, whilst also addressing the complex nature of work with different client groups. Art therapists often have to work in professional isolation, which is undoubtedly exhausting but can also be dangerous within the therapeutic relationship. Lack of support can lead to cynicism, silence and unethical practice when complex dynamics go unaddressed. Silence is not what adult survivors of abuse need, as this is what keeps them from forming healthy understanding of themselves and others. Silence will not protect children from evil and fear and it will not teach us what we need to know about perpetrators and how they operate. Art therapists working with survivors, adults or children, are witnesses to crime perpetrated against children. This can be a frightening, lonely place, which may ultimately lead to public exposure or appearing as an actual 'witness' in court.

Sensory impacts of abuse work can also have a detrimental effect on us physically and psychologically when left unattended. The power of art therapy, which we instinctively know works with many clients in processing disturbing imagery, will also work for us when we prioritise a commitment to it.

The HPC (Health Professions Council) now stipulates that art therapists, in order to maintain health and fitness to practise must engage in their own art making. This means we must speak our own language in order to connect with our clients. Creativity allows us to process fear, mess, despair and tolerate the unknown. It also allows us to be playful, uncertain, courageous, and insightful. Survivors will recognise all of this within us thereby feeling empowered to address their own developmental needs through play, humour and creativity. If we can play, hope and imagine then we know that empowerment and change is possible. Survivors may see that we have faith in the work we do and begin to see us on equal terms. Art therapists know their own inner resource and the abilities, which make the profession unique. Maintaining connection to our artist selves may be what it takes to sustain us in difficult and often lonely work. It may also be the crucial element in protecting us from vicarious traumatisation.

References

Bacon, H. & Richardson, S. (2000). Child sexual abuse and the continuum of victim disclosure. In: Itzin, C. (ed) *Home Truths About Child Sexual Abuse.* pp 235 – 276. London: Routledge

Bacon, H. & Richardson, S. (2001). *Creative Responses to Child Sexual Abuse.* London: Jessica Kingsley Publishers

Bannister, A. (2003). *Creative Therapies With Traumatised Children.* London: Jessica Kingsley Publishers

Bass, E. & Davis, L. (1988). *The Courage To Heal.* London: Cedar

Burt, H. (1997). Women, art therapy and feminist theories of development. In: Hogan, S. (ed) *Feminist Approaches to Art Therapy.* pp 97-114. London: Routledge

Cardena, E. & Speigal, D. Predictors of Post Traumatic Stress Symptoms Among Survivors of the Oakland/ Berkeley, California, Firestorm. *American Journal of Psychiatry 151* (1994). pp 888-894.

Case, C. (1994). Art Therapy In Analysis: Advance/Retreat. In The Belly Of The Spider. *Inscape, (1)*

Case, C. & Dalley, T. (1992). *The Handbook of Art Therapy.* London: Routledge

Courtois, C. (1998). *Therapy for adults molested as children: Beyond Survival.* New York: Norton

Davis, J.M. & Frawley, M.G. (1991). Dissociative processes and transference-counter transference paradigms in the psychoanalytically oriented treatment of adult survivors of childhood sexual abuse. *Psychoanalytic Dialogues, 2 (1)*, pp 5-36

Dudley, J., Gilroy, A., Skaife, S. (2000). Teacher's, Student's, Client's, Therapist's, Researchers. In: Gilroy, A. and McNeilly, G. (eds) The Changing Shape of Art Therapy, pp 172-199. London: Jessica Kingsley Publishers

Edwards, D. (1994). On reflection: A note on supervision. *Inscape (1)*

Hagood, M. (2000). *The Use Of Art In Counselling Child and Adult Survivors of Childhood Sexual Abuse.* London: Jessica Kingsley Publishers

Hall, L. & Lloyd, S. (1989). *Surviving Child Sexual Abuse.* London: Falmer Press

Health Professions Council. (2003). *Standards of Proficiency. Arts Therapists.* London.

Herman, J.L. (1992). *Trauma And Recovery.* London: Pandora

Hogan, S. (1997). *Feminist Approaches to Art Therapy.* London: Routledge

Gilroy, A. (2004). On Occasionally Being Able To Paint. *Inscape 9 (2),* pp72-78

Greenwood, H. (2000). Captivity And Terror In The Therapeutic Relationship. *Inscape, 5 (2),* pp 53-61

Itzin, C. (2000). *Home Truths about Child Sexual Abuse.* London: Routledge

Learmonth, M. (1994). Witness And Witnessing In Art Therapy. *Inscape, (1),* pp 19-22.

Marmar, C.R., Weiss, D.S., Schlenger, W.E., Fairbank, J.A., Jordan, K., Kulka, R.A. & Hough, R.L. Peritraumatic Dissociation of Posttraumatic Stress In Male Vietnam Veterans. *American Journal of Psychiatry 151* (1994): pp 902 – 907

McCann, I.L. & Pearlman, L.A. (1990). *Psychological trauma & The Adult Survivor.* New York. Brunner/ Mazel

McNiff, S. (2004). *Art Heals: How Creativity Cures The Soul* Boston: Shambhala Publications

Moon, C.H. (2002). *Studio Art Therapy.* London: Jessica Kingsley publishers

Nelson, S. (2001). *Beyond trauma.* Edinburgh: Edinburgh Association For Mental Health

O'Brien, F. (2003). Bella and The White Water Rapids. *Inscape 8 (1)*

Pearlman, L.A. & Mac Ian, P.S. (1994). *Vicarious traumatisation in therapists: An empirical study of the effects of trauma work on trauma therapists.* Submitted for publication

Pearlman, L.A., & Mac Ian, P.S. (1994). *Vicarious traumatisation in therapists: An empirical study of the effect of trauma work on trauma therapists.* Submitted for publication

Pearlman, L, A. & Saakvitne, K.W. (1995). *Trauma And The Therapist.* New York. W.W. Norton & Company, Inc.

Racker, H. (1968). *Transference and Counter transference.* London: Hogarth and Institute of Psycho-Analysis

Rogers, M. (2002). Absent Figures: A Personal Reflection On The Value Of Art Therapist's Own Image Making. *Inscape, 7 (2),* pp 59-71

Schaverien, J. (1990). The Triangular Relationship (2) Desire, Alchemy And The Picture: Transference And Counter transference In Art Therapy. *Inscape, Winter 1990* pp14-19

Waldman, J. (1999). Breaking The Mould. *Inscape, 4 (1)* pp 10-19

Warner, S. (2000). *Understanding Child Sexual abuse.* Gloucester: Handsell Publishing

Woodward, J. (2000). The uses of therapy: understanding and treating the effects of childhood abuse and neglect. In: Itzin, C. (ed) *Home Truths About Child Sexual Abuse.* London: Routledge

SIMONE ALTER-MURI

ART IN TIMES OF WAR AND POLITICAL CONFLICTS

Humans have an innate need to create. The Minoan pottery and miniature replicas of buildings are examples of the amazing need not only to create utilitarian items but to make objects of beauty. Dissaynake (1998) has documented that making marks is an activity common to all people. Since ancient times, people from all cultures have drawn, carved and scratched on rocks, stones and wood as a form of communication. People create art not only in times when resources are scarce, but also create art from a need for expression. Self expression is especially important when individuals feel that they have no power and are not heard. This manuscript focuses on art that children and adults create during some of the most difficult of times, even in times of war and political conflicts.

Children all over the world create art. Art making plays a valuable role in culture and society. Art provides personal fulfillment and a form of non verbal communication that can strengthen the presentation of ideas and emotions. Until about age six, children's art from many places in the world looks similar. All young children draw what they know rather than making an exact interpretation of the physical world. In other words, young children tend to draw objects or people bigger or smaller because of their relationship to that person or object.

Researchers in children's art development discuss the differences in the art produced by children from some Middle Eastern and African countries versus the art produced by most children in Western cultures. These differences such as the Islamic torso according to (Wilson & Wilson, 1982) consist of a rectangular shaped torso with a fused neck and the half moon face. They are not usually apparent until the child is older than age seven. Wilson and Wilson (1984) found a link between culture and artistic development. The drawings of children are affected by the influences of the culture and of objects in their world.

Art is very important to healing. Creating a piece of art can assist the artist to be in the present, to have a few moments while they are creating to remove themselves from their pain. Art can empower children to make sense of difficult situations. There is a paradox seen in this art created in times of profound misery; there is often a ray of hope as well as depiction of despair that emerges in the art.

As an art therapist and an art educator I feel obligated to pay homage to the pioneers of these professions and to acknowledge that there is a role for art education even in the most difficult of times. During World War II in the Jewish ghettos and later in the concentration camps, there were several Jewish art educators who continued to teach art even when they were starving and had no traditional art materials. Friedl Dicker-Brandeis was one of the most prominent art teachers from Vienna who perished in Auschwitz and taught art in the Jewish ghettos and concentration camps. She was an art educator and a political activist who was arrested for her work (Hurwitz, 1991). Although she was able to secure a visa to Palestine, as a Jewish educator she refused to leave the children who needed faith in the face of terror. Dicker-Brandeis also encouraged the children to draw and motivated then to use metaphors from the Old Testament to create a sense of hope. Edith Kramer, (Zwiauer, 1997) one of the founders of the art therapy field in the United States, was a student of Dicker-Brandeis when she was a child in Vienna at the beginning of the Anschlus. Friedl was described by Kramer and as a humble person. When an extra morsel of food was offered in return for her teaching, Friedl refused to take accept it (Zwiauer, 1997). Many children in the Terezin camp created art under her guidance. From my observations of art created during and after the Holocaust from the collection at the Jewish Museum in Prague, many of the drawings contained drawing with black outlines around objects. Black outlines could indicate the need to create a boundary, the need for control of the object that is drawn. The art by victims and survivors may also include objects drawn very lightly.

The book "*I Never Saw Another Butterfly*" (Volakova, 1994) includes art and poems of children who were in Terezin and worked with Friedl Dicker-Brandeis. Dicker-Brandeis taught adults as well as children and encouraged them to keep their minds active through the creative process.

Art can document events and serve as an act of resistance. When looking at the art of Holocaust survivors, researchers have discovered that a common trait is to recreate the same theme in their art over and over again (Schaverien, J., 1996). This repetition of themes, colors, lines, and imagery often occurs for many years. Ellie Wiesel eloquently described that there are no words in any language that can describe genocide; when words fail visual images fill in the gap (Costanza, 1982).

The Vad Vashem art collection has over 3,000 works of art by European Jewish victims and survivors of the Holocaust. According to Shalev (1997) preserving even a small part of a prisoner's identity was important for survival. Creating art was a means to preserve one's identity. I was amazed when during a visit to the Buchenwald concentration camp I encountered a large exhibition of drawings and paintings created by victims and survivors of the Nazi regime. Some of this art was produced during the Jewish prisoners' struggle to survive in the concentration and work camps. There were different ways that the inmates obtained meager art supplies. Art materials were obtained by "favors" from SS officials who wanted to have portraits drawn of their families from their photographs to Nazis who wanted the artists to document the "lost" race or artists who drew with whatever materials they could find including dirt, coffee grinds on whatever scraps of paper were found. (Hurwitz, 1991).

The art was saved by different means. For example, it was hidden in the barrack that housed typhus patients, buried wherever possible, or snuck out of the camp by Nazi soldiers who were able to do some favors. The art of daily life in the camps depicted by thirteen year old Helga Weissova-Hoskova was created in the Terezin concentration camp. (Weissova, 1998). Helga was able to get art materials smuggled to her from the adult artists who worked on technical drawings, graphs, and maps. In her book she discusses the consequences by the SS if they found out that prisoner's drawings were made about the conditions of the camp, both the artist and his or her family would be murdered or sent to other concentration camps. Before being deported to Auschwitz she gave her drawings to an uncle who hid them (Weissova, 1998). Her art was very striking and powerful. Graphic representation can fill in the gap when words fail, (Costanza, 1982). No matter how silent a work of art can be, art has an amazing capacity to evoke feelings.

Besides the content of the art, the colors, lines, use of space and amount of energy in the art created by children and adolescents in the Holocaust is interesting. At first glance there might be nothing unusual about this art but upon closer examination there is a need for a sense of order that is often expressed by patterning in the drawings (Grossman, 1975). The colors are often somber and dull and there is shading which could correlate to anxiety. When people are drawn the faces rarely smile, and often guns, fighting, and violence are depicted. Children draw what they perceive and as a child matures their visual concepts become more detailed and more complex (Arnheim, 1974). This art brings the conflicts to our conscience; it mandates us to look, to not forget and it even prompts us to help.

Sometimes the artist depicts drawings that can be perceived as peaceful. However, even in these "peaceful" drawings there are clouds, birds or crows that may foreshadow a sense of helplessness or feelings of suicide. Although some of the drawings depict violence, pain, brutality and despair, this art records and documents daily events, and can depict images of hope, resiliency and faith. In the Zucherberg war home in Switzerland where children and adolescents were transitioned after liberation from the concentration camps, children who had an easier time dealing with their trauma were those children who were motivated to draw or write about their experiences (Knigge, 1997).

Although there are many examples of art that depicts war and politically caused violence, I have focused my investigation of art created by children and young people from different areas of the world from World War II until the current situation in Sudan, Africa. As an American, I am presenting this topic of art in times of war with humbleness regarding the situations that occurred in Hiroshima, Vietnam, El Salvador and Iraq.

Many times societies, especially American society, are not ready to accept the visual documentation of the horrors of sanctions, political unrest or war. This was true in the case of art by Holocaust survivors, and the art of American veterans. In the United States, it took many years before a home could be found for the National Vietnam Veterans Art Museum. After over 10 years of looking for a site, Chicago, Illinois, was the only city willing to fund this venture and gave the collection a small storefront on the outskirts of the city to start the museum (Sinaiko, 1998). The art in the Vietnam Veterans Museum was mainly produced after the war by veterans; however the museum also exhibits the art of Vietcong civilians and soldiers (Sinaiko, 1998). Another of the numerous examples of this issue is the story of Alfred Kantor. Kantor a survivor of Auschwitz created a visual journal of his experiences. After his liberation from Auschwitz he tried to publish his work. Even after immigrating to America he did not find acceptance of his memoirs. His work was finally accepted for publication in the 1970's. Kantor's art served as a visual document and as a place where he could record his feelings and put some small closure on those feelings by the act of drawing.

Thomas Geve was thirteen when he was liberated from Auschwitz. After his liberation in a displaced person's camp, he produced many drawings depicting how the Nazis tried to eliminate the humanity of the prisoners and their personal attributes (Geve, 1997). He tried to publish his memoirs of his experiences of being in four concentration camps. In 1949 he was rejected by publishers in England who felt that it was not the right time for the public to hear this information (Geve, 1997). In 1958 he published a book entitled *"Youth in Chains"*. This book was a literary description of the drawings he created immediately after his liberation from Auschwitz. After it was reviewed by the editors, he was told that it would only sell if he translated the pictures into words (Knigge, 1997).

Art is important in coping with trauma and during times of war and political unrest. Art can be a link to a former identity before a crisis and can provide a bridge to the future. No matter how silent a work of art, art has an amazing capacity to talk. It has all been said, yet all remains to be said.

The art of the children who were displaced during the Spanish Civil War was described by Geist and Caroll (2002). These children drew their memories of life before the war as a means to remember the past (Alter-Muri, 2004). Children drew their terrors and their fears during the war. The Spanish Republic in Exile was aware of the impact of war on children (Geist and Carroll, 2002). In the temporary shelters organized for refugee children, basic supplies were given and children were encouraged to draw. In 1937, three thousand children's drawings were exhibited in Valencia, Spain. The collection and exhibition of the art was used to help to raise funds for the displaced children's relief effort in Spain (Geist and Carroll, 2002).

Michirio Yoshida was a young solider in Japan who turned to art as a vehicle for healing and expression after he witnessed the smell and horror of Hiroshima. Currently in his 70's, Yoshida described that art was a force in the face of uncertainly and trauma and inhumanity to man that he could trust (Yoshida, 2002). His current art combines landscapes with non-traditional figure painting and vibrant colors. He blends symbols from the landscape of his native country with the directness of his message (M. Yoshida personal communication, November, 2002).

Phyllis Rodin visited Japan after Hiroshima and she worked with adolescent girls who survived and had lived in a boarding school. These girls found pieces of material that survived the bombings and with the charred and torn pieces of materials from curtains, bedcovers and clothes they created fabric collages, making something of beauty from something that was a memory of pain (P. Rodin, personal communication, October, 2003).

Art therapists look at drawings and often distinguish certain symbols, styles of drawing, directions of strokes or the pressure of the mark that may fit into research about trauma. However, sometimes children may be emotionally numbed and tend to draw pleasant pictures, or drawings of earlier times. Other times children draw their memories of the past and things of beauty. Children's drawings during traumatic times can show resilience, an ability to express strengths, wishes, hopes and their abilities to live with traumatic events.

The art by children in El Salvador regarding the violence that occurred there depicts another common theme in the art of children during war. It depicts the need to reach out to anyone anywhere who can help. Often older children tend to write on their drawings pleading for the violence to end. In 1980 and 1981, over

1,000 civilians that attempted to go to escape the violence in El Salvador and go to Honduras were tortured and killed. (Vornberger, 1986). The book: "*Fire from the Sky*" depicts examples of art from Salvadorian children who were hungry and witnessed killings, rapes and brutality of their families and friends were able to escape to refugee camps. The art by these children serves as a testimonial, a visual journal of their reality, and as a hope for a time when flowers continue to bloom (Clements, 1986).

The art from children in Bosnia also serves as an example of how art can be created as a message to society from children who are helpless in political battles. Europeans are currently commemorating the 10th anniversary of Srebrenica where 20,000 Muslims were killed by Serbs. In contrast to children who experienced the Holocaust, the art by Bosnian children shows the emphasis of the need to create pictures of peace. Examples of drawings that depict peace include the drawings collected in Zagreb, Croatia, by members of the Student Organization Advocating Peace (S.O.A.P.) in 1994. There are no people depicted in their drawings of houses, churches and gardens. The elements of two often opposite elements are apparent in the sun and the clouds. The S.O.A.P. organization brought young Bosnian refugees sponsored from the Dora foundation to the United States (R. Mac Crostie, personal communication, June 15, 2005).

A Friendly Bond is a child-to-child art exchange between children in Western Massachusetts and the children in Baghdad, Iraq. This art collected by Claudia Lefko was collected before the war, during the time of the American sponsored sanctions in 2001. She returned to Iraq after the war in 2004. The art collected in 2001 was created by children in Al-Mansour Pediatric Hospital (C, Lefko, personal communication, March 2005). The art from after the war was collected in displaced persons camps. This art depicts what children tell us about their worlds. They know the lies, the essence of wars and the realities of their lives. Children's art may show stylized drawings, repetitive patterns, outlining, the use of traced or stereotyped images, drawings of power images, superheroes, comic book figures or their art may reflect a drawing that seems regressed. These drawings are very powerful and what is striking is how many drawings do not depict the brutality that surrounded them.

The organization, Doctors Without Borders has collected over 100 drawings by children in a refugee camp in Dafur, Sudan. In these drawings collected by a humanitarian worker in 2004 from Dafur, Sudan, we can see images of the children's reality. Currently in Dafur (Ahmed, 2005) the Sudanese government using Arab militias, acts of rape and organized starvation tactics are systemically killing, torturing and destroying villages and crippling several African communities (Graham, 2005). There are approximately 1.6 million forcibly displaced people and violence continues to exist in the Internationally Displaced Peoples' Camp (Save Dafur.org 2005, Retrieved June2, 2005 from http;//www.savedafur.org). Depicted in these drawings of planes, village life during war, or United Nations refugee camps, there is a chaotic use of composition and line quality in the drawings. There seems to be a need for order in these drawings. Often a need for order occurs during times when things are hectic, disordered and out of control in life. Some of these drawings contain a picture of United Nations tents for refugees. These tents are plain canvas;

however, the children's drawings depict the tents having beautiful colors and designs that are similar to the patterns and colors of their garments. These drawings are powerful statements that words do not justify.

One of my graduate students worked with children from Somalia who were fleeing from violence and were able to flee to refugee camps. These children and their families received refugee status to immigrate to the United States. The children did not have any experience with marking instruments and were not aware of the concept of drawing. Although this art work according to developmental theories may appear regressed, one may also conjecture about the influence of trauma in their art.

Viewing and creating art in response to political conflict can create a forum where dialogue can occur (Alter-Muri, 1998). How can we use this art to think about issues in our world? The very process of creating art prompts children to tell more than they would if they just talked. The art brings to our conscience several human needs; to express sadness, pain and empathize, to bear witness and the need and responsibility to know and to react to what is happening to all of our children. This art is an example of how powerful visual images are and how art cuts through cultural, language and political boundaries to speak to the language we all know, the language of our hearts.

References

Alter-Muri, S. (1998). Beyond the melting pot: Postmodernist theories and art therapy. *Art Therapy: Journal of the American Art Therapy Association*, 15, (4), 245-251

Alter-Muri, S. (2004). Teaching about war and political art in the new millennium. *Art Education: The Journal of the American Art Education Association*. 57, (1), 15-20

Ahmed, M. (2005). *In honor of international woman's day: Exhibit of children's art from Dafur*. Press release published by American Friends Service Committee, Amherst, MA.

Arnheim, R. (1974). *Art and visual perception*. Berkeley, CA: University of California Press

Clements, C. (1986). Introduction. In Vornberger, W. (Ed.), *Fire from the sky: Salvadoran children's drawings*. (pp 1-13). New York: Writers and Readers Publishing Cooperative

Costanza, M. (1982). *The living witness: Art in the concentration camps and ghettos*. New York: The Free Press

Dissaynake, E. (1998). *Homo aesthetics: Where art came from and why*. Seattle, WA: University of Washington Press

Geist, A. & Carroll, P. (2002). *They still draw pictures. Children's art in wartime from the Spanish Civil War to Kosovo*. Chicago, IL: University of Illinois Press

Geve, T. (1997). About myself, about my pictures. In Knigge,V. *There are no children here: Auschwitz, Gross-Rosen, Buchenwald: Drawings of an art historian*. (pp. 26-28) Gottingen,, Germany. Wallstein-Verlag.

Graham, K. (2005). Child's-eye view of a hellish place. *Philadelphia Inquirer*. p.20

Grossman, F. (1975, January). *Creativity under conditions of extreme stress: A psychological study of children's concentration camp art*. Paper presented at the International Conference on Stress and Adjustment in Times of War and Peace. Tel Aviv, Israel

Hurwitz, A. (1991). *Friedl Dicker-Brandeis: The art educator as hero. In Seeing through "paradise". Artists and the Terezin concentration camp*. Boston, MA: Massachusetts College of Art

Knigge, V, (1997). With the eyes of a child historian and engineer. In Knigge, V. (Ed), *There are no children here: Auschwitz, Gross-Rosen, Buchenwald: Drawings of a child historian.* (pp.12-18).Gottingen, Germany: Wallstein-Verlag

Schaverien, J. (1998). Inheritance: Jewish identity, art psychotherapy workshops and the legacy of the Holocaust. In Dokter, D. (Ed). *Arts Therapists refugees and migrants: Reaching across borders,* (pp. 155-173). London and Philadelphia, PA.: Jessica Kingsley Press

Shalev, A. (1997). In Knigge, V. (Ed.), *There are no children here: Auschwitz, Gross-Rosen, Buchenwald: Drawings of a child historian.* (p 25.) Gottingen, Germany: Wallstein-Verlag

Sinaiko, E. (1998). *Vietnam: Reflexes and reflections. The national Vietnam Veterans Art Museum*: New York: Abrams

Violence and suffering in Sudan's Dafur region. Retrieved June 2, 2005, from http://www.savedafur.org/.

Volavkova, H. (Ed.). (1994). *I never saw another butterfly: Children's drawings and poems from Terezin concentration camp.* (2nd edition). New York: Schocken Books.

Vornberger, W. (1986). *Fire from the Sky: Salvadorian children's drawings.* New York: Writers and Readers Publishing Corporation

Weissova, H. (1998). *Zeichne, was Du siehst: Zeichnungen eines Kindes aus Theresienstadt/Terezin.* Gottingen Germany Wallestein Verlag.

Wilson, B. & Wilson, M. (1982). *The case of the disappearing two eye profile. Or how little children influence the drawings of other little children.* Review of Research in Visual Art Education, 15, 19-32

Wilson, B & Wilson, M. (1984). *Children's drawing in Egypt. Cultural style acquisition as graphic development.* Visual Arts Research. 10, (1), 13-26

Yoshida, M. (2002, October). Art by Yoshi. Retrieved October 11, 2002 from http://www.artbyyoshi.com/.

Zwiauer, C. (1997). *Edith Kramer: Malerin and Kunsttherapeutin zwischen den Welten.* Vienna, Austria: Pincus Verlag

ALEKSANDRA SCHULLER

ART AS A VEHICLE: PERFORMING ARTS AND ARTS THERAPIES BETWEEN RITUAL AND AESTHETICS

Throughout its history, European, western theatre was primarily perceived as dramatic theatre, i.e. as the staging of the dramatic text, operating within the domain of art. In the beginning of the 20th century however, the theory and practice of theatre started to deal with the following issues: the thesis on the ritual origins of theatre and the need to determine the essence of performing as art.

1. The leading members of the *Cambridge Ritualist School* – Jane Harrison, Gilbert Murray and Francis Cornford – developed a hypothesis on the ritual origins of the ancient Greek drama which was thought to have derived from the Dionysus rituals in the 6th century BC (Harrison, 1912; Murray, 1921; Cornford, 1914). The *Cambridge Ritualists* built their premises on the supposed existence of the pre-Dionysian ritual which praised the Spring-daimon (*eniautos daimon*), death and the resurrection of god (such as Osiris, Tamuz, Adonis or Persephone) and the change of vegetation cycles. The Dionysus ritual was thus thought to be derived from the Spring-daimon ur-ritual and the Dionysian dithyramb from the ritual dance (*sacer ludus*) which presented the *aiton* (the mythical narrative) on the divine power of the Dionysus. Their speculative hypotheses, albeit refuted by later researchers (Pickard-Cambridge, 1927, and Rozik, 2003), nevertheless had a surprising "ideological" impact on the theatrical practice and theory. Moreover, they established a somewhat vague connection between theatre and ritual that has found its way into the present general perception of the theatre. Their theses defined theatre as an artistic medium which in addition to its aesthetic function also possesses a somewhat indeterminable, but strong and "magical" link to the numinous – the transcendental.

This paper is not aimed primarily at questioning the idea on the ritual origins of theatre, but strives to detect reasons for its tenacious presence within the western theatre and culture. This could perhaps be explained by the fact that the supposed ritual character of theatre regards not only the structural analogy of the theatre and the ritual but implies the existence of something that transcends the aesthetic form: it suggests that theatre creates ritual community, ritual space and time where a person can be realized both as the ritual *homo religious* and *homo ludens*. The latter could also account for the longing that (post)modern people transfer onto theatre: finding meaning (in one's life), participating in a "primordial community" and (re)inventing a "ritual connection" with what goes well beyond their (ordinary) context/world. From this perspective, theatre is perceived as a medium – a (wo)man's link with the numinous, sacred.

2. The practice and theory of theatre in the beginning of the 20th century was marked by a tendency towards its autonomy as independent art. In order to

escape the suffocating relationship with literature (dramatic texts) and to find its identity, the western theatre had to find, or else invent, its own specific character which would distinguish it from other arts. The forerunner of theatre reformers was Richard Wagner's *Gesamtkunstwerk* (*total artwork*). In his *Das Kunstwerk der Zukunft* (1849), Wagner defined performing as an aesthetic context with artistic autonomy that was created within the act of performing itself, which, in turn, became a place for creative co-existence and interaction of various arts. Initiated on various levels by theatre reformers such as Edward G. Craig, Adolphe Appia, Konstantin S. Stanislavski, Vsevolod E. Meyerhold and Antonin Artaud, the process towards the autonomy of theatre began with the renovation of the relation between the text and performance: theatre no longer wished to be perceived as merely the embodiment of dramatic literature and strove to become autonomous art (not necessarily a mimetic activity) defined by performing, the presence of the actor, performer and the scenic space. The latter is not necessarily separated from the audience and conceived solely within the Italian box, but becomes an active part both of the performing and the relationship between the audience and the performer, who are consequently no longer separated by the active/passive role distinction, but can both actively participate in the performing process. These directions were adopted by the historic avant-gardes in their attempts to break the conventional methods of staging in western dramatic theatre: futurist performances, *syntheses,* (also Russian constructivists' actions and the expressionistic cabaret events) strove to erase the traditional genre distinctions, asserting condensation and quickness of action, unbridled creativity, active socio-political commentary and provocation (see F.T. Marinetti's manifesto *The Variety Theatre* (1913); *The Futurist Synthetic Theatre* (1915) by F.T. Marinetti, Emilio Settimelli and Bruno Corra; Enrico Prampolini's manifesto: *The Futurist Stage* (1915) in Appolonio 1973: 126-131, 183-196, 200-202). They attack the passive role of the traditional spectator and try to transform the audience, together with performers, into creators of performance events which aim at breaking the aesthetic and social conventions of the *passéist theatre* (see *The Futurist Synthetic Theatre* manifesto in Appollonio 1973: 183-196) built on the staging of dramatic texts.

Avant-garde actions were generated by the need for active transformation of social context, which involves the tendency for the renewal of the man and community as well as, according to futurists, the total deconstruction of the existing world of *passéist* and the utopia of the new beginning from the" barbaric chaos". They call for life and art more natural, primordial, authentic and vivid than the existing one; all that is old has to die and give way to a new quality of life (F.T. Marinetti's *Manifesto of Futurism* (1909) in Appolonio 1973: 23):

> "Take up your pickaxes, your axes and hammers and wreck, wreck the venerable cities, pitilessly!"

The struggle for the autonomy of the western theatre in the early 20th century was thus not only an escape from the hegemony of the dramatic text, but was also evident in numerous attempts to (re)define the ontological status of theatre, its identity in the field of art and society in general. But how is it possible to determine the element that places performing arts on the junction of the aesthetic and the ritual? Can that surplus quality which many theoreticians have termed ritual, proto-aesthetic or sacred ever be realized within performing in the domain of art, the aesthetic?

In his *Le théâtre et son double* (1938), Antonin Artaud defines the theatre of cruelty as a means for the crucial reform of the western theatre as well as man and society in general. His vision was to establish theatre as the space of initiation allowing for radical ethical transformation of individuals and the entire western culture. For Artaud such theatre exclusively provides space for the *active metaphysics* which he sensed vividly in eastern, Balinese theatre and felt was completely extinguished from the European theatre, suffocated by words, banal psychology and empty aesthetics. With his idea of the *theatre of cruelty,* using the metaphor of *plague* to describe its destructive as well as constructive force (tearing down the emptiness and renewing creativity and freedom within western people), Artaud actually proposed the idea of theatre as a therapeutic tool, which follows the principles of a *ritual process* (Turner, 1982) and initiates the decay of life-inhibiting social and personal structures and leads through the destructing phase of creative chaos into the renovation of ethical, spiritual and creative dimensions of individuals and society.

In the 60s and 70s, Artaud's theoretical endeavours resounded widely among the numerous theatrical practitioners such as Jerzy Grotowski, Eugenio Barba, Richard Schechner and Peter Brook who research(ed) the possibilities of establishment or revitalization of the ritual elements of theatre. Similar tendencies marked the work of the first performance artists who categorically rejected the mimetic aspect of the traditional theatre, its dependence on the dramatic text and its leisurely functioning within the mechanisms of cultural and social institutions. They replaced the traditional notions actor/representation with the performer/presence pair and focused on the research of *organic presence* (Grotowski in Richards, 1995: 66-67) which requires supreme mastering of skills, accompanied by an extremely disciplined and dedicated research of the unutterable; that which eludes words and can arise through theatre.

The work of Jerzy Grotowski, theatre director and researcher, could be described as the journey from the aesthetic, *Art as presentation*, towards the attempt for a (re)invention of ritual, *Art as vehicle* (Grotowski, 1995): when theatrical frame had proven to be inadequate and limiting, he stopped creating theatre performances and committed himself solely to practical research aimed at developing precisely structured *Actions* – a result of long-term physical and vocal work of his performers. *Actions* were no longer aimed at the public, but became the research polygon for the development of skills, psycho-physical and spiritual potentials of those who actively participated in the working process. Grotowski defined his notion of performer with these words (Grotowski, 2001a: 376):

> "*Performer,* with capital letters, is a man of action. He is not somebody who plays another. He is a doer, a priest, a warrior: he is outside aesthetic genres. Ritual is performance, an accomplished action, an act. Degenerated ritual is show. I don't look to discover something new but something forgotten.

something so old that all distinctions between aesthetic genres are no longer of use."

Grotowski defined himself as a *teacher of Performer* (Grotowski 2001a: 376) in the traditional sense of the word: as a master who passes his knowledge on to the apprentice, follows and supports his spiritual development and the acquiring of artistic skills. This ancient method is today still being practised in the Eastern theatre, where Artaud sensed the possibility of transcending the aesthetic by stressing the spiritual component of knowledge transmission, that is, the unutterable which transcends the passing down of the craftsmanship. Grotowski stressed that such work is based on the interpersonal *one to one* relation, i.e. a personal relationship between two people, known in particular for its dedication to work and the spiritual link between teacher and student. The process of passing on artistic skills is therefore also the process of spiritual growth of both the *teacher* as well as the *Doer* (who works on him/herself) – the apprentice.

Primarily an individual's spiritual quest, such a work has a strong personal component: the participants have to show not only an exceptional working discipline, but also the ability to work in an environment where most of the factors that could threaten the "organic presence" of their structures are not present. Grotowski was well aware of the obstacles performers face in their working processes, among them the desire to please the audience and the "easy" working attitude he called *tourism* or *dilettantism* (Grotowski, 2001a, Grotowski, 2001b; and Richards 1995: 33-51). Unfortunately, this often leads to ready made formulas or may even end in the "creative death" of the performer. The principle of Grotowski's work therefore must have been the fact that "the peak of the sacred" is not where the lights are: the bright light is too often blinding for the seeker, making him/her stray away the essence. Seen in this perspective, then, his decision to stop creating theatre performances proves to be completely in tune with the new course of his research.

Actions which Grotowski developed with his performers were primarily a creative tool used by the *Doers* in their personal processes and had no ambition to be presented in public in the form of theatre performance: a space that is public by definition, which constantly creates a specific interaction between audience and performers, theatre perceived as art hinders (though not completely and necessarily) the performer's "organic presence" (Grotowski, 1995: 122):

We can say "Art as a Vehicle", but also "objectivity of ritual" or "Ritual Arts". When I speak of ritual, I am referring neither to a ceremony nor a celebration, and even less to an improvisation with the participation of people from the outside. Nor do I speak of a synthesis of different ritual forms coming from different places. When I refer to ritual, I speak of its objectivity; this means that the elements of the Action are the instruments to work *on the body, the heart and the head of the doers*.

However, in spite of this seclusion from the public, the *Workcenter of Jerzy Grotowski and Thomas Richards* (who continues, with Mario Biagini, Grotowski's research) has a tradition of inviting individuals to witness their *Action/s*. Having the opportunity to observe their work, I can attest to its high quality in terms of its artistic and spiritual value: with some reserve, I would define it as "a personal ritual". It is evident that the extremely concise structure of *Action* enables the *Doers* to pursue a continuous development of their vocal, physical and spiritual potentials. Nevertheless, I did not feel as if I were taking part in a "ritual". However, if the Witness and the Doer establish synchronicity, which cannot be predicted, the "ritual" meeting of two sacred inner spaces can actually take place. Since the sixties, numerous performance artists have turned to the spiritual traditions of the non-European cultures in their quest for the ritual component. One of their main motifs was doubtlessly the search of the primordial spiritual experience that would fill "the empty space" in western theatre and in western culture itself. Performance artist Marina Abramoviæ described her own fascination by the notion of art in the non-European cultures (Abramoviè, 1995):

"[..] their art is a part of general ritualistic complex. They use it as a tool. Only in a disconnected society like ours, the western society, art is called art, it's isolated and not a part of the whole system."

It is thus impossible to separate the persistent tendencies to find or create "the ritual" within theatre, art and daily life from the spiritual condition of our postmodern culture, described by Marina Abramoviæ with the evocative term "disconnected society". This term, I believe, also explains the recent boom of various syncretic forms of "new spirituality" in the West: the inflation of "techniques", "therapies" and spiritual practices, provided by "qualified teachers and healers", which has drawn on the militant business approach to occupy the vacated space of the ritual in our society. The cunning business of pop-culture enables them to offer us instant "enlightments" in the form of various "primordial rituals", termed for example "ancient, medieval or shamanic".

In what relation to the "ritual question" can we place arts therapies? At a first glance it might seem that they alone represent the ground for the ideal process that theatre is (or never even has been) able to provide:

1. The creative-therapeutic process creates a certain "ritual community" (in group therapy) or "ritual bond" (one-to-one relation, based on confidence between the therapist and the client). Both involve a process relationship of support, stimulation and particular sort of learning (self-development) that involves many layers of the client's personality. In optimal conditions, the therapeutic potential of creativity enables the client to restructure, improve or even eliminate certain problems and inhibitions that had prompted him/her to enter into therapy. In a way then, arts therapies and also other forms of psychotherapies can offer grounds for a "ritual transformation" of the individual or collective.

2. Certain "ritual" features are also evident in the formal structure of the therapeutic process. The arts therapies processes have the potential to lead the client through three basic ritual phases: firstly through *initiation*, where the client voluntarily enters the creative-therapeutic relationship and accepts its rules. What follows is usually a longer phase of *transformation*. Through the creative-therapeutic process, the client gradually develops his/her creativity. S/he possibly

also becomes cognizant of certain matters that gain relevance through the therapeutic process and considers deep aspects of his/her personality or specific problems that s/he encounters in daily life. The final phase could be termed *reintegration* – the establishment of the new level of the clients' personal integrity; which can regard a certain aspect of their personality and activity. Or it may even reflect in the change of clients' life circumstances, that is in the quality of expressing their creativity and in their communication and relationships with the external world.

3. Arts therapies could be said to bring about what Marina Abramoviæ (Abramoviæ, 1995) exposes as an important spiritual quality, speaking (in the quote) of the notion of art in indigenous cultures. The subject of her discussion is not the traditional Western understanding of art but, first and foremost, the art as one of the basic attributes in a man and as creativity (to define it as artistic is therefore optional and secondary). Creativity is not a privilege of a certain group (artists) nor does it separate communities into artists and receivers. It is not estranged from the everyday life – on the contrary, it is there for everyone to recognize it as a tool which enables a unique way of (self-)expression. Creative therapeutic practice poses no criteria or value imperatives to individual creativity that are otherwise inherent in the western perception of art. In this way, they create "the ritual space and time" for the opening and the free flow of creativity.

In fact, the success of a therapy depends on a number of factors, which are connected with both the level of the therapist's qualification and sensitivity as well as the client's ability and readiness for a long and often unpredictable personal development. Of course, we should mention external circumstances as well: the relatively young field of arts therapies is still in the process of developing its working methods and research strategies. It is, maybe just for this reason, even more important to stress that the practice of arts therapies actually operates as the "ritual process" because it addresses, researches and tries to develop the individual's inner "sacred space". It does so by helping to create and support the process of activation of each person's creative forces. Here, enormous importance is attributed to the professional expertise of the therapist (the mastering of the art medium with which s/he works, as well as psycho-therapeutic knowledge) which are prerequisites that allow him/her to develop the required sensibility with which s/he can sense and recognize specific needs of the individuals with whom s/he enters into the therapeutic process.

References
Abramovic, M. (1995). *Cleaning the house.* 1st edition. London: Academy editions
Appolonio, U. (1973). (ed.). *Futurist manifestos*. London: Thames and Hudson
Artaud, A. (1938). *Le Théâtre et son double.* 1st edition. Paris: Gallimard
Cornford, F. M. (1914). *The origin of attic comedy.* 1st edition. London: Edward Arnold
Grotowski, J. (1995). From the theatre company to art as vehicle. In Thomas Richards, *At work with Grotowski on physical actions,* 115-135. 1st edition. London & New York: Routledge
Grotowski, J. (2001a). Performer. In Richard Schechner, Lisa Wolford (ed), *The*

Grotowski sourcebook, 376-380. 1st paperback edition. London & New York: Routledge

Grotowski, J. (2001b). Tu es le fils de quelqu'un. In Richard Schechner, Lisa Wolford (ed), *The Grotowski sourcebook*, 294-305. 1st paperback edition. London & New York: Routledge

Harrison, J. E. (1912). *Themis. A study of the social origins of greek religion.* 1st edition. Cambridge: Cambridge University Press

Murray, G. (1912). Excursus on the ritual forms preserved in greek tragedy. In Jane Ellen Harrison, *Themis. A study of the social origins of greek religion*, 341-63. 1st edition. Cambridge: Cambridge University Press

Pickard-Cambridge, A. W. (1927): *Dithyramb, Tragedy and Comedy.* Oxford: Clarendon Press

Richards, T. (1995). *At work with Grotowski on physical actions.* 1st edition. London & New York: Routledge

Richards, T. (1997). *The edge-point of performance.* 1st edition. Pontedera, Documentation Series of the Workcenter of Jerzy Grotowski

Rozik, E. (2003). The ritual origin of theatre: a scientific theory or theatrical ideology?. The Journal of Religion and Theatre, Vol.2, No.1, 105-140. http://www.rtjournal.org/vol_2/no_1/rozik.html

Schechner, R. & Wolford, L. (2001). (ed.). The Grotowski sourcebook. 1st paperback edition. London & New York, Routledge

Schumacher, C. & Singleton, B. (1989). (ed.): *Artaud on theatre.* 1st edition. London: Methuen

Turner, V. (1982). *From ritual to theatre. The human seriousness of play.* 1st edition. New York: PAJ Publications

Wagner, R. (1895). The art-work of the future. (Das Kunstwerk der Zukunft, 1849). In Richard Wagner's *Prose Work*, Vol.1, 69-213. Transl. William Ashton Ellis. London: Kegan Paul, Trench, Trubner & Co http://users.belgacom.net/wagnerlibrary/prose/wagartfut.htm (The Wagner Library)

SABINE C. KOCH

EMBODIMENT AND CREATIVE ARTS THERAPY: FROM PHENOMENOLOGY TO COGNITIVE SCIENCE

> "Art and science are two sides of the same coin.
> Art is a passion pursued with discipline
> science is a discipline pursued with passion".
> (A.Sackler cited after Goodill, 2005:165)

This article introduces interdisciplinary embodiment approaches from cognitive linguistics, and psychology and relates them to creative arts therapies. Creative arts therapies (CATs) have acquired increasing acceptance and application in recent years. The professional fields are prospering internationally, accompanied by numerous qualitative and a smaller number of quantitative research studies which altogether almost unanimously support CATs' effectiveness. CATs work well for all clients for whom the verbal channel is not the primary means of expression. Assessment and therapy can proceed entirely or at least to a major part in the nonverbal realm. It has, however, continuously been emphasized that it remains unclear how exactly many creative arts therapy interventions work. New findings in neuroscience and cognitive science, particularly those compiled within recent embodiment approaches, increasingly shed light on the mechanisms underlying CAT. Some embodiment approaches go so far as to proclaim a paradigmatic change beyond the cognitive paradigm in favour of the inclusion of the phenomenal, lived, subjective body into behavioural sciences' major theorizing. Potential and limitations of the embodiment perspective in relation to the creative arts therapies are discussed.

The End of the Cartesian Body-Mind Split

Creative arts therapies have always assumed the union of body and mind as a basic underlying principle of their work (e.g., Laban, 1960; Kestenberg, 1975; Loman & Brandt, 1992). Conversely, only now are the cognitive sciences on the verge of reconciling the body and the mind (e.g., Damasio, 1994). This new trend is reflected in the emerging embodiment approaches. Embodiment approaches almost unanimously developed on the basis of and in the legacy of Merleau-Ponty's phenomenology of perception (1962) – the first philosophical approach that put the body in the centre of its theorizing. Ever since Merleau-Ponty's groundbreaking work on the ontological and epistemological meaning of the body for our human condition, the reconciliation of body and mind emerged in many scientific disciplines. Embodied theories have their roots in philosophy (Fuchs, 2000; Hurley, 1998; Merleau-Ponty, 1962; Zaner, 1964), anthropology (Lock & Scheper-Huges, 1987; Csordas, 2002; Strathern, 1996), artificial intelligence research (Clark, 1999) and cognitive linguistics (Lakoff & Johnson, 1980; 1999), but nowadays also include arts and art-related research, communication research, dynamic systems approaches, educational sciences, linguistics and language-related research, psychology, robotics, sociology, sports, and other fields (for an overview of major theories see Table 1; cf. Koch, 2005). One of the main characteristics of embodiment theories is that they take the body as the existential ground for perception and action; they collapse such dualisms as body and mind, subject and object (Sax, 2002), perception and conception (e.g., Lakoff & Johnson, 1999), and perception and action (e.g., Hurley, 1998; v. Weizsäcker, 1940/1996). They assume a perceptual, modality-specific way of knowledge representation (as opposed to an abstract, symbolic way), a way that leads via the sensory-motor system and uses this system for thinking through embodied simulations (Barsalou, 1999; Barsalou, Niedenthal, Barbey, & Ruppert, 2003; Gallese, 2003; Glenberg, 1997; Pfeifer & Bongard, 2006). Embodiment approaches are furthermore closely related to approaches of situated cognition (e.g., dependency of cognition on cultural context) and dynamic systems approaches (e.g., Thelen, 1995; 2000). Overarching literature speaks of humans as situated, embodied, dynamical agents (cf. Beer, 2000). Whether embodiment approaches offer a simple shift in cognitive psychology or a full paradigmatic change remains yet to be determined (cf. Clark, 1999). The following pages focus on theoretical developments in cognitive linguistics and psychology, and address some connections to creative arts therapies research.

Cognitive Linguistics: Concepts and Language are Grounded in the Body

"Our ability to move in the ways we do and to track the motions of other things gives motion a major role in our conceptual system. The fact that we have muscles and use them to apply force in certain ways leads to the structure of our system of causal concepts. What is important is not just that we have bodies and that thought is somehow embodied. What is important is that the peculiar nature of our bodies shapes our very possibilities for conceptualization and categorization." (Lakoff & Johnson, 1999: 19).

In their 1999 book "Philosophy in the Flesh" Lakoff and Johnson define an embodied concept as "a neural structure that is actually part of, or makes use of, the sensorimotor system of our brains. Much of the conceptual inference is, therefore, sensorimotor inference" and not just preceded by or followed by sensorimotor inference (Lakoff & Johnson, 1999:20). They state that the embodied mind hypothesis radically undercuts the distinction between perception and conception. In an embodied mind, the same neural systems engaged in perception or in motion play a central role in conceptualization and reasoning. This implies that *movement is a direct part of reasoning*. Lakoff and Johnson emphasize that replacing traditional disembodied with embodied concepts is a gain for science, and how it is in line with the most recent neuroscience and cognitive findings. In their view, traditional scientific thought misses that *"what has always made science possible, is our embodiment, not our transcendence of it, and our imagination, not our avoidance of it."* (Lakoff & Johnson, 1999: 93). It is exactly the human embodiment, the human experience, and the use of metaphor and imagination that makes science possible. The authors' theory on metaphor as a central human capacity could benefit from creative arts therapists' knowledge on how metaphor on a nonverbal body-level and art-related level is part of that capacity.

Philosophy	Merleau-Ponty, 1962; Hurley, 1998	Perception is grounded in the body Unity of perception and action
Anthropology	Lock & Scheper-Huges, 1987; Csordas, 1988, 2002	The phenomenal body Culture is grounded in the body
Linguistics	Johnson, 1987; Lakoff & Johnson, 1999	Concepts are grounded in the body Language/metaphor is grounded in the body Unity of perception and conception
Neurosciences	Gallese, 2003	Embodied Cognition/Simulation
Artificial Intelligence	Clark, 1997; Pfeifer & Bongard, 2006	Intellect/being is grounded in the body
Cognitive Science	Varela, Thompson & Rosch, 1991	The embodied mind
Social Psychology	Barsalou, Niedenthal et al., 2003; Niedenthal et al., 2005	Cognition is grounded in the body Attitudes/emotions are grounded in the body
Memory Research	Glenberg, 1997	Memory is grounded in the body
Developmental Psychology	Thelen, 1995; 2000	Development is grounded in the body Primacy of Motion

Table 1: Overview of major embodiment theories

Cognitive Psychology and Neurosciences: Cognition and Emotion are Grounded in the Body

"Minds awaken in a world. We did not design this world, we simply found ourselves within it. We awake to ourselves and the world we inhabit. (...) We explicitly call into question the assumption – prevalent throughout cognitive science – that cognition consists of the representation of a world that is independent of our perceptual and cognitive capacities by a cognitive system that exists independently of the world. We outline instead a view of cognition as embodied action". (Varela, Thompson, & Rosch, 1991: XX).

Varela, Thompson and Rosch (1991) were the first authors to introduce embodiment approaches into cognitive psychology. Their approach is revolutionary. They state that cognitive science has hardly brought forth any applicable knowledge, and therefore it was time to change this trend. Since their original work, embodied mind theories gain influence in the context of explaining situated social cognition and behavior (e.g., Jeannerod, 1997; Niedenthal, Barsalou, Winkielman, Krauth-Gruber, & Ric, 2005). Action simulation is an integral part of embodiment theorizing. Empirical evidence for action simulation comes from Rizzolatti, Fadiga, Fogassi, & Gallese (2002) study on "mirror neurons" and subsequent research into similar "hard wired evidence". Rizzolatti et al. (2002) have shown that in apes observation of a grasping movement, led to the same activation in motor centers as in the individual that was actually performing the grasp, just less strong. Hormonal and endocrinal findings also suggest convergent evidence for the central relevance of the body as an organ of perception, internal communication, memory, and other human capacities (cf. Pert, 1997). Meanwhile a strong body of convergent evidence has accumulated in favor of cognitive simulations while perceiving motor activity (Barsalou, 1999) of the interconnectedness between perception and action (Hurley, 1998), on the sensory-motor qualities of thought. This is shown by the activation of the same sensory-motor pathways while thinking about the activity as if actually performing the activity (Gallese, 2003; Rizzolatti et al., 2002). For CATs this means evidence for functional mechanisms in relaxation and mental imagery exercises.

Cognitive Developmental Psychology: Human Development is Grounded in the Body

The notion that development is grounded in the body is not new, ever since Piaget's influential work, it is the state-of-the-art knowledge and the ground that cognitive developmental psychology builds upon. Lately, Ester Thelen from Indiana University described the dynamics and situatedness of human development and human motion in infant stepping ability (Thelen and Smith, 1994; Thelen, 1995; 2000; similarly, Kelso, 1996, for adult rhythmic finger motions). She found evidence for the influence of motor behavior on the cognitive and affective development of the young infant. She writes about rhythms as fundamental properties of infant movement. Nava Lotan a DMT researcher from Israel adapted Thelen's new approaches for her work on behavior patterns of small children with the Kestenberg Movement Profile (Lotan & Yirmiya, 2002).
In a similar vein, Pauen and Träuble (2002) describe the *primacy of motion* in human cognitive development. Motion perception is a basic cognitive process. The ability to distinguish animate from inanimate objects is one of the first cognitive functions we acquire in our lives (Pauen & Träuble, 2002). To recognize intention from motion is psychologically and evolutionarily important at the most elementary level of social cognition (Blythe, Todd, & Miller, 1999; Krämer, 2001). Motion is a major cue we use to infer intentions and motivations, and to make causal attributions (Heider, 1958; Heider & Simmel, 1944).

Social Psychology: Social Cognition, Affect, and Human Interaction are Grounded in the Body

Preverbal motor development does not happen in the individual space, but in the interpersonal space. We are social beings and social psychology has contributed a new line of body-based research culminating in the *social embodiment approach* of Barsalou, Niedenthal, Barbey, and Ruppert (2003). By *embodiment* Barsalou et al.

(2003) mean that "states of the body, such as postures, arm movements, and facial expressions, arise during social interaction and play central roles in social information processing" (Barsalou et al., 2003:43). Social information processing means cognitive processing (or thinking) related to social situations. Four types of embodiment effects have been reported by social psychologists. First, perceived social stimuli next to cognitive states produce bodily states as well. Second, perceiving bodily states in others produces bodily mimicry in the self. Third, bodily states in the self produce affective states. Fourth, the compatibility of bodily states and cognitive states modulates performance effectiveness (Barsalou et al., 2003). Movement therapists might be strongly reminded of the empathy theory of Theodor Lipps (1903; cf. Wallbott, 1991) for the first three types of findings. The social embodiment approach bundles single empirical results and other body-based research strings and propose an alternative theoretical account for the workings of mind and memory with reference to recent results in the neurosciences. Embodiment theories offer a new view on knowledge representation. While traditional theories assume that a symbolic system "redescribes" sensory, motor, and introspective states, resulting in amodal descriptions, embodied theories of cognition proclaim the following:

"embodied theories represent knowledge as partial simulations of sensory, motor, and introspective states (...). When an event is experienced originally, the underlying sensory, motor, and introspective states are partially stored. Later, when knowledge of the event becomes relevant in memory, language, or thought, these original states are partially simulated. Thus, remembering an event arises from partially simulating the sensory, motor, and introspective states active at the time. (...) Depending on the situation, embodiment may range from simulation, to traces of execution, to full-blown execution. (...) these embodiments are not merely peripheral appendages (...) of social information processing – they constitute the core of it. (Barsalou et al., 2003:44).

Most embodiment effects are unconscious and occur automatically (Dijksterhuis & Bargh, 2001; Zajonc & Markus, 1984). Emotional contagion is one example (Hatfield, Cacioppo, & Rapson, 1994), the effects of approach and avoidance motor effects on attitude formation are another one (Cacioppo, Priester & Berntson, 1993; Neumann & Strack, 2000). Wilson (2002) and Niedenthal et al. (2005) distinguish online and offline embodiment. Online embodiment refers to a present situated embodiment effect where cognitive activity operates directly on real-world environments or vice versa. Offline embodiment refers to effects from memory, where cognitive activity that is de-coupled from real-world environments. For example, sitting in the classroom being called upon by the teacher and not knowing the answer to any of her questions might cause cold sweat, a dry throat, gaze aversion, and an increased heart rate (online). Imagining this situation may have the same bodily effects (offline). This distinction has implications, for instance, for CAT work with traumatized patients.

Clinical Psychology and Psychotherapy: Healing is Grounded in the Body
Clinical practice is increasingly involved with nonverbal techniques, basically without being conversant with their explicit way of working (e.g., EMDR, NLP, body feedback, mirroring, passing, etc.). Authors such as Damasio (1994), LeDoux (1995), and Schore (1994) have indicated important directions in clinical thinking. There is, however, no explicit embodiment approach in clinical psychology and psychotherapy research. Even though the saluto-genetic approach (Antonovsky, 1997) and trauma-related approaches (e.g., van der Kolk, 2003) are closely linked to concerns in embodiment and creative arts therapies, mindfulness-based approaches come possibly closest (Baer, 2006). CAT research could be contributing to the understanding of the common principles at work behind all therapies by looking at the therapeutic intervention techniques applied by therapists of any school, and organizing them along the lines of embodiment theories. Evidence for clinical relevance of embodiment research is presently again coming from social psychological research: McIntosh, Reichmann-Decker, Winkielman and Wilbarger (2005) compared autistic subjects to typical subjects. On the basis of the mirror neuron theory and the amygdala theory in explaining autism, they found that particularly social mirroring is impaired in autists. The treatment implied by this research is the use of mirroring interventions to create reciprocity – interventions dance therapists have been using ever since they worked with autists (Adler, 1969) – that are now science based.

Fundamental Questions
Is the world centerless, and is it just us searching for a center, an inner organizer? Or is the existential ground given in form of our bodies? Can we really explain all perceptual and memory phenomena on the grounds of embodiment or are embodiment theories just a constraint for specific cases? i.e., is the sensory-motor simulation occurring in all cases or are there still other forms of processing information and of being? Is embodiment a new paradigm that will replace cognitive sciences or will it find its place as a part of it? In the progression from cognitive sciences to embodied sciences the mind is increasingly viewed as part of the body. There are at present many attempts to find the neurological, endocrinological, or hormonal traces of the mind or consciousness. This is *not* the return to a disenchanted view on life. On the contrary, it possibly reconciles the century-long analytical separation of body, mind, and world.

Conclusions
Embodiment approaches offer new scientific perspectives for creative arts therapies. Most embodiment approaches compile empirical results that are suited to support CAT practice, to stimulate CAT research, and to explain how CATs works. Particularly, the cognitive science model of modality specific knowledge representation (Barsalou et al., 2003) lays a foundation for CAT theory development and provides a rationale for CAT's functioning.

Embodiment approaches claim that the typical partition of the cognitive system into a variety of neural or functional subsystems is often misleading. It blinds us to the possibility of alternative, more explanatory views that cut across the traditional body/mind/world division (cf. Clark, 1997). For cognitive science this means that researchers need to rethink critically their subject matter. For creative arts therapists with their more holistic approach their task will be to formulate diligently and thoroughly their embodiment ideas and make them available to other scientific communities. The potential is a better visibility and a more explicit formulation of CATs theory in the light of a new paradigm. The danger of the embodiment view is a too one-sided focus on the body, as mentioned above.

In an embodiment perspective, all cognition and affect is grounded in the body's present and past. Mind and body are not two interrelated entities but a living inseparable whole. Cognition (including perception, memory, and language) and affect are grounded in the body and are describable in terms of its functions. Embodiment approaches strengthen the theoretical underpinnings of the bodily basis of thought and affect. Theories of embodied cognition attribute new scientific value to experience-based approaches and validate major theoretical assumptions in CAT. In turn, CAT can offer its well-developed experiencially-based assessments and theories with a high degree of differentiation. Research at this interface will be relevant wherever the manipulation of embodiment is intended to stimulate healing, improvement of symptoms, or freedom from symptoms. This applies to all creative art therapies, all forms of body psychotherapies, and physiotherapy. All of them work with the body as an instrument of resonance and central relevance.

References

Adler, J. (1969). *Looking for me.* A film documenting Adler's work with autistic children. Center for Media and Independent Learning, 2000 Center Street, Berkely, CA, 94704

Antonovsky, A. (1997). *Salutogenese: zur Entmystifizierung der Gesundheit* [Salutogenesis: The demystification of health]. Tübingen: DGVT

Baer, R. (2006). Mindfulness-based treatment approaches: Cluinician's guide to evidence base and applications, London: Elsevier

Barsalou, L.W., Niedenthal, P.M., Barbey, A.K. and Ruppert, J.A. (2003). Social Embodiment. In BH Ross (Ed.), *The psychology of learning and motivation: Vol. 43* (pp. 43-92). San Diego, CA: Academic Press

Barsalou, L.W. (1999). Perceptual symbol systems. *Behavioral and Brain Sciences, 22,* 577-660

Beer, R.D. (2000). Dynamical Approaches to cognitive sciences. *Trends in Cognitive Sciences, 4,* 91-99

Blythe, P.W., Todd, P.M. and Miller, G.F. (1999). How motion reveals intention. Categorizing social interactions. In G Gigerenzer, P Todd, & the ABC Research Group (Eds.). *Simple heuristics that make us smart* (pp. 256-285). Oxford: Oxford University Press

Cacioppo, J.T., Priester, J.R. and Berntson, G. (1993). Rudimentary determinants of attitudes II: Arm flexion and extension have differential effects on attitudes. *Journal of Personality and Social Psychology, 65,* 5-17

Clark, A. (1997). *Being There. Putting brain, body and world together again.* Cambridge: MIT Press

Clark, A. (1999). An embodied cognitive science. *Trends in Cognitive Science, 3,* 345-351

Csordas, T.J. (2002). *Body Meaning Healing.* New York: Palgrave MacMillan

Damasio, A.R. (1994). *Descartes' error: Emotion, reason, and the human brain.* New York: Putnam

Dijksterhuis, A. and Bargh, J.A. (2001). The perception-behavior expressway: Automatic effects of social perception on social behavior. In M.P. Zanna (Ed.), *Advances in Experimental Social Psychology: Vol. 33* (pp. 1-40). San Diego, CA, Academic Press

Fuchs, T. (2000). *Leib Raum Person.* Stuttgart: Klett-Cotta

Gallese, V. (2003). The manifold nature of interpersonal relations. The quest for a common mechanism. *Philosophical Transcripts of the Royal Society of London, 358,* 517-528

Glenberg, A.M. (1997). What memory is for. *Behavioral and Brain Sciences, 20,* 1-55

Goodill, S.W. (2005). *An Introduction to Medical Dance/Movement Therapy. Healthcare in Motion.* Philadelphia, Jessica Kingsley Publishers

Hatfield, E., Cacioppo, J.T. and Rapson, R.L. (1994). *Emotional contagion.* Paris, Cambridge: University Press

Heider, F. (1958). *The Psychologie of Interpersonal Relations.* New York: Wiley

Heider, F. & Simmel, M. (1944). An experimental study of apparent behavior. *American Journal of Psychology, 57,* 243-259.

Hurley, S.L. (1998). *Consciousness in Action.* Cambridge: Harvard University Press

Jeannerod, M. (1997). *The cognitive neuroscience of action.* Cambridge, Blackwell Press

Johnson, M. (1987). *The body in the mind. The bodily basis of meaning, imagination, and reason.* Chicago: University of Chicago Press

Kelso, S.C. (1996). *Dynamic Patterns.* Cambridge: MIT Press

Kestenberg, J.S. (1975). *Parents and Children.* Northvale: Jason Aronson

Kestenberg-Amighi, J.K., Loman, S., Lewis, P. and Sossin, K.M. (1999*). The meaning of movement. Developmental and clinical perspectives of the Kestenberg Movement Profile.* Amsterdam: Gordon & Breach

Koch, S.C. (2006). Interdisciplinary Embodiment Approaches. Implications for Creative Arts Therapies. In SC Koch & I Braeuninger (Eds.). *Advances in Dance/Movemnet Therapy. International Perspectives and Empirical Findings.* (pp. 17-28) Berlin: Logos

Krämer, N.C. (2001). *Bewegende Bewegung. Sozio-emotionale Wirkungen nonverbalen Verhaltens und deren experimentelle Untersuchung mittels Computeranimation.* [Moving Movement]. Lengerich, Germany: Pabst.

Laban, R. (1960). *The mastery of movement.* London: MacDonald & Evans

Lakoff, G. & Johnson, M. (1999). *Philosophy in the flesh. The embodied mind and its challenge to Western thought.* New York: Basic Books

Lakoff, G. & Johnson, M. (1980) *Metaphors we live by,* Chicago: University of Chicago Press

LeDoux, J. (1995). Emotions. Clues from the brain. *Annual Review of Psychology, 46,* 209-235

Lipps, T. (1903). *Leitfaden der Psychologie (Kap. 14: Die Einfühlung,* pp. 187-201). Leipzig: Wilhelm Engelmann

Lock, M.M. & Scheper-Hughes, N. (1987). The mindful body: A prolegomenon to future work in anthropology. *Medical Anthropology Quaterly, 1,* 6-41.

Loman, S.T. & Brandt, R. (eds.). (1992). *The body-mind connection in human movement analysis.* Keene, NH: Antioch New England Graduate School

Lotan, N. & Yirmiya, N. (2002). Body movement, presence of parents and the process of falling asleep in toddlers. *International Journal of Behavioral Development, 26,* 81-88

McIntosch, D.N., Reichmann-Decker, A., Winkielman, P. & Wilbarger, J.L. (2006). When the Social Mirror Breaks: Deficits in Automatic, but not Voluntary Mimicry of Emotional Facial Expressions in Autism. *Developmental Science, 9,* 295-318

Merleau-Ponty, M. (1962). *Phenomenology of perception.* London: Routledge.

Neumann, R. & Strack, F. (2000). Approach and avoidance: The influence of proprioceptive and exteroceptive cues on encoding of affective information. *Journal of Personality and Social Psychology, 79,* 39-48

Niedentha, P., Barsalou, L.W., Winkielman, P. Krauth-Gruber, S. & Ric, F. (2005). Embodiment in Attitudes, Social Perception, and Emotion. *Personality and Social Psychology Review, 9,* 184-211

Pauen, S. & Träuble, B. (2002, April). *Causal attribution of animate motion in 7-months-olds.* Paper presented at the biannual meeting of the International Conference on Infant Studies, Toronto, ON, Canada

Pert, C. (1997). *The Molecules of Emotion: Why You Feel the Way You Feel.* NY: Scribner.

Pfeifer, R. & Bongard, J.C. (2006) How the body shapes the way we think. London: MIT Press.

Rizzolatti, G., Fadiga, L., Fogassi, L. & Gallese, V. (2002). From mirror neurons to imitation: Facts and speculations. In A.N. Meltzoff & W. Prinz (Eds). *The imitative mind: Development, evolution, and brain bases* (pp. 247-266). New York: Cambridge University Press.

Sax, W. (2002). *Dancing the Self. Personhood and Performance in the Pandav Lila of Garhwal.* New York: Oxford University Press.

Schore, A. (1994). *Affect regulation and the origin of the self.* Hillsdale: NJ, Erlbaum

Strathern, A.J. (1996). *Body Thoughts.* Ann Arbour, MI: University of Michigan Press

Thelen, E. & Smith, L. (1994). *A dynamic systems approach to the development of cognition and action.* Cambridge: MIT Press

Thelen, E. (1995). Motor development – A new synthesis. *American Psychologist 50,* 79-95

Thelen, E. (2000). Grounded in the world: Developmental origins of the embodied mind. *Infancy, 1,* 3-28

Van der Kolk, B.A. (2003). Posttraumatic stress disorder and the nature of trauma. In MF Solomon & DJ Siegel (Ed.). *Healing trauma. Attachment, mind, body, and brain* (pp. 168–195). New York: Norton

Varela, F.J., Thompson, E. & Rosch, E. (1991). The embodied mind. Cognitive Science and Human Experience. Cambridge: MIT Press

Wallbott, H.G. (1991). Recognition of emotion from facial expression via imitation? Some indirect evidence for an old theory. *British Journal of Social Psychology, 30,* 207-219

Weizsäcker, Vv (1940/1996). *Der Gestaltkreis. Theorie der Einheit von Wahrnehmen und Bewegen* (6te unveränderte Auflage). Stuttgart: Thieme. (Originally published in 1940)

Wilson, M.. (2002). Six views of embodied cognition. *Psychonomic Bulletin & Review, 9,* 625-636

Winkielman, P. (2005). Embodied emotional responses as exemplified in impairments such as autism. Presentation at the Biannual Conference of the European Association of Experimental Social psychology (EAESP) 19.-23.July, in Würzburg, Germany

Zaner, R.M. (1964). *The problem of embodiment. Some contributions to a phenomenology of the body.* DenHaag: Nijhoff

Zajonc, R.B. & Markus, H. (1984). Affect and cognition: The hard interface. In C. Izard, J. Kagan & R.B. Zajonc (Eds.). *Emotions, cognition and behavior* (pp. 73-102). Cambridge: Cambridge University Press

V
DEVELOPMENT IN TRAINING AND EDUCATION

ALISON LEVINGE

LISTENING TO THE MUSIC OF THE WORDS AND THE WORDS BEHIND THE MUSIC: REFLECTIONS ON THE SELECTION AND ASSESSMENT PROCEDURE FOR STUDENTS APPLYING TO A MUSIC THERAPY TRAINING PROGRAMME

I would like to begin this paper with a short vignette, describing an experience which I had in my first years as Head of Programme and which impacted on my thinking with regard to the selection procedure for potential students wishing to train on the Music Therapy course, at the Royal Welsh College of Music and Drama, Cardiff, Wales.

Both my office and the music therapy teaching room are based on the 3rd floor of a small building named a Conservatoire. The rooms on this floor have been designated as music practice rooms. However, due to the increasing lack of space, certain of them have been commandeered for other purposes, my office being one. Therefore, whilst busy at my computer, or in discussion with students or staff, I will be serenaded by the various sounds emanating from practising musicians.

Some time ago, on a day when there were interviews and auditions arranged for the music therapy training course, I was due to assess the candidates with the then Head of Music. As I was setting down the corridor from my office to the audition room, I heard some music playing. Clearly someone was practising. However, on hearing their music, immediately I felt that this was not just any music student and that, for some reason, I became convinced that it was a music therapy candidate. It was not immediately obvious why I should believe that this particular music belonged to someone who was about to audition for a music therapy training.

Having completed the first audition, the second candidate entered the room with her accompanist. She settled herself, announced her programme and began to perform. I immediately recognized the music and its performer as being the musician I had heard practising previously. After she had completed her music audition the verbal interview took place.

Following the candidate's departure, the Head of Music and I began by discussing her musical performance. My colleague was very enthusiastic, describing the candidate as an extremely skilled performer, with a high standard of musicianship. The fact that she had also worked for the BBC, appeared to give credence to his assessment. It was clear that she had made a significant musical impression upon him. However, in vivid contrast, during her performance I had found myself feeling very uncomfortable. Her music had penetrated my being and left me feeling that it was difficult to be close to the sound and, consequently, to her. In fact, I felt as if I needed to move a significant distance away in order to be able to listen. This was not related to the volume of the music, and there was no doubt that the candidate possessed a high level of musicality and technical skill. On arriving at the point when a decision regarding the acceptance or rejection of the candidate was being discussed, it was clear to me that the Head of Music wanted to offer a place. Feeling under pressure, and against my better judgment, I took this person on to the training course.

On reaching the half-way point of the first term, this student asked to speak to me. Following Reading Week, which had provided a space to think, she explained that she had come to realize that this course was not for her. We spent some time discussing the issues, which had lead her toward considering this option, and eventually mutually agreed that to leave the training was the most appropriate action to take. The student spoke of how she had found the experience valuable, but had come to realize that this pathway did not lead in a direction which was right for her. I am pleased to say that we were able to part amicably.

This experience had taught me, that through my own training and subsequent clinical practice, I had learnt to listen to music in quite a different way, and in one which was clearly different to that of a trained musician. Using music therapeutically and specifically for the purposes of making a relationship, rather than for performance, had it seemed enabled me to attune to an-other at levels which go beyond the externalized musical expressions. Therefore, I began to think more carefully about what kind of information I might receive through this way of listening and how it could be used more fully in the understanding of a candidate taking part in the selection procedure.

I am aware that up to this point of the paper, I have been describing only one element of the selection process. That is the music. However, I am equally aware of the fact that we use also words in the procedure, in particular during the interview. Therefore, it became important for me to also think about the part words play and how they might relate to the musical expressions. Reflecting on the selection procedures in the UK overall, it is usual that a musical assessment named audition, and a verbal assessment named interview are carried out. On some training programmes, these two elements are conducted one immediately following another, whereas on others, the two procedures may be carried out quite separately. Some training programmes may make their choice based on the musical performance alone. In other words, if the candidates have not reached the required standard musically, then they do not proceed to the next stage. Others use both processes before arriving at their decision.

My own experience has lead me to believe that what is important is not only how a candidate is assessed, but also the order in which the different elements of the process are carried out. Therefore, although the music is central to the process, I would say that it is not this element alone which provides us with a picture of the candidates' potential for becoming music therapists. Also, it is not the only source which informs our thinking with regard to their ability to use their music interactively. As well as the musical language, the selection procedure has to include the language of words. When we use both languages certain tones, colours, impressions and images will be created. However, I believe that the sound picture we eventually hear will be dependent upon the ways in which the two languages are combined or connected. Considering how they are woven together in the process, helps us to reach a more complete picture of the candidate.

There is a healthy debate amongst music therapists which evolves around the question of whether in the therapeutic process, it is within the music alone that development takes place and changes occur. Some music therapists believe in the need for words in order to facilitate integration of the feelings which arise both out of and within the musical exchanges in the therapeutic relationship. Nevertheless, for all music therapy trainings, music is at the heart of the programme. In the teaching, the different elements of this language of sound and its application in a therapeutic context are explored both musically and theoretically – the ultimate aim being to create music therapists rather than more experienced musicians. Students will not only learn to use their medium in order to connect with and relate to an-other, but they will also have to learn to listen or receive the others music in ways which do not just connect to the external or more obvious musical expressions. The aspect of the personality into which a music therapist may tune, has been given names such as the 'music child', or the 'musical personality'.

In considering our particular selection procedure, although we acknowledge that music is central to the process, we also believe that it is the specific context in which it is performed and played which makes its impact different from its use in a therapeutic setting. More significantly, we have also come to realize the particular significance of how the psychotherapist relates to the music, as well as to the words of a candidate.

Arising from one of the reviews of the admission procedure and influenced by the early experience of selecting students with the Head of Music, it became clear that it was more relevant to have a music therapist to assess the musical component, rather than a highly trained musician. I now consider that this has become not just important but essential. Currently, the actual personnel involved in the selection of candidates, are the music therapist responsible for teaching Clinical Improvisation, a psychotherapist, the Programme Leader and a group music therapist. The music therapist will formulate what we as musicians describe as the musical profile and the psychotherapist a personal or psychological profile. From the musical expressions a sound picture will be created, whereas in the interview quite different information may be revealed.

Candidates are required to perform a piece of music on their principle instrument, one on their second and to sing a song which they consider comfortable for their voice. They are then asked to improvise on a given theme, and more recently also to improvise freely with the music therapist. At some point in the day, they also take part in a music group and are eventually interviewed by a psychotherapist. The fact that they will play two kinds of music, that is, precomposed and improvised, allows the panel to tune into the candidate at different levels. All the music is played in the presence of the Music Therapist, that is a musical linguist and the psychotherapist, who could be described as a verbal linguist.

The decision to include the psychotherapist in the musical component of the process occurred following a discussion which she initiated. Having originally interviewed the candidates without hearing their music, the psychotherapist became aware that an important area of information was missing. She said that listening to and experiencing the music live and in the moment had provided her with information, which she felt could not be gained in the interview – that is, through the words alone. Considering that the language of words is the main tool of psychotherapy, then her comment may seem rather strange. However, the elements which we appear to be considering, are, I believe, what might be named as the music behind the words, and the words behind the music. During the selection procedure, the music played by the candidate in the performance element of the process, are the notes composed by another. These notes are learnt and then interpreted and represented to the panel. At this stage of the selection procedure, they are not the candidate's own notes or equivalent words. Yet in my experience, nevertheless, it is possible to hear something which I would describe as expressions which are at another level. Behind the written music, the notes played connect to the person or self of the performer herself, and go beyond the character of the composer expressed in the style of the piece. As I listen to the candidate's performance, I become aware of what I am being made to feel, not as a trained musician, but as a musical person. In other words, I feel as if I am listening to the music behind the music. The second part of our selection procedure involves improvisation and it is in this music that a more primitive musicality may be expressed, or avoided – particularly if the candidates have played how they think an improvisation should sound. Between the two played musical elements, is the song. This particular form of musical expression connects more directly with the representation of the musical personality, and can reveal a more core aspect of the candidates. The highly developed technical competencies in the playing of their principal instrument are usually moved aside when they sing. At this stage of the procedure, we are listening to a voice within, which has not had the refinement of years of practice and teaching, yet expresses something of an inner self.

Experiencing as well as hearing the different languages spoken, played or sung within the selection procedure, can provide different perspectives from which we can come to understand a candidate's personality. As I have already described, at the heart of the selection process is a consideration of the relationship the candidates have with their own musical language. This is assessed in four ways: firstly, through observing and experiencing directly their musical expressions; secondly, through observation of the ways in which they actually use this language in the different kinds of musical conversations and dialogues; thirdly, through listening to how they reflect in words upon what they have created and expressed in their music; finally, and following a space, hearing what the candidate has made of their different musical experiences, in both the context of the musical element as well as the psychotherapy interview. By encouraging the candidates to reflect on their musical experiences using words, allows the psychotherapist to understand how they are processing the music. This means that the audition, that is the music, and the interview, the words, come together to make a whole experience.

An example of how this interweaving of music and words helps to illuminate further our understanding of a candidate occurred following the improvisation which she had completed. Having been given the choice of a picture, or the subject "Feeling Upset", she had chosen to improvise on the latter. As she played, I wrote down the word mourning, whilst my other musical colleague wrote sad. Following the candidate's departure, we discussed her music. I was struck by how I had been so specific about the impression created by her improvisation. For me it was not just sad, as my colleague had suggested, but had a quality which felt more intense. The psychotherapist took these different impressions to the interview. They began this part of the procedure by asking the candidate to reflect on the different musical experiences she had had during the day. In thinking about the first improvisation, the psychotherapist asked the candidate to describe what she had been trying to express. During the candidate's explanation, she happened to refer to a number of bereavements which she had experienced during the last few years, quickly adding that this had not been in her mind during the improvisation. It seemed that, although the impact of these experiences had not been in the forefront of the candidate's mind at the time of playing, something of the feelings relating to the bereavements had nevertheless been conveyed in the music. The music behind the music, had expressed a deep sense of loss, that went beyond both ordinary sadness and the theme provided of "Feeling Upset".

In our primitive and more unconscious states of mind we are without language and in a place where strong and powerful feelings and experiences exist. Therefore, it is often difficult to find the words to describe the emotions and sensations experienced at this level, or even to connect consciously with this place. During the psychotherapy interview, it would appear that directly experiencing the musical expressions in the musical part of the procedure enabled the psychotherapist to reach a different area of the candidate's psyche and had provided her with an opportunity to understand the capacity of this candidate to integrate the intellectual with the emotional aspects of herself.

Returning to the story with which I began this paper, and reflecting upon my experience of discovering a potential candidate practising, I am left wondering what it was that I had recognized, or with what phenomena had I resonated? Perhaps the element of her music to which I had connected, was the wounded part of her being. In other words, in her music she had expressed a vulnerable and more primitive element of herself. Often, those who enter the therapeutic profession may be seeking their own healing – a phenomenon common amongst therapists. In their clinical practice they may go on to use those parts of themselves which have been hurt or damaged in order to connect with their client, whether consciously or unconsciously. These aspects of ourselves are only of therapeutic value, however, if they have been reasonably integrated into our psyche. I would suggest that it was something of the wounded aspect of this candidate, which I had heard being expressed behind the doors of the practice room.

During the selection procedure, we are asking the candidates to be creative and to play, as well as perform, their music. However, we are also asking them to play with their thoughts. Winnicott (1991:64) emphasized the fact that play was rooted in formless functioning, and likened this to being in a neutral zone. Bringing together the words and the music, helps to create a space in which the interweaving of feelings, thoughts, sensations, emotions and expressions can happen. Music is a medium based in time, is ever moving and fundamentally relational. Music can therefore be viewed as a bridge, or a pathway going between what is inside and what is outside, what is conscious and what is unconscious.

Candidates are often very nervous when they come for interview. All the old familiar feelings and sensations connected to their previous experiences as performers may return. Their defenses are raised. Bringing together the experiences of the music and the words can help to reach behind the battlements. The space created in which it is possible to play with sounds and play with words, can be one which links inner and external reality. In my story at the beginning which I related in words, I had connected with a place within, which allowed me to feel something of that candidate's vulnerability. Her sound had even called out through a closed door. This vulnerability had not felt integrated, and consequently became projected outside into the passing world. At the time, and in the audition, I think that what I had been able to do was to allow myself to hear this vulnerability – unlike the Head of Music who appeared only to hear the technical musical skill.

In the selection procedure, combining the verbal and musical experiences, albeit with the psychotherapist being silent in the musical space, and the music therapist silent in the verbal space, I believe creates a mutual space. This space is one in which the coming together of the two mediums forms an overlap, which in turn creates a different kind of space and therefore ultimately a different kind of understanding.

Freud (1912:115-6) in the following few lines, may provide us with a useful analogy for what might be going on during the selection procedure:

> "…..(the analyst) must turn his own unconscious like a receptive organ toward the transmitting unconscious of the patient. He must adjust himself to the patient as a telephone receiver is adjusted to the transmitting microphone. Just as the receiver converts back into sound waves, so the doctor's unconscious is able, from the derivatives of the unconscious which are communicated to him, to reconstruct that unconscious, which has determined the patient's free associations."

References

Freud, S. (1912). *The Dynamics of Transference* London: Hogarth Press

Winnicott, D.W. (1991). *Playing and Reality*, London: Penguin Books

PÄIVI-MARIA HAUTALA

PERMISSION TO BE SEEN: ART THERAPY IN FINNISH EDUCATION SETTINGS

Research Premises

Even though students with learning difficulties are being helped in many ways, Finnish schools have an increasing number of young people with various symptoms and special needs requiring support. Thus, novel ways of helping, teaching and integrating these young people into the school environment are needed. Art therapy and art therapeutic teaching have been tested as one of these ways. However, art therapy has not yet been researched in Finland.

A youth's growth process includes the search for and the development of an individual identity, which may suffer from despair and anxiety. Mood swings and changes are typical in all stages of adolescence. Sometimes such mood swings can be experienced as depression or may develop into such. On the other hand, crises bring about the possibility of change. As a method of support, art therapy and art therapeutic activities offer means to build an outline of one's self and to set its boundaries. With the help of art therapy, an adolescent can gather his/her strength and build a more complete self-image, as well as find his/her way to adulthood and a commitment to education as well as to everyday life.

As a theoretical basis for my research I will be using David A. Kolb's (1984) model for experiential learning, which is based on his research of Dewey's, Piaget's and Lewin's models for action research. In the research of art therapy and art therapeutic education, I will utilize Kolb's conclusion that both learning and convalescence are processes based on experience and thus cannot be considered solely on the basis of the outcome. Kolb's model is well suited to art therapy and art therapeutic activities, in which the learning process is a cycle with four stages (see diagram 1). This learning process requires the presentation of dialectically opposed coping methods. In experiential learning, two dimensions can be detected: understanding experience and transforming experience. In this continuum, learning and convalescence vary from concrete experience of events to more abstract conceptualization, and from active experimentation to reflective observation (Kolb 1984: 25–38).

According to Kolb, learning is an individual's holistic process of acclimatization and adaptation to the world. This process is strongly represented in art therapeutic education, because learning, and, similarly, art therapeutic education encompass transaction between the individual and the environment. It is precisely the therapeutic framework which supports this transaction and enables it. The environment, here a therapeutic space, is formed by experience of the circumstances which are interactive with the individual's objectives, needs and abilities. A therapeutic space is seen as a holding situation, in which the therapist is strongly present and gives the client, in this instance the learner, sufficient space to express his/her various emotions. In the learning process, knowledge is created through transformation of experience. Thus, through analytical thought, the understanding of one's own life and identity is strengthened. In art therapeutic

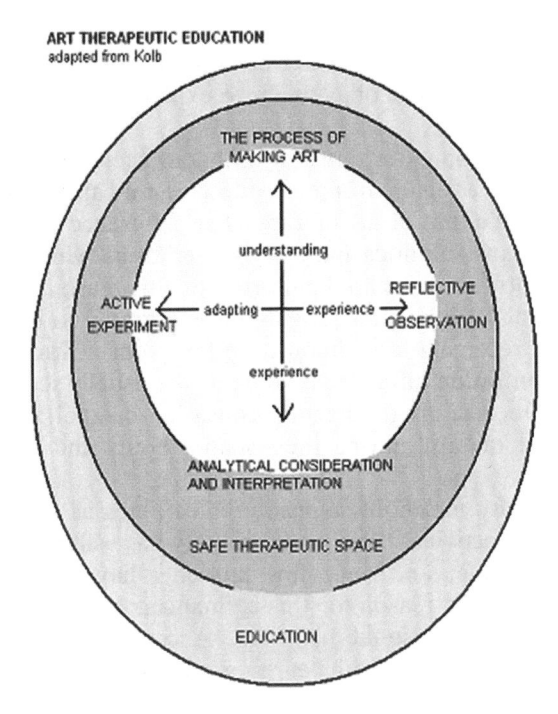

Diagram 1. Art therapeutic education, paraphrasing Kolb (1984).

education, the picture is unpredictable and surprising. The picture is created on paper, like a dream, from the subconscious. The picture is interpreted by the artist. This analytical contemplation changes the learner's experience, and teaches them something distinct and new about themselves. Interpretation and analysis help the learner to view things from new perspectives. The therapeutic space is a requirement for this process.

Research methods
My research is a qualitative study based on semi-structured thematic interviews and it has also hermeneutic characteristics. The goal is to conceptualize the experiential significance of the phenomenon in question. The goal is to put an already known fact into practice. My work as a therapist is the basis for my research. My research method is thus partially ethnographic.
The primary data for the present study will be gained from interviews and questionnaires to art therapists operating in Finnish schools. I sent questionnaires to twenty-one therapists facilitating art therapy in schools. With these questionnaires, I reached fourteen art therapists. From them I also gathered data using thematic interviews. Using the data from these interviews, I studied how art therapeutic activities are integrated into the school setting. The therapists work at different educational levels from basic education to vocational training. I charted the art therapists' methods and practical work in a school setting.

Research results

This study focused on building a model of how art therapy and art therapeutic education work in practice. The objective is to explain, define and understand the phenomenon in question.

The results of the questionnaires directed to the art therapists working in schools indicate that the school as an environment differs significantly from the traditional psychiatric operating culture of art therapy. The difference is manifested, among other things, in concepts, methods and cultural traditions, which become relatively strong as they conform to the school culture. For this reason, the art therapeutic method in the school setting is linked with and integrated to the students' needs. Students typically receiving art therapy suffer from learning difficulties, or attention and concentration difficulties. Students are usually sent to art therapy by their teachers and receive art therapeutic education on their teachers' initiative. Usually they attend therapy during their school hours and only rarely outside school time.

Art therapeutic activity in schools typically takes place as a group activity, less often as an individual activity. Therapeutic activity has usually been implemented for one year at a time, and very few students have received longer-term therapeutic education. The reason for this is financial: lack of funds and, in some cases, deficiencies in operational planning. According to the art therapists, permanent results for students with learning and concentration difficulties can only be achieved with a minimum of 2-4 years of therapeutic activity.

The art therapists define art therapy and art therapeutic education mainly on the basis of their own educational background. The different schools of thought in art therapeutic education include the psychodynamic, cognitive, behaviorist, expressive and Steiner-pedagogical schools. The educational background of the therapist is the main factor guiding the therapist's operational model. A defining factor stronger than the therapist's frame of reference, however, is the school setting itself. Its influence on the therapeutic activity, its quality and quantity, is significant. The school setting proved to be considerably inflexible, persistent and slow to embrace new methods and ways of thinking.

According to the art therapists, they are expected to work flexibly within the constraints of the school setting. Art therapy in schools appears to be art therapeutic activity rather than traditional, orthodox psychodynamic art therapy. Art therapists' activities in schools are rarely referred to as therapy or art therapy groups; therapists themselves prefer to call their activities art groups, creative expression groups or picture groups. This practice illustrates well the unfamiliarity of therapy in the school setting. The word 'therapy' involves a great deal of stereotypical connotations which may in part label the students into a kind of patient context or general otherness.

For the therapists operating in schools, the greatest problems were communication difficulties and problematic interaction circumstances, or even the lack thereof, with other members of the school staff. However, good interaction and collaboration are explicit conditions for successful education. The community's support is one of the principles of successful art therapeutic work. Art therapeutic work has been better integrated into education in those schools in which the teachers and other staff members have been familiarized with the principles and rules of art therapeutic education, than it has been in those schools where this is not the case. This kind of familiarization is most successful when it is based on action and experience; art therapeutic work, in which the staff members themselves participate in. The goal is also to create an educational model for teachers for academic supplementary education in order to guarantee the supportive work environment and to extend the cooperation to help the learners therapeutically.

For cooperation, increasing knowledge and the therapeutic process, it is important that the art therapist takes part in staff meetings, which deal with students' well-being and learning (Moriya 2000: 27). A particular communicative problem may arise from the small amount of information concerning the student-drawn pictures, required by the therapeutic doctrine. The pictures function as a medium of therapeutic activity and thus fall under therapeutic confidentiality. Keeping this information between the therapist and the therapy group sometimes creates negative associations and suspicion in the community. Is the activity somehow secret or improper, when it is kept outside public knowledge? The school world is used to assessing learning results on the basis of the results of a process. Works of art are thus regarded as these kinds of demonstrations of learning. This approach is in direct conflict with the therapeutic view and regulations that consider the process more important than the product.

A therapeutic picture is seen as a sensitive interpretation of emotion, that can express things in multiple levels and in which the client can find new, personally significant meanings even years later. These kinds of new meanings may appear, for instance, after defences are dissolved, whereupon, among other things, understanding deepens as feelings of anger are identified. The learner may, after several years, notice that they have depicted these emotions in their works, but have denied their existence at the time of creating the picture. It may have been too early to process these emotions verbally, but they have become visible in the picture.

In many schools, the art therapist is merely a weekly "guest star". As a member of the staff, the art therapist could contribute his/her own individual perspective to the staff meetings and so diversify the support given to each student. Since the art therapists mainly work part-time, it is difficult for them to attend the staff meetings. In these cases it would be important that the therapist communicates at least with the student and the student's homeroom teacher, curator or principal, who could act as a contact person and present the therapist's views in the staff meetings.

Art therapeutic activities in schools are funded by various project funds, such as the European Social Fund of the Finnish National Board of Education, special needs teaching funds and the funds of National Pensions Institute. Funding is allocated on an annual basis, and thus tends to be rather short-term, considering the students' long-term need for special support.

The way art therapists in England view and define the school culture as an art therapeutic community is similar to that of their Finnish colleagues. Funding is difficult to obtain, and usually depends on various projects. One exception to the usual means of funding was a project funded by the Finnish police forces. In this project, young people with various criminal backgrounds were rehabilitated into society with the help of special training. This curriculum included art therapeutic activities.

Conclusions

Art therapy must adapt itself to the needs of the school in order to achieve good conditions for activity supported by the community. School staff members should be informed of the school's therapeutic limits and regulations, and this should take place before the therapeutic activity itself is introduced into the school environment.

The contribution of the present study for developing education is a model of supplementary education for teachers. Its objective is to familiarise special teachers and class teachers with therapeutic education so that the method could be adopted for the benefit of learners from various age groups. In this model, the art therapist acts as a work instructor for teachers rather than as a therapeutic teacher. The supplementary education model (see Diagram 2) is one way of expressing what kind of education teachers should receive about art therapy and art therapeutic education.

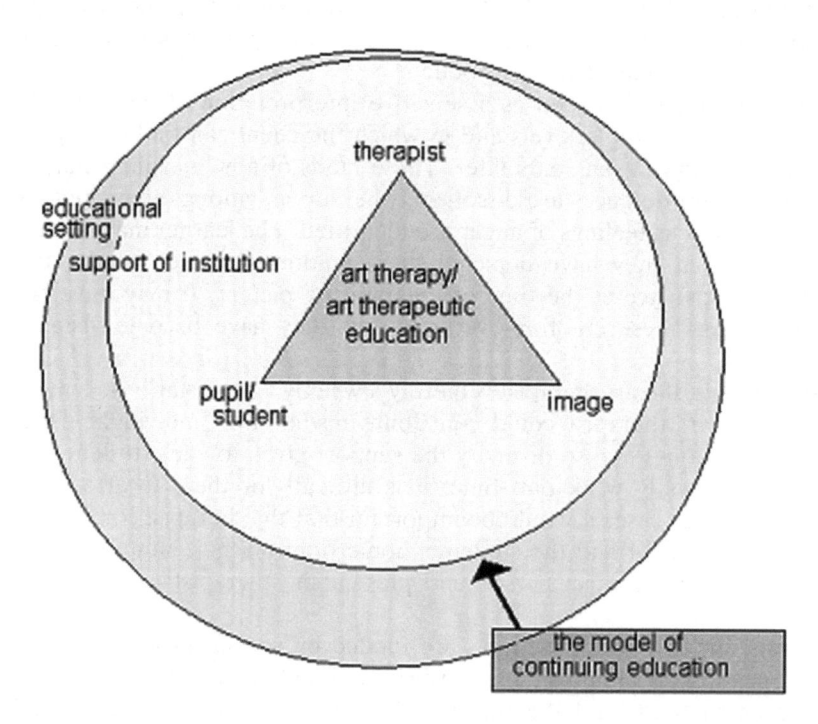

Diagram 2. Supplementary education models.

It is important that the education focuses on the specific nature of the school culture in maintaining the therapeutic boundaries: how the school community could achieve the best possible circumstances to commence the therapeutic processes that provide help for learners of various ages and enrich the educational environment. It is also important that the supplementary education familiarises the teachers with the triangle of therapeutic education: how the symmetry between the learner, the teacher and the picture works, and how the institution's support can strengthen this interactive, creative learning and convalescence.

References

Aaltola, J. (1992). *Merkityksen käsite ihmistutkimuksen ja kasvatuksen perusteiden analyysin lähtökohtana.* Jyväskylän yliopisto. Kokkola Chydeniusinstituutti

Alasuutari, P. (1993). *Laadullinen tutkimus.* Tampere: Vastapaino

Cattanach, A. (1999). *Process in art therapies.* London: Kingsley

Heikkinen, R.-L. & Laine, T. (1997). *Tutkimuksen polulla.* Helsinki: Kirjayhtymä

Hirsjärvi, S., Remes, P. & Sajavaara, P. (1997). *Tutki ja kirjoita.* Helsinki: Kirjayhtymä

Huhmarniemi, R., Skinnari, S. & Tähtinen, J. (toim.). (2001). *Platonista transmodernismiin.* Suomen Kasvatustieteellinen Seura

Kinnunen, M., Perälä, A. & Rautio, P. (1991). *Projektitutkijan opas.* Helsinki: Valtion painatuskeskus

Kolb, D.A. (1984). *Experiential learning. Experience as a source of learning and development.* Englewood Cliffs, Nj: Prentice Hall

Kuula, A. (1999). *Toimintatutkimus: kenttätyötä ja muutospyrkimyksiä.* Tampere: Vastapaino

Lehtovaara, M. (1994). *Dialogisuus, reflektointi ja ihmisen maailmassa oleminen.* Tampere: Suomen fenomenologinen instituutti, 213-234

Linnainmaa, P. ym.kaikki kirjoittajat (1999). *Mielenterveystyö ja opetus –matkalla kohti muutosta.* Helsinki: Kirjayhtymä

Moon, B.L. (1998). *The Dynamics of art as therapy with adolescents.* Springfield, IL: Charles C.Thomas.

Moriya, D. (2000). *Art therapy in schools. Effective intergration of art therapists in schools.* Israel

Nussbaum, M. (2001). *Upheavals of thought. The intelligence of emotions.* Cambridge: University Press

Sava, I. & Vesanen-Laukkanen, V. (toim.). (2004). *Taiteeksi tarinoitu oma elämä. Opetus 2000 -sarja.* Jyväskylä: PS–kustannus

Seeskari, D. (2004). *Lasten ja nuorten taideterapia kasvamisen voimavarana. Kirja kerrallaan.* Helsinki

Skaife, S. & Huet, V. (1998). Art psychotherapy groups. Between pictures and words. London: Routledge

Stepney, S. (2001). *Art therapy with students at risk.* Springfield. IL: Charles C. Thomas

Tuomi, J. & Sarajärvi, A. (2002). *Laadullinen tutkimus ja sisältöanalyysi.* Helsinki: Tammi

Vehviläinen, J. (2000). *Ammattipajan kautta tutkintoon? Ammatillisen oppilaitoksen innovatiiviset työpajat–ESR –projekti.* Opetushallituksen moniste 8. Helsinki.

Vehviläinen, J. (2001). *Innolla ammattiin? Opetushallituksen moniste 21.* Helsinki.

MEZZI FRANKLIN

A STUDY INTO THE INDIVIDUAL'S AND THE DIRECTOR'S EXPERIENCE OF TRAINING AND PRESENTING FORUM THEATRE

This paper is based on research carried out as part of Masters Study at the University of Plymouth, U.K (Franklin, 2005).

Introduction
Forum Theatre is a dynamic theatrical tool that acts as host for individuals to explore real life situations of oppression and to debate a resolution (Dwyer, 2004; Jackson,1997). Despite this, there appears to be no literature that reports on the lived experience of individuals training for and presenting Forum Theatre. This study explored the experience of amateur actors training and performing Forum theatre and the potential impact of these experiences on the director's approach and technique.

The aim of this paper is to identify new areas of technique that could improve the director's practice and future Forum Theatre training. The situation here explored in the Forum Theatre is that of dilemmas in palliative care. Palliative care is defined as:

> Holistic care that promotes quality of life for people whose disease is not curable but for whom the prognosis of life expectancy is uncertain. The focus is on optimising quality rather than quantity of life.
> (National Council for Hospices, 2002:11).

Situations of perceived oppression may occur in palliative care due to the emotive and often distressing nature of the speciality (Maeve,1998).
There is evidence-based research that confirms that Forum Theatre improves individual practice, relating to the situation explored (Taylor, 2002). However, this evidence relates only to the audience's experience of performance (Day, 2002; Franklin, 2001; Fursland, 2001). Boal (1997) gives a clear explanation of the training exercises for preparing actors to present Forum Theatre. However, he fails to report on the experience of the individuals undertaking this instruction. Forum Theatre can be presented in two ways.

- A trained group of actors can present the situation of perceived oppression to the individuals who live it.
- The individuals experiencing the oppression present scenarios depicting the oppression to each other (Boal, 2003).

Theoretical Framework
The conceptual framework of this research has been based on Mezirow's transformational theory of adult learning, which suggests that adult individuals uphold a personal belief system that informs any further learning (Mezirow, 1991; Merriam and Caffarella 1999; Taylor, 2004). Understanding the needs of the adult learner led to encompassing Landy's model of role. This model informed the director's process of developing the characters in the scenarios (Landy, 1993). Improvisation methods were used to teach the individuals how to respond to new scenes, whilst remaining in character (Johnstone,1997). Of equal importance was the researcher's understanding of the life of a group of adult learners. The role of the group leader is crucial to understanding group dynamics.
This research questions the individual's experience of participating in training to present Forum Theatre and the potential impact of these experiences on the director's approach and technique.

Method
The research is a qualitative study using a phenomenological method of enquiry (Husserl, 2002). A phenomenological method includes self-revelation by the participants; listening, interpreting, and producing a meaningful critical written account of the phenomenon by the researcher (Coyle and Sculco, 2004; Kleiman, 2004). Verification was obtained from using Husserl's system of epoche, or bracketing (Husserl,2002).

Design
Semi structured, in depth interviews were chosen to elicit information following the training and performance. Data was analysed using Moustakas' stepped approach (Moustakas, 1994).
The following research questions were posed:

1. What has been your experience of learning how to work in the medium of Forum Theatre? (Probe: did the practical experience evoke any personal feelings?)
2. What is your experience of embodying the role of your character? (Probe: did you personally relate to any of the roles that you embodied during the portrayal of the character?)
3. What is the experience for you of portraying individuals facing dilemmas in life threatening illness?
4. Have you learned anything about yourself, and what in particular stimulated this learning?
·Is there anything else you want to tell me about the experience of your Forum Theatre training?

Horizontalisatoin of statements
Statements relating to the research interview questions were scrutinized and isolated into clusters of themes which describe the individual's experience of the phenomenon.

Audit trail
An audit trail was written into the procedure to inform and verify the analytic process (Bong, 2002; Etherington, 2004). Trustworthiness was sought, through seeking confirmation from the individuals that the transcripts were an honest account of the taped interview.

Self-reflection
The researcher reflected on the meaning of the experience and asked the following questions of herself (Moustakas, 1994).

- Did the interviewer influence the contents of the subject's descriptions?
- Were there conclusions in the analysis that could have been derived, but were not picked up by the researcher?

Procedure
The group met for two hours once a week for seven weeks. The sessions were based on an eclectic model using Johnstone's improvisation techniques and Boal's structured Forum Theatre training games (Johnstone, 1997; Boal, 1997). Each training session included an introduction to the session, practical application of the training, and time for process and reflection at the end of the session (Meldrum, 1999). The group had the opportunity to present Forum Theatre to each other in order to experience the role of the spectating audience and actors performing the theatre.

Following the training period performances were presented to health care professionals working in palliative care. Semi structured interviews were carried out fourteen days after the cessation of the training and recorded on a tape machine.

Results and Data Analysis
The challenge of qualitative research is reflexivity, the recognition of the researcher's influence on the research process and the findings (Coast et al, 2004; Etherington, 2004; Jenkyns, 1996). These influences can be used as a strength through recognition of the subjectivity of the researcher as a starting point in the search for truthfulness (Atkinson, Coffey, and Delmont2003).

This viewpoint may support the researcher's influence on the research process, but it does not address the influence of director role in the Forum Theatre training for the group. The director may influence the group both from experience of the phenomena being acted and the style of direction and training. This may have a positive or negative impact on the group and this was not addressed in the research questions.

Results showed that there were unexpected differences in the reported experience of the actors that appeared to be gender related. In question 4, for example, the male positive and negative response focuses on the development of the actor through exploration of role. By contrast, the female response focuses on personal growth and challenges of a personal level. This is a consistent pattern of response from the genders to this question.

In the significant statements from the research questions, the male responses related to the theatrical experience of performance and the actor's relationship with the audience. In the female formulated meanings, the emphasis was the group's relationship, and personal reflection. The females identified this as an important part of the process of training.

The formulation of meanings was further narrowed into meaningful clusters of themes that were common to both male and female participants. Forum Theatre was recognised as a very different form of dramatic interchange where group co-operation was crucial to the success of the work.

Humour
A common experience reported was the recognition of humour in the training sessions. Whilst some of the individuals identified concerns regarding the place of humour in this training, others felt it was beneficial, particularly when building on role interpretation.

Character
The females related to difficulties with the subject matter because of personal experiences that coloured the role interpretation. There was real doubt experienced by some actors regarding ability to portray truly the character they had been asked to play. This may have been linked to tension between actor and director concerning roles the actor had been asked to play

Discussion
Five themes were identified in the clusters derived from the formulated statements:

- Learning to work in the medium of Forum theatre.
- Embodying the role.
- Portrayal of individuals facing dilemmas in life threatening illness.
- Personal learning relating to Forum Theatre.
- Further comment on the Forum experience.

These themes can be related back to the original research questions because the experience of the individuals and the researcher are addressed within them (Moustakas, 1994).

Learning to work in the medium of Forum theatre
All the amateur actors reported that Forum Theatre was unique and unlike any form of theatre they had experienced (Boal, 1997). However, during the actual training, the actors expressed doubts as to whether the Forum Theatre would work or that the director would be able to facilitate the process. The timing of these concerns appeared to relate to the storming phase in the group process (Squirrell, 1998). In this study, the concerns of the individuals were resolved when they performed to the health care professionals. This may have been achieved by the director continuing to focus on the conceptual framework of adult learning and ensuring time for group discussion and reflection. Trying to solve all the group's problems for them at this stage could have resulted in the director

assuming the role of rescuer, which may have encouraged the group to embody the role of victim (Landy, 1993).

The amateur actors recognised that the emphasis of the performance was to empower the audience to control the drama (Boal, 1997). This relationship with the audience is unique to Forum Theatre and is based on Brecht's concept of political theatre (Muller-Scholl, 2004). Other forms of theatre present improvised scenarios to a participating audience, but the actual resolution to the performance is pre-planned (Engelberts, 2004). This understanding of the impact of the audience on Forum Theatre was not realised by the actors until the performances. This may be an important point to consider when developing training in Forum Theatre.

The actors reported that concern for personal performance, was superseded by the desire to support fellow performers, which was interpreted as teamwork. This phenomenon has been described as the alchemical metaphor in the life of the group, when the group's structure is based on support and empathy (Noak, 2002). This would indicate that the evolving relationship within the group is significant. Although this was highlighted in the literature, it was not part of the research question. Further investigation into this phenomenon in future training may reveal more findings.

Embodying the role

Individuals reported that initially the level of ability to engage with the role was directly related to common themes of life experience between themselves and the role. However, using one of Stanislvaski's (1999) methods, transferring an emotion from their own experience to inform the role, was not helpful. What did appear to help the actors was the improvisational work that studied different stages in the lives of the characters they were portraying. For example, M 1, stated that the role being enacted became much clearer to M 1 when the improvisation exercise took the scenario back in time, to a point before the situation effecting the character had happened. This may have positive implications for future practice. It indicates that improvisation, using different moments in time in the story to be enacted, can help the individual to embody the emotional experience they wish to portray. Boal (2003) changed his practice because he felt that performers needed to experience the oppression to enact it. The research results suggest that, with appropriate training, it is possible to empathise with the lived oppression. Improvisation has long been used as a team building exercise, and to develop acting skills (Engelberts, 2004). However, this has not included improvising scenes that precede the story being presented in the Forum Theatre as a way to embody the role.

Disagreement over role portrayal resulted in conflict within the group between director and individuals. Brook (1988) describes this as the shifting point. This is the realisation of the differing opinions of the actor and director. Although the director may have a more panoramic view of the scenario, it is important to remember that the actor may have more insight into the character (Brook, 1988). This may have impacted tension on the performance and the reflective experience of both director and performer. Whilst these differences of opinion may not be resolved, it appears that by ensuring time for process and discussion at the end of the training session, there is opportunity for individuals to express concerns. There was concern expressed by all the individuals relating to the ability to disengage from a role. This was related to the time spent on stage maintaining character. For the director, this may pose a dilemma. It is crucial to the credibility of Forum Theatre for the performers to remain in role on stage, but safety measures must be in place to support them. When this is not appropriately addressed this may have a very negative effect on the person in role (Forrester, 2000).

Portrayal of individuals facing life-threatening illness
There was recognition by the individuals, that palliative care is a stressful area of healthcare, where dilemmas are the basis for debate and ethical principle (Magnan, 2002). Subjects reported that they felt an individual did not need to have experienced the dilemma in order to relate to the problem. Emphasis was placed on a joint witnessing, by the actors, of the emotion within the situation being enacted. This appeared to have a cathartic effect on the group. This experience underpins the philosophy of Greek theatre, which has been embodied by social/ political theatre (Van Erven, 2001).
The ability of the subjects to recognise this catharsis as a positive experience was identified through the process of reflection at the end of the sessions. This is an important process of transformational learning (Apt, 2004).
As the training sessions developed, the group began to form into a mutually supportive unit (Elwvyn, Greenalgh and MacFarlane, 2001). It appeared from the reflection at the end of the sessions that the real life experience of one individual was an enriching experience for the rest of the group. Boal, (1997) does not incorporate reflecting on role representation in his training. This may be an important epilogue to include in the ending of sessions.
Palliative care is an emotive subject and can raise individual fear relating to the future and mortality (Froggatt, 2004). The subject matter was reported as challenging and exhausting, by the group, but not unacceptably distressing. It may have been that allowing time for concerns to be raised encompassed this. There may also have been an influence of the researcher using the role of a palliative care nurse to explain aspects of palliative care to the group. The significance of this is that an individual who did not have palliative care expertise may not be able to replicate this research.

Personal learning experience relating to Forum Theatre
All subjects reported that as a group, they had become co operative and reported this as a positive experience (Mackert, 2005). The amateur actors noted that this co-operation extended into performance. Whilst it was highlighted as an important part of developing a training session, there was no question relating to this in the research.
All the amateur actors reported that when performing, the true character enacted was upheld, despite working with changes introduced by the audience (Dwyer, 2004). The ability to accomplish this was attributed to the improvisation work in the training. Some individuals admitted that, initially, they had felt reticent about engaging with the improvisation because they felt they lacked experience in

comparison with others in the group. These individuals felt that the encouragement from the director to take risks and feel supported helped to overcome this. Improvisation should therefore be planned in such a way that the performers do not feel vulnerable in front of the other members and the director (Dunmore, 2005).

Further comment on the Forum Theatre experience
The importance weighted to the games, as a building block for the group process was not recognised by the actors until the interviews. One individual stated that the games helped to build on trust within the group (Cattanach, 1994).
The actors recognised the role of the audience in Forum Theatre. One member stated that the learning that took place was two-fold. The audience taught the performers about working not only with the dilemma, but also, with Forum Theatre because of their committed engagement to the performance.
The individuals in this research did not share the same testimony as the audience, and this was a challenge for them. What was not taken into account was the director's experience in palliative care. The scenarios were based on real life experience of this role. This may have made the director credible to the *spect-acting* audience. This in turn may have made the performers credible.

The director's influence
The style of the director may have helped inform the actor's understanding of Forum Theatre. The stringent workshop training focused on improvisation techniques to help develop the ability to be spontaneous and work with changes suggested by the audience when in performance mode. It could be argued that this influenced the actor's perception of Forum Theatre training because of the reference to improvisation and the benefit of using this theatrical tool by the actors.
The director worked within the situation of oppression that was being acted out. This may have had a controlling effect on the group because of the concerns from the director to support the group as they worked through the story of a person with life limiting illness. It is hard to say whether this was a blessing or a curse because there was a real need to ensure the group was adequately supported when exploring issues concerning life and death. However this needed to be qualified by objective reasoning that ensured the group was still being treated as an adult commodity of learning which should be respected, concerning individual decision making.
When considering the findings of the research questions it would appear that:

1. The group benefited from the teaching style of the director, which focused on improvisation to inform understanding of Forum Theatre.
2. The fact that the director worked in the situation of oppression that was being dramatised in the Forum theatre, made it credible both to the actors and *spect-acting* audience.

In this research the director only focused on role and role interpretation and improvisation techniques as a conceptual framework for learning the art of Forum

Theatre. There are many other theatrical tools that can be used in Forum Theatre training. This research does not explore the director's specific teaching techniques and the action on the training for the actors. It appears from this research that the director's style of training had a very positive effect on the groups' ability to understand and present Forum theatre.

The developing group process was thematic in the training and became a normal part of the life of the group (Chesner and Hahn 2002). Improvisation skills training and role interpretation were a cause of tension between the director and the individuals. The possible value of improvisation as a vehicle for change in role interpretation was not recognised during the training sessions. There was disbelief concerning whether Forum Theatre would work which lasted up until the moment of presentation.

Limitations

The sample selected was not representative of the total population because it represents a particular group of individuals. Different employments were not taken into account and it could be argued that this group of individuals represented a specific section of society, because they shared the common theme of involvement with amateur theatre.

The interpretation of the questions varied with the individuals, and this may have influenced the results. For example, question one asked specifically about the experience of learning to present Forum Theatre, but the majority of cases the individuals related the experience to performance. The emphasis on learning through training may have been the researcher's preconceived idea. Further, it is not possible to define whether the individuals were saying what they really experienced or what they thought the researcher wanted to hear.

The problem with an interview is the fact that the memory is a continuously developing phenomenon. Social and psychological experiences will influence the memory as a present lived experience (Atkinson, Coffey, and Delmont 2003). For example, one interviewee stated that they had not learned anything new about themselves. Later in the same interview, they recognised a coping strategy relating to role distancing which they identified this as a new personal learning experience. This needs to be recognised in research.

Implications For Practice

Future training will include work on role using improvisation methods. Whilst it is crucial to provide time for performers to de-role at the end of a session, one structured approach may not suit all. Protected time will be included at the closing of each session for reflection and feedback. This research has highlighted that knowledge of facilitating challenging situations in groups is necessary to promote a credible director. It has established that it may be possible for individuals to perform a subject that is not familiar to their life experience, if the following criteria are met:

- The director has expert knowledge of the perceived oppression or dilemma.

- The training period incorporates explanation of the oppression and opportunity to reflect and discuss the phenomenon.

Conclusion

This qualitative study has shown that for the amateur actors in this research the experience of learning to present Forum Theatre required both training and live performance. Results showed that, during the training period, it was crucial for the actors to explore through drama the oppression issue to be presented to the *spect-acting* audience. In this study, this was achieved through the development of the characters to be portrayed in the presentation. Improvisation techniques enhanced the development of role.

The engagement of the audience with the performance was recognised as essential to the success of the Forum Theatre. Teamwork and support of each actor was more important than individual performance.

The director's role is pivotal to the success of the presentation if it is a subject not familiar to the actors. If the director has experience of the situation of oppression, the Forum Theatre presentation is likely to be accepted as credible by the *spect-acting* audience.

Individuals emphasised the value of the group in relation to training to present Forum Theatre. This indicates that it is important for the director to understand the group process in undertaking this training. The individuals in this study appeared to respond positively to the conceptual framework of adult learning, which informed their experience. The main concerns expressed related to whether Forum Theatre would work when it came to the live performance. These doubts remained until the first performance. This is a challenging situation for the director to work with. This final point suggests that, when individuals are experiencing training to perform Forum Theatre, they need a performance to an audience to authenticate the experience.

References

Apt, B. (2004). Advocating a Critical Reflective Approach. Retrieved, May 5th 2004 from the World Wide Web. http://www.bath.ac.uk

Atkinson, P., Coffey, A. & Delmont, S. (2003). *Key Themes in Qualitative Research. continuities and change.* Oxford: Altrama Press

Boal, A. (1997). *Games for Actors and nonactors.* London: Routledge

Boal, A. (2003). *The Rainbow of Desire.* London: Routledge Press

Bong, S.A. (2002). Debunking Myths in Qualitative Data Analysis. Qualitative Social Research. Vol.3 (2) 1-22. Retrieved November 24th 2004 from the World Wide Web:- http://www.qualitative-research.net/fqs

Brook, P. (1988). *The Shifting Point.* London: Methuen

Cattanach, A. (1994). *Play Therapy. Where the Sky Meets the Underworld.* London: Jessica Kingsley Publications

Chesner, A. Hahn, H. (2002). *Creative Advances in Groupwork.* London: Jessica Kingsley Publications

Coast, J., Mcdonald, R. & Baker, R. (2004). Issues arising from the use of qualitative methods in health economics. *Journal of Health Services Research and Policy.* Vol. 9 (3) 171-176

Coyle, N. & Sculco, L. (2004). Expressed desire for hastened death in seven patients living with advanced cancer: A phenomenological Inquiry. *Oncology Nursing Forum.* Vol. 31. (4) 699-706

Creswell, J.W. (1998). *Qualitative inquiry and research design.* London: Sage

Day, L. (2002). Journal of Moral Education Studies. Oxford, United Kingdom: Retrieved 2nd June 2004 from the World Wide, http://www/datastarweb.com

Dunmore, S. (2005). Recommended Guidelines for Ethical and Responsible Behaviour by Theatre Directors. Retrieved January 5th 2005 from the World Wide Web. http://www.simon.dunmore.btinernet,co.uk

Dwyer, P. (2004). *Research in Drama Education.* Vol. 9. (2) 199-210

Elwyn, G., Greenalgh, T. & Macfarlane, F. (2001). *Groups. A guide to small group work in healthcare, management, education and research.* Oxford: Radcliffe Medical Press

Engelberts, M. (2004). "Alive and Present": Theatresports and Contemporary Live Performance. *Theatre Research International.* Vol.29. (2) 155-173

Etherington, K. (2004). *Becoming a reflexive researcher. Using ourselves in research.* London. Jessica Kingsley Publications.

Forrester, A.M. (2000). Role-playing and dramatic improvisation as an assessment tool. *The Arts in Psychotherapy.* Vol. 27. (4). 235-243.

Franklin, M. (2005) A Study into the individual's and the director's experience of training and presenting Forum Theatre. Submitted to the University of Plymouth (UK) as a dissertation towards the degree of Master of Arts by advanced study in Drama-therapy. Plymouth University Library, Unpublished

Franklin, M. (2001). Acting on Dilemmas in Palliative Care. *Nursing Times.* Vol. 97 (49). 137-138

Froggatt, K. (2004). *Palliative Care in Care Homes for Older People.* National Council for Hospices. London

Fursland, E. (2001). At the learning stage . Forum Theatre as a Type of Interactive Drama. *Nursing Standard.* Vol.15. (39) 16-17.

Greenhalgh, T. (2001). How to Read a Paper. London: British Medical Journal Publishing Group.

Husseral, E. 2nd Ed. (2002). *Ideas pertaining to a pure phenomenology and to a phenomenological philosophy.* Translated by Rojcewicz R. Schuwer, A. The Netherlands: Kluwer Academic Publishers.

Jackson, A. (1997).Translator's introduction. In Boal, A. (1997). *Games for actors and nonactors.* London: Routledge

Jenkyns, M. (1996). *The Play's the Thing. Exploring Text in drama and Therapy.* London: Routledge

Johnstone, K. (1997). *Impro. Improvisation and the Theatre.* London: Methuen. Publications.

Kleinman, S. (2004). *Phenomenology: to wonder and search for meanings.* Nurse Researcher. 11 (94) 7-19

Landy, R. J. (1993). *Persona and performance, the meaning of role in drama, therapy and everyday life.* London: Jessica Kingsley

Mackert, M.J. (2005). Group Functions and Development. Retrieved from the World Wide Web. January 5th 2005. http://www.umkec.edu/medpharm/

Magnan, M. (2002). The dilemma of therapy. *European Journal of Palliative Care.* Vol. 9. (5). 197-201.

Maeve, M. K. (1998). Weaving the fabric of moral meaning: how nurses live with suffering and death. *Journal of advanced Nursing,* Vol. 27. 1136-1142.

Meldrum, B. (1999). The Theatre Process in Dramatherapy. In Cattanach, A (1999) *Process in the Arts Therapies.* London: Jessica Kingsley Publications

Merriam, S. & Caffarella, M.R. 2nd ed. (1999). *Learning in Adulthood. A comprehensive guide*. San Francisco: Jossey-Bass.
Mezirow, J. (1991). *Transformative dimensions of adult learning*. San Francisco: Jossey-Bass Publications
Moustakas, C. (1994). *Phenomenological Research Methods.* London: Sage Publications
Muller-Scoll, N. (2004). Theatre of Potentiality. Communicability and the Political in Contemporary Performance Practice. *Theatre Research International.* Vol. 29 (1). 42-58.
National Council for Hospices and Specialist Palliative Care (2002). Definition of Supportive and Palliative Care Briefing Paper. London. N.C.S.P. Publications.
Noak, (2002). Working with trainees in Experiential Groups. In Chesner,A. & Hahn,H (2002). *Creative Advances in Groupwork*. London: Jessica Kingsley Publications
Squirrell,G. (1998). *Becoming an Effective Trainer*. London: Russell House Publishing
Stanislvasaky, K. (1999). *An actor's handbook.* Hapgood, E. translation London: Methuen
Taylor, P. (2002). Afterthought: Evaluation Applied Theatre. Applied Theatre Researcher. Vol. 6/3. 1-9. Retrieved December 5th from the World Wide Web. http://www.gu.edu.au.
Van Erven, E. (2001). *Community Theatre, global perspectives.* London: Routledge
Woodward, F.J. (2004). An argument for a qualitative research approach to hypnotic experiencing and perceptually orientated hypnosis. *Psychological Reports*. Vol. 94. 955-966

BRIGITTE ANOR

THE FASCINATING DIALOGUE BETWEEN PHOTOGRAPHY AND THERAPY:
The Phototherapy Institute in Jerusalem

The Phototherapy Institute in Jerusalem was established based on the conviction that photography is a fascinating language which deserves to be introduced into the world of education and therapy.

1. The unique nature and significance of Photograph
a) Photography is a bridge between reality and subjectivity
Photography is unique among the spectrum of the arts because of its capacity to **frame** easily **reality** and to **stop time** selectively. We can freeze a moment of our life, remember it, cherish it or not and then work with it. But the significance of the photographic image depends on a perceptual phenomenon: the **subjectivity** of the photographer and, later, of the viewer is a part of the dialogue with the photographic image.

b) A photographic image is a concrete object
Photos are tangible objects that have become an integral part of our daily lives. We can carry them; we can show them to our friends.
The quality of permanence that is inherent in a snapshot allows us to touch our memories, feelings and personal stories which form our identity.

c) Photography is a stimulus
Working with photography encourages observation, sensitivity, analysis and the development of innovative ways of thinking.
The use of photography generates an emotional experience that fosters personal, inter-personal and professional development.

d) Photography is a bridge to Intermodal Therapy
Photo Therapy is a new and unique modality in the field known as the Expressive Art Therapies. Working with photography facilitates observation, analysis and the growth of inventive ways of thinking. Participants at the Institute develop skills in photography and the integration of other arts, as both intelligent viewers and as creators.
It is easy to use photographic language as a bridge to other artistic modes of expression:
Photography can, for instance, be a source of inspiration for **creative writing** and a starting point in the creation of a **visual** presentation. A photograph image can be the initial scene from which we begin a **psychodrama**. We can also use a photo an inspiration for **dance** and **music**.

2. The Program

Our three year Program is based on the belief that the photographic image itself and the act of taking pictures have the power to enable any individual to undergo change.

Our students are trained to work with diverse populations such as children in special education, patients in psychiatric hospitals, old people and so on.

Our students come from various professional backgrounds: photographers, psychologists, art therapists and educators who are interested in personal enrichment and in the integration of new tools in their work.

The Master's degree Program, affiliated to the European Graduate School, EGS, Switzerland, integrates also in-depth study of therapeutic methods, psychology, and communication theories. These studies enrich the dialogue between the photo-therapist and those who choose to be helped by Photo Therapy.

The program is built around two approaches:

a) The analysis of photographic image: that is the level of reception and interpretation.
b) The active use of the camera: understanding of the psychological power of taking pictures.

a) Using the first approach, students are asked to bring along photos as stimuli for telling their life story.
Significant photos force them to take a deeper look into the "story of their lives".

There are three types of photos involved in this process:
– Students bring photographs of them selves to speak about self image. This category may simply serve as witness to the different stages in their lives but this can be much more complicated and awake questions relating to self-representation.
– They bring family photos to depict at first sight a more or less official and happy version of the family chronicle but, sometimes, if they dig a bit further, they find beyond it lost and hidden stories: secrets, lies, and family mythology.
– Photos from the media are also a part of their life story: such photos are part of the collective memory; they connect to social groupings and illustrate the interaction between the personal and the collective stories.

These photographic images can play many diverse roles (Anor, 2003). These roles range from the submissive to the unruly:
– In the more or less submissive roles the photographs can organize and illustrate experience, giving a chronological structure to life. They can support and enrich the pre-existing structure of a life story. Photos also allow the subject to crystallize a story into a narrative that can be shared with others.
– In their resistant roles photos can reflect the confusion and imbalance inherent in the human condition. They awaken in the subject the need to rethink his perspective on the world, on himself and others. In an unexpected way, they can provoke spontaneous associations belonging to the world of the unconscious, or serve as a creative springboard.

Sometimes, a photographic image can stimulate someone to re-consider the story of his life.

This material is supported by a theoretical structure dealing with narrative identity (Ricoeur,1985); with the theme of interpretation in general (Gadamer, 1965); and with the relationship between the photo and the viewer in particular (Barthes, 1980).

b) The second approach of photography is at a production level: to improve the photographer's abilities and to analyze the meaning of taking pictures. This is the active use of the medium: taking pictures, developing and fostering artistic understanding and skills.

- The camera helps the person **to control** his field of vision. The camera gives power to the user.
- It is also interesting to notice how sometimes; by framing reality the photograph gives some **coherence** to the world which surrounds the user.
- The camera is a **protective accessory**; it allows freedom of movement. It gives to the user an exterior position as observer, tourist, somebody who came, saw, and left.
- The camera is also a certificate of guarantee of the individual's having "been there". With a camera the subject bears **witness** to his field of vision.

Both approaches, photography **in** therapy (photographic images as stimuli) and photography **as** therapy (the active use of taking pictures) create a powerful emotional experience that brings about individual and professional enrichment.

3. The school

The Phototherapy Institute was created in the framework of the Musrara School of Photography, Media & New Music in Jerusalem. Musrara neighborhood, perhaps more than any other place, symbolizes the complexity of the Israeli experience: a neighborhood situated at the divide between West and East Jerusalem, overlooking the walls of the Old City.

The school sees the artistic process as a facilitator of change and a force for bridge building and the reduction of social gaps. Students represent a cross-section of Israel, comprising secular and religious, Jews and Arabs, native-born Israelis and new immigrants.

From its inception the Musrara School strove to become a unique institution of higher learning in Israel – open to its environment, innovative and connected to the pulse of society. It works to strengthen the connection between art, the community and the wider society.

References

Anor, B. (2003). *Les différents rôles de l'image photographique dans la narration de notre vie: du docile au réfractaire*, Doctoral dissertation, Suisse: EGS

Ricoeur, P. (1985). *Temps et récit,* 3 volumes, Paris: éd. point Seuil

Gadamer, H-G. (1965). Wahrheit und Methode: Grundzuege einer philosophischen Hermeneutik, Tuebingen
Trad: Gadamer, H-G. (1996). *Vérité et méthode: les grandes lignes d'une herméneutique philosophique*, Paris: Seuil.
Barthes, R. (1980). *La chambre Claire, Note sur la photographie,* Paris Cahiers du cinéma, Gallimard-Seuil

THE CONTRIBUTORS

Simone Alter-Muri
PhD. Professor and founder of graduate and undergraduate programs in Art Therapy/Art Education, Springfield College. She has lectured and published internationally. She was the Massachusetts Art Educator in Higher Education for 2003. (**United States of America**).

Brigitte Anor
Ph.D. in Expressive Arts Therapy. Fonder, director and teacher of the Photo Therapy Institute, Musrara – Jerusalem. Doctoral thesis: *The different roles of the photographic image in the narration of our lives.* (**Israel**).

Michael Barham
State-registered arts therapist (dramatherapy), a registered supervisor with BADth and until recently a council member of the Health Professions Council (HPC). He is Dean of Human and Life Sciences at Roehampton University. (**United Kingdom**).

Ralf Bolle
Prof. Dr. med., is a specialist in psychotherapeutic medicine, psychiatry and psychotherapy, psychoanalyst (CG Jung), lecturer and teaching-analyst at the CG-Jung-Institut, Stuttgart and responsible for the sector of "psychotherapeutic medicine" at the University of applied Sciences Art Therapy, Nürtingen, teaching therapist of the German Society for Guided Affective Imagery and Mental Techniques in Psychotherapy and Psychology. (**Germany**).

Martin Cope
MA, Registered Dramatherapist/Performing Arts Practitioner based in Wales. Extensively travelled. Specialisms: individual, group and 'planned environment' therapy for adolescents. Developing narrative, anthropological, musical, ecopsychological and circus approaches to therapy. Owner/Director of new woodland initiative 'Hiraeth' where therapy, arts, psychology, education and ecology unite. (**United Kingdom**).

Katerina Couroucli-Robertson
M.A., Reg. D.T.A., Dramatherapist, PhD candidacy in Dramatherapy at Roehampton University, UK; Teacher in Special Education; Full member of the British Association for Dramatherapists and the Health Professions Council; Founder member and president of the Panhellenic Professional Association of Dramatherapy and Playtherapy. She works as a Dramatherapist and supervisor at the Herma Dramatherapy centre and at the Athyrma training centre. She also runs a music and theatre group consisting of people with different handicaps, for V.S.A. HELLAS. (**Greece**)

Mezzi Franklin
RN Dip Cancer nursing; Cert Ed; B. Phil Complementary Therapies; Masters in Dramatherapy. Employed as hospital Macmillan CNS with lead for developing education for palliative care in the hospital. Has developed and integrated approach to palliative care education using Forum Theatre to help individuals challenge and explore dilemmas in cancer care with particular reference to teaching communication skills in breaking bad news. (**United Kingdom**).

Erna Grönlund
ADTR, Ph.D, Professor Emerita in Dance Education at the University College of Dance, former leader of the Swedish Graduate Dance Therapy Program. Her speciality is dance therapy for children and adolescents with deep emotional disturbances. (**Sweden**).

Nita Gyllander Vabö
Registered dance therapist and supervisor at the University College of Dance. She started as a dancer, then studied to be a dance teacher and a dance therapist. She specializes in dance therapy for children and adolescents. (**Sweden**).

Päivi-Maria Hautala
Diaconate in the parish of Askola, 1980-1985. Teaching since 1992, main subjects; health services, art and creative expression. MA, University of Helsinki, 2001. Diploma in Art Therapy, Satakunta Polytechnic, Pori/University of Hertfordshire, 1998-2001. Art Therapist, Vammala, psychiatric hospital and policlinic 2001. Teaching 2004, Satakunta Polytechnic Studying at the University of Jyväskylä, aim: PhD, 2006. Art Exhibitions in Finland, Canada and Austria since 1989. (**Finland**).

Violeta Hemsy de Gainza
Well known in music education. She is a pianist, music teacher, president of the LatinoAmerican Society of Music Education, author of a number of books on music pedagogy and on music therapy. She was professor at the Universities of La Plata and Santiago, and in different conservatories of music. She has worked in close relationship with the development of music therapy in Argentina. (**Argentina**)

Phil Jones
PhD, MA. Childhood Studies, Carnegie Faculty, Leeds Metropolitan University co-author and co-editor of 'Childhood' (Pearson 2007), author of 'The Arts Therapies' (Routledge 2005) and 'Drama As Therapy' (Routledge 1996). He has held positions of Course Leader and Principal Lecturer on Foundation, Postgraduate and MA courses in Drama, Art and Dance Movement Therapy and has lectured widely on the arts therapies. (**United Kingdom**).

Sabine C. Koch
PhD, M.A., DTR, psychologist and dance/movement therapist at the University of Heidelberg, Germany, works in Personality and Social Psychology, and Gender and Communication Research. She is specialized in video-microanalysis of verbal and nonverbal communication pattern and movement analysis with the Kestenberg Movement Profil (KMP). (**Germany**).

Christine Lapoujade
PhD in psychology, Course Coordinator of the department of Arts Therapies (music-therapy, dance and drama-therapy and art therapy) at the University Descartes – Paris 5, founder member of ECArTE, member of the Executive Board and Chair since 2002 to present. (**France**).

Edith Lecourt
Psychologist, music therapist, Freudian psychoanalyst, and clarinettist. She is professor of clinical and pathological psychology at the University Paris-Descartes. She is Adjoint-Head of the Institut of Psychology of this University, and co-head of the Department of Art Therapies; course leader of music therapy. She is author of many books and articles some translated into English, Italian, Spanish and Portugese. (**France**).

Alison Levinge
PhD, is currently Course Leader for the MA and PGDip training programme in Music Therapy, at the Royal Welsh College of Music and Drama, Cardiff, Wales. Her main research interest is in early development and, in particular, the mother baby relationship. She is also chair of the profession's Supervision Committee. (**United Kingdom**).

Pauline McGee
Pro-active in campaigning work and developing support services for children and adult survivors of sexual abuse in Scotland. Currently teaching on Art Therapy MSc course at Queen Margaret University College, Edinburgh. (**United Kingdom**).

Pauline Mottram
BA (Art) HDip Ed, PGDip AT, MA by Res. She has many years' art therapy experience in Adult Mental Health, Learning Disabilities and in Art Therapy Education. She is registered for PhD (Critical Psychology). Since 2003 she is Course Leader of the MSc Art Therapy Programme, Edinburgh, UK. (**United Kingdom**).

Peter Rech
PhD, is an artist and art therapist. He holds the Chair for Art Education and Art Therapy at the University of Cologne, is Director of the Cologne School of Art Therapy and founder and editor of the review *Art & Therapy*, corresponding member of the new Lacanian school. (**Germany**).

Barbro Renck
DrPH, MPH, RN, senior lecturer and director of higher studies in Public Health, Karlstad University. She is a psychiatric nurse and has worked for many years as a leader in psychiatric care within a child and adolescent clinic. (**Sweden**).

Aleksandra Schuller
PhD, Lecturer at Cultural Studies/Anthropology Department, Faculty of Humanistic Studies, University of Koper and guest lecturer/collaborator of Arts Therapies Postgraduate Programme, Faculty of Education, University of Ljubljana. Performance Artist and Researcher (performance studies and drama theory, theories of play and creativity, arts therapies). (**Slovenia**).

Sarah Scoble
Programme Leader MA in Dramatherapy and MA (Upgrade) in Dramatherapy, School of Applied Psychosocial Studies, University of Plymouth. Previously, Head of Centre for Performing Arts and Media, South Devon College. Member of Executive Board of ECArTE since 1995 (Co-ordinator 1995 to 2002; Vice Chair 2002 to present. Dirtector of ECArTE European Arts Therapies conferences 1995 to present). (**United Kingdom**).

Peter Sinapius
1985–1991: Studying fine arts at the University of fine arts in Kassel and the San Francisco Art Institute, further art therapies at the University of Cologne. 1992–2003: art therapist. Since 2003: Professor for art therapies and painting at the University of applied sciences Ottersberg. (**Germany**).

Mathilde Tubben
Dramatherapist (RDT) and psychologist, who is working in the Dutch Ambulant Psychological Health Care in Amersfoort (Riagg Amersfoort & Omstreken). She is also a lecturer and supervisor in Drama Therapy and a member of the Department of Social Work and Arts Therapies at the CHN University in Leeuwarden. The national norming and validation study, concerning the observation-instrument, 'the building of a hut' is a graduation study (PhD) at the University of Utrecht. (**The Netherlands**).

Jan Van Camp
Psychoanalyst (Belgian School of Psychoanalysis) working at the University Psychiatric Centre KU, Leuven. He is also a lecturer at the College of Science and Art (campus Lemmensinstituut), college for Masters degree in music, and trainer and supervisor at the post-graduate training programme for psychoanalytic psychotherapy at the Catholic University in Leuven. In the last few years he has published on the significance of music for thinking about and handling psychopathological phenomena. (**Belgium**).

Lambros Yotis
MD, PhD. Psychiatrist and Dramatherapist (PGDip), with studies and professional work in theatre. Since 1990, he has been working in mental health and rehabiliation in Athens, Leros and London. As a Dramatherapist, he has developed a model of therapeutic performance – making with clients with schizophrenia and he has completed a PhD in this field (2002, University of Hertfordshire). He is currently working at the University Mental Health Institute in Greece and he is directing a professional Playback Theatre company. (**Greece**).

Vicky Zerva-Spanou
MA in Play Therapy; lecturer of Play Therapy at the Hellenic Institute of Play Therapy and Drama Therapy; Dramatherapist supervisor for professionals; full member of the British Association of Play Therapy (B.A.P.T.) and the Hellenic Professional Association of Play Therapists – Drama Therapists. (**Greece**).

Lia Zografou
She holds a Post-graduate Diploma (1999) and an MA (2004) in dramatherapy from the University of Surrey, Roehampton. She is a dramatherapist and supervisor in private practice in Greece. (**Greece**).

AUTHOR INDEX

Alter-Muri, Simone	172
Anor, Brigitte	219
Barham, Michael	42
Bolle, Ralf	28
Cope, Martin	78
Couroucli-Robertson, Katerina	140
Franklin, Mezzi	208
Grönlund, Erna	103
Gyllander Vabö, Nita	103
Hautala, Päivi-Maria	202
Hemsy de Gainza, Violeta	120
Jones, Phil	13
Koch, Sabine C.	186
Lecourt, Edith	120
Levinge, Alison	196
McGee, Pauline	162
Mottram, Pauline	54
Rech, Peter	69
Renck, Barbro	103
Schuller, Aleksandra	179
Sinapius, Peter	64
Tubben, Mathilde	110
Van Camp, Jan	2
Yotis, Lambros	91
Zerva-Spanou, Vicky	131
Zografou, Lia	149